PAIN IS THE PITS!

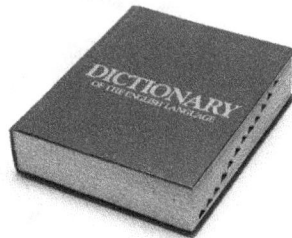

The Pits slang

an extremely unpleasant, boring, or depressing place, condition, person, etc.…the absolute worst.

Usage 1: When you are alone, Christmas is the pits.

Usage 2: When you are in pain…
       …PAIN is the PITS!

PAIN IS THE PITS!

A Pain Management Program to Answer America's Opioid Crisis

Peter A. Kechejian, MD, CPE

Pain Management Specialist
& Certified Pain Educator

NOTICE

Medicine is an ever-changing science. As new research and clinical experience broaden our knowledge, changes in treatment and drug therapy are required. The authors and the publisher of this work have checked with sources believed to be reliable in their efforts to provide information that is complete and generally in accord with the standards accepted at the time of publication. However, in view of the possibility of human error or changes in medical sciences, neither the editors nor the publisher nor any other party who has been involved in the preparation or publication of this work warrants that the information contained herein is in every respect accurate or complete, and they disclaim all responsibility for any errors or omissions or for the results obtained from use of the information contained in this work. Readers are encouraged to confirm the information contained herein with other sources. For example and in particular, readers are advised to check the product information sheet included in the package of each drug they plan to administer to be certain that the information contained in this work is accurate and that changes have not been made in the recommended dose or in the contraindications for administration. This recommendation is of particular importance in connection with new or infrequently used drugs.

PITS PROGRAM, LLC

Copyright © 2022

All Rights Reserved

Printed in the United States of America

Library of Congress Control Number: 2022917616

ISBN Numbers
Paperback: 979-8-9870071-0-5
Audio: 979-8-9870071-2-9

www.painisthepits.com

TABLE OF CONTENTS

CHAPTER 6 *Continued*

INTRODUCTION

If you plan to live the one life you have never getting injured in a slip-and-fall or a car accident, never developing any kind of arthritis, never hurting your back or neck at work, and never planning to get too old that you cannot do every activity you desire... *then this book is not for you.* On the other hand, if you are like the one hundred million Americans today, including myself, who realize that they suffer from some sort of chronic recurrent or persistent pain, then this book can be an answer to your pain and suffering. This book can offer you an easy to understand and follow *lifetime wellness program* for the management of your pain!

All of us living with chronic pain know it is a daily struggle that can turn into a lifelong challenge. Staying functional and comfortable for many years after diagnosis of certain pain conditions requires paying attention to details and staying on track in a pain management program. Keeping chronic pain under control is critical, because constant and intense pain can cause greater health problems, and these potential negative circumstances need to be avoided. Excessive levels of pain also impair our ability to carry out activities of daily living, setting the stage for loss of normal daily function, heightened depression and anxiety, more dependence on those around us, and a general sense of loss of self-esteem. Quality of life is impaired when we can no longer do the everyday tasks such as working, taking care of family, and recreating.

The good news, however, is that physicians today know more about how to diagnose and treat pain to minimize or prevent these quality-of-life issues. As a result, more people with chronic pain are keeping their jobs, and traveling all over the country, goals that were impossible for many in the past.

As a board-certified **pain management specialist** and **certified pain educator** for America, I have now created a national educational pain management program for all of us who hurt. The name of this program is the **Pain is the PITS Program**, or what will be known as the **PITS Program**. The aim of the program—the **"Holy Grail"**—is to optimize what I call your, **PITS Pain and Quality-of-Life Score**, or **PITS Score** (see **APPENDIX A**). The higher your **PITS Score**—*maximum 120 points*—the better your pain control and quality of life. The overall goals of the program are to keep patients staying functional, controlling pain, avoiding depression, keeping active with friends and family, and ultimately feeling better and living their lives.

Office check-ups, or **PITS *stops*,** are an important part of the program, because loss of functional status and comfort can be detected earlier rather than later, and adjustments in patient care using the **P-I-T-S *treatment protocol*** can be implemented. Unfortunately, many people do not fully know about the availability of pain management services, and how to incorporate evaluation and management into their busy schedules. Many people never get referred by their doctors or other healthcare professionals for an initial evaluation, or do not know family, friends, or colleagues who have had successful pain management evaluation and treatment. The **PITS Program** provides a unique educational integrative care protocol for our vast community of pain sufferers. It also helps to educate referring physicians for treatment options, other than just prescribing opioid medications.

The **PITS Program** will answer the critical question of what to do with all the narcotics and the *opioid* *crisis* as it relates to pain therapy. All the chronic opioid use to treat pain has come with a price. All too often, the management of pain involves the prescription of an opioid, which in turn, can become less effective through time and become highly addictive. This has created a multitude of additional problems, well beyond the treatment of the original symptoms. The **PITS Program** will provide an integrated more balanced approach to treatment options for chronic pain. So, the primary goal of the **PITS Program** is to maximize a patient's comfort, function, and quality of life, without the need to keep escalating opioid narcotic levels for pain treatment therapy.

Adoption of the **PITS Program** will help to:

- keep chronic daily pain within tolerable levels
- increase patient awareness and adherence
- lower risk of losing functional mobility
- reduce depression and anxiety
- decrease long term healthcare costs

Now let me begin to describe how the **Pain is the PITS Program** came into existence, and why I am so passionate about offering it to America!

It is with great hope and anticipation for change that I am writing this book on pain management and wellness for all of America. It is especially timely considering America's current opioid crisis and pain epidemic, which affects all levels of society without any prejudice. After twenty-five years of academic and clinical practice, it became clear to me that *two major factors were critical for successful pain management*:

First, it is important to establish and follow a comprehensive multidisciplinary integrative pain management program, *balancing* an assortment of assessment and treatment methods.

Second, it is equally important to continuously *educate* patients about their specific pain condition assessment and treatment options, so they can best comprehend, develop, and adjust their own individualized program with their pain management team through time, as needed.

This level of understanding and participation in an adjustable pain relief wellness program will reduce reliance on opioid therapy as a sole source for pain relief. The reduction in opioid prescriptions will lower the opportunity for abuse and unintentional addiction. This is what works best for the management of chronic pain care over a lifetime.

My academic and clinical pain management expertise, and the eventual development of my **Pain is the PITS Program**, did not come easy through the years—but I was very fortunate. As hard as I worked to achieve this pain knowledge and experience, and now my national **PITS Program** goal, I was fortunate to be one of the first anesthesiology pain management physicians to be fellowship-trained in interventional pain management back in the early 1990s, when credentialing of this medical specialty fellowship training was just being introduced. So, I got a great start on what is now this whole rapidly growing pain management field of medical care in America.

After my anesthesiology residency and pain management fellowship, I found an academic position in a Long Island County hospital teaching anesthesiology and pain management to resident doctors and patients for seven years. After my formal academic teaching years, I was fortunate to get an academic and clinical pain management position in a large private anesthesiology group at multiple hospital sites, in the North Shore-Long Island Jewish Healthcare System (now Northwell Health) in Nassau County, Long Island. Ten years later, I moved on to a clinical private practice in Suffolk County, Long Island, teaming up with another pain management physician. Here I spent seven more years focusing my office and surgical center work on safe, outpatient, minimally invasive medical and interventional pain management techniques for the treatment of chronic pain disorders. It was also during this time that I had the opportunity to do several years of professional media work, developing the **PITS Program** into what it is today. Now, for the last three years, I have been working with a large private orthopedic group in offices on Long Island, focusing on the care of acute and chronic neck and back spine pain conditions.

Through this twenty-five-year journey on Long Island, and after thousands of successful pain management stories in my practice, I have finally put all the steps together to create a universal educational clinical care pain program that could reach millions of patients that suffer from any type of pain, to help guide them to improved wellness. The hope, and now a clear realization, is that this program, the **Pain is the PITS Program**, will be tremendously useful to patients and healthcare professionals all over the country in helping them formulate an integrative pain management program that would best fit a specific type of pain—whether it is acute from an injury or after a surgical operation, pain from a bad neck or back, chronic headache or arthritis pain, or pain from a cancer-related condition—essentially for *any pain*—you will see!

After all my academic and clinical years of experience, I realized that the key to the **PITS Program** was to develop a simple and straightforward educational pain management assessment and treatment protocol and fit this program into a universal model for the country. The *acronym* **P-I-T-S** stands for both the *assessment and treatment* of pain. Hopefully, this acronym will be nationally recognized someday, and be used to *instantly put together a "thought pattern"* of pain management care.

Assessment: The assessment part of the **PITS Program** is divided into *four sections*, which follow the **P-I-T-S** *acronym*, and involves a detailed evaluation of the patient's pain and overall quality of life. This can either be a self-assessment process or accomplished through a professional consultation interview. At this time, the **P–Physical Function** of the patient is determined, along with the **I–Intensity of Pain** they are experiencing. As a patient's history is developed, the assessment continues to include the **T–Thoughts and Behaviors** for determining their mental and emotional state, and finally **S–Social Interactions**. Looking at these four areas of your life provides a simple yet comprehensive *snapshot* assessment, to discover your strong and weak areas, which can then help guide and tailor your future treatment options.

Now there are three categorical assessment questions for each of these sections, with each question answered on a 0–10 scale, which when scored and added up, leads to the **Pain and Quality-of-Life Score**—the **PITS Score**. The **PITS Score** allows the patient's pain condition to have a baseline assessment, which can then be monitored on a weekly basis or monthly, if preferred. This provides a consistent assessment of pain and quality of life that patients can self-perform as part of the **PITS Program**. Patients can then implement an appropriate treatment program, either on their own or in consultation with a pain management team, and adjust the treatment program as necessary with the periodic **PITS Score** reevaluations, as they move forward with the overall care plan. Remember, the higher your **PITS Score** the better you are doing!

Treatment: The treatment portion of the program is determined after the initial assessment, and is started at a patient's own direction for milder pain or done with informed professional pain management team input and direction, as is often the case for more severe pain conditions. Treatment options are divided into *four sections* of care, which again follow the **P-I-T-S** *acronym*, with choices of treatment offered depending on the severity of pain and the root cause of that pain. At this time, **P–Pills** or medications, are considered in a carefully controlled and monitored fashion, especially when it comes to using opioids. The second option is **I–Injections,** or a series of injections, if necessary, to help with the pain of a herniated disc, or an inflamed joint, or a muscle spasm, as examples. The third treatment option is **T–Therapy**, often considered the most important option, and recommended in conjunction with other treatment options, and includes physical, psychological, sleep, and complementary therapy approaches. The final treatment option is **S–Surgery**, which is usually recommended when patients fail to get adequate relief with the other three options. Again, this provides a *snapshot* of your current treatment options at any given time, and gets you thinking about future treatment options as needed.

These multidisciplinary integrative treatment options are set forth in the **PITS Program** as a clinical pathway protocol toward optimizing a patient's **PITS Score**, and therefore, improving their overall comfort and quality of life. All the new pain patients seen in my office each week are placed in this program concept, where their pain care is individualized to their specific comfort and functional level goals. In a comfortable outpatient environment, patients are taught how easy and straightforward the care plan aspect can be by remembering, that for *any pain*, you always ask yourself using the **P-I-T-S** *acronym*: *"Is there a **pill** for it, an **injection** for it, a **therapy** for it, and is there a **surgery** for it?"*—it really is that simple! Patients return for evaluation, many monthly, if necessary, to determine if their management program is working to their satisfaction, and to adjust the care plan as needed. It is important to remember, that if a patient has a chronic pain situation, the focus of the **PITS Program** is on *management* of pain, rather than the *cure* of chronic pain which is rare.

Highlights of the P-I-T-S Program

The **PITS Program** has shown to be a *great time saver* for patients, and helps coordinate more comprehensive care strategies, with just *one* initial evaluation. It turns out, many patients have previously been to numerous doctors and through numerous different medications and therapies, but nonetheless are still experiencing significant pain.

Another advantage of the program is that it *reduces stress*, knowing that your pain care team is going to take the pain seriously, like any other serious medical disease such as diabetes or high blood pressure. Keep in mind, the key behind all the treatment options, is that all these options cover the three basic pain management care approaches as needed to help patients reach their individual goals—*medical pain management* (medications and therapy), *interventional pain management* (injections), and finally *surgical pain management* (operations), if necessary.

Most of the **P-I-T-S** *treatment protocol* is based on *conventional medical care. Complementary techniques* like acupuncture, massage, and yoga, are also very important for patients to consider when treating chronic pain in a multidimensional wellness program, because many patients do not get enough relief with just conventional pain care management alone. Thus, we often combine conventional and complementary care, to form what is called *integrative medical care*. An integrative model offers patients the best of both

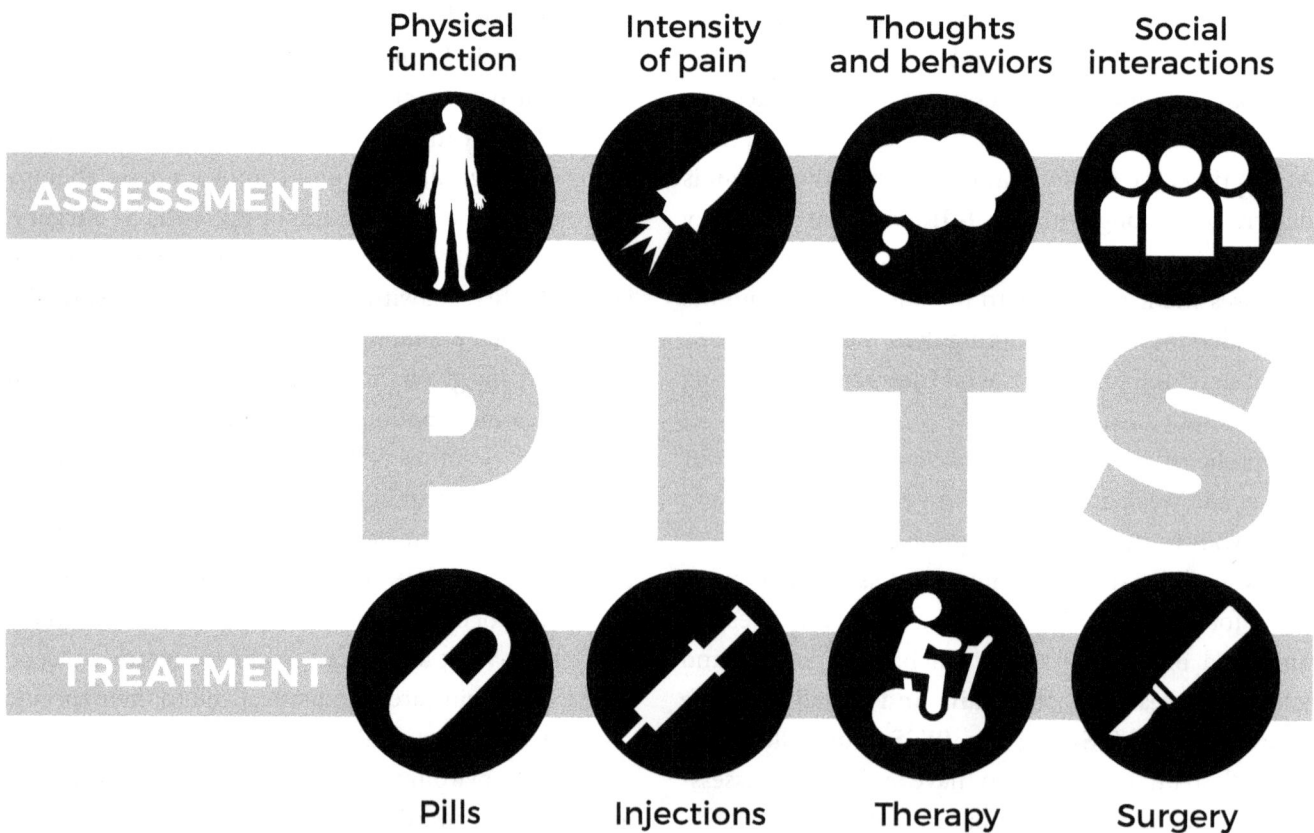

| Physical function | Intensity of pain | Thoughts and behaviors | Social interactions |

ASSESSMENT

PITS

TREATMENT

| Pills | Injections | Therapy | Surgery |

approaches. Most patients appreciate the many options available for pain care, once someone explains how it all works, and answers their questions.

So, you will learn that following a multi-disciplinary plan for chronic pain, with many options of care, is *always better* than just following a uni-modality plan, with just one option of care. The philosophy of constantly increasing and repeating the same treatments of opioids, injections, and surgery is not a solution, and in fact, is part of the problem with opioid addiction in America today. Some doctors keep prescribing the same course of treatments, even when the patient says, "*They have stopped working.*" The new generation of pain management specialists have realized that just pills were not enough to help patients, just injections were not enough, just doing therapy was not enough, and just having surgery was not always the right answer. In my experience, it is the balanced approach to integrative clinical management, and having a strong educational focus to pain care, which works best for most patients in a wellness program, especially when you customize the treatment plan to the individual where *they tell you that it is actually working.*

Historically, in January 2001 the United States Congress proclaimed the first decade of the new millennia as the *Decade of Pain Control and Research.* This proclamation tasked the medical community with studying and improving the poor job that America had been doing in addressing and treating acute, chronic, and cancer pain issues. At that time, one of the big concerns was that a lot of patients were being undertreated with opioid narcotics. So, you can imagine what happened in the years that followed with the escalation of *opioid pain killer* prescriptions and pill amounts. Even with the best intentions, the country got in trouble with patient overdoses, doctor shopping issues, drug diversion concerns, and so forth—it happened.

Persistent pain causes long term physical, mental, and emotional damage—no doubt—but the **PITS Program** approach will help alleviate all three, and at the same time help reduce America's healthcare costs.

Now, many pain management practices are finally reducing the issuance of opioid prescriptions as a primary course for pain relief, in terms of dosage amounts and frequency. They have begun utilizing more non-narcotic pain medications, more therapy-based approaches, and more interventional injection-based pain control methods. The reality is that many pain management specialists still use a fair number of opioid narcotics in controlling pain, especially when other strategies have not been successful. However, today we are putting relative limits on doses and frequencies, and conducting mandatory monitoring protocols with opioid narcotic prescribers and suppliers. We follow state prescription monitoring programs, we require periodic office urine drug testing when using long-term opioids, and provide patient opioid risk assessments. *We now guide patients toward more therapy and injection-based care and even recommend surgery, if necessary, rather than just keep escalating opioid narcotic levels.*

Again, it is *all about balance and making sure that patients move forward with their pain care,* in their ultimate quest for a satisfactory level of comfort and function, and their overall quality of life. Everyone who reads this book will discover the **Pain is the PITS Program** is the simplest yet comprehensive, straightforward, understandable and effective *"best practice"* wellness program pathway for any type of pain.

The **Pain is the PITS Program** is my educational and clinical care vision to help advance the latest teachings in pain management for the country. Again, I found that as important as it is to treat the patients, it is equally important to teach the patients. I think most pain patients appreciate that pain treatment plans can be more successful if they better understand their specific options, and the scope of their overall treatment program. The ultimate goal is to maximize their **PITS Score** so they can realize their optimal comfort and function levels and have the best possible quality of life.

So, I hope you agree that the **PITS Program** is a much needed and timely national patient-oriented educational pain management program for America. More and more patients and families will gain access to this knowledge and start reducing the chronic pain burden in their daily lives. I will teach America about the **PITS Program** and show them how it works—after all, *not only am I the creator of the program, but also, a patient!* It can be similar to a typical weight loss program, where you first weigh in, buy food products if you desire, go to the all-important support meetings, get motivated, then reach and maintain your goal of weight loss through time.

When it comes to a *"pain loss"* program, there is no universally known national pain program to learn and follow, which is why I established **P-I-T-S**. Picture this—a patient first takes their **PITS Score** assessment, selects treatment options by themselves and with their pain management team as needed, buys pain relief products as desired, goes to **P-I-T-S** *Question-and-Answer Meetings* for support and to get motivated and learn to take a proactive approach, then eventually reaches and maintains their acceptable pain relief and quality-of-life goals through time—see the similarity between the two program approaches? When patients follow educational worksheets in a program with certain goals in mind, follow a point score, and are motivated to stay on track, then the desired outcome should happen—just give it a chance!

Today there are an estimated 100 million pain sufferers in the United States, with an annual cost of over $600 billion in all the pain care itself, not to mention all the resultant disability. Moving forward, America needs further significant change in how we assess pain and treat acute and chronic pain. Improvements must really come from all the major stockholders, including the government, healthcare providers, the medical profession academia, and the patients themselves. The **Pain is the PITS Program** is designed to adjust the way America thinks about pain assessment, and how to best treat pain in an integrative **P-I-T-S acronym** fashion. If *we all get it there*, it will become the premier educational pain management wellness program in the country, with the universally recognized ***P-I-T-S philosophy of care!***

CHAPTER 1

Pain is a Disease

As an anesthesiologist and pain management physician caring for patients over the last twenty-five years practicing on Long Island, I eventually realized that I was part of an initial group of highly trained doctors that helped advance the modern-day specialty of *Pain Medicine and Interventional Pain Management* in this country. I feel very honored and privileged to have had the opportunity to study and learn under many wonderful scholars and clinicians. Today, the field of pain management has grown to include other specialties, including physical medicine and rehabilitation (physiatry), as well as neurology and psychiatry. All three of these American Medical Association (AMA) approved medical specialties have come together to form what is now the current multidisciplinary pain fellowship training for aspiring pain management doctors today. It is a growing focus of pain care medical training today for physicians, to help those who suffer from chronic persistent intractable pain, so patients can seek out the best care possible.

One of the big shifts in thinking in this country was not just treating pain as a *symptom*, but rather, thinking of it as an actual *disease state*, especially as it applies to chronic persistent pain. Similar to addiction, which has long been classified as a disease, pain was viewed by previous generations as a weakness with stronger people having higher thresholds for pain. This is no longer the conventional wisdom. There can be actual permanent neurologic changes in the brain and spinal cord of chronic pain patients, as demonstrated using functional-MRIs and other tests, and it all happens as a direct result of chronic persistent pain sensations bombarding the nervous system!

Acute pain most often will resolve through time within days, weeks, or perhaps months—but chronic pain does not. Chronic pain can linger for years, or a lifetime, and serves no useful purpose. It is a *pathological manifestation* of a disease state. Statistics show that eight out of every ten visits to a doctor in America involve the patient experiencing some sort of pain, and more than half of those pain-related doctor visits, are due to chronic recurrent pain. This is a real disease problem from my perspective.

It took many years for government agencies, the medical profession, and patients and insurance payers, to accept pain management as a disease-model of care with its own distinct set of pathophysiological processes and treatments. Through advanced academics, research, and clinical studies, and learning more and more about how pain is transmitted in the body and brain, with the help of neuroimaging and neuro-chemical analysis, the field of pain management is now well established as a sub-specialty of medicine. Currently, physicians must first be *board-certified* in their primary area of medicine, whether it is anesthesiology, physiatry, neurology, psychiatry, and so forth, and then do a *fellowship* year of additional training specifically in pain management. Maybe in the future, the field of pain medicine will become its own specialty, where students who finish with medical school can apply to enter directly into a pain medicine residency training program—time will tell.

I was fortunate enough to be board-certified in anesthesiology and interventional pain management early on in my career. One of the goals of this book is to be a *"how-to-do"* guide to help educate patients, and the general medical community, about current and emerging pain assessment and therapy options, and how specific pain management teams can better support both patients and non-pain trained health professionals.

Ideally, the **Pain is the PITS Program** helps people adopt a new lifestyle with reduced pain. It will become commonplace and represent a different way of thinking about and dealing with pain in our everyday lives. The program's primary focus is to provide an educational philosophy of care, which offers both a clinical pathway and an interactive tool (the **PITS Pain and Quality-of-Life Score**) for the assessment and treatment of chronic recurrent and persistent pain in America. *It is all about pain awareness and treatment options!*

An Institute of Medicine (IOM) survey in 2011 revealed that there are more than one hundred million Americans suffering from a recurrent or persistent pain state. That is one in three Americans based on current U.S. population estimates. All of these people are potential benefactors of the **PITS Program**. In the past, we know that the treatment of pain of all types created other problems in the form of opioid abuse, misuse, and addiction.

But we also know that many Americans suffer from untreated pain and have no pain management plan in their lives. Some of these people think that pain is an inevitable part of life, or they believe that as you get older you must endure the body's natural breakdown. Many that suffer have gone through multiple doctors, pain medications, and injections, for naught. Many have even had surgery to alleviate their pain, but they still hurt, and have lost hope that they will ever find a solution to their chronic pain. There usually is not just one solution, which is why they still feel pain. They need a comprehensive series of solution-based strategies, which will focus on the symptoms with a broad integrative approach. That is what the **PITS Program** can do for all these patients.

Pain is as much a disease as cancer, and possibly more debilitating. This does not have to be the case. As mentioned earlier, persistent and untreated pain leads to a vicious cycle of poor, non-restorative sleep, and

mood disorders, such as anxiety and depression. If a patient knows that they are part of a pain management program that customizes a wellness strategy just for them, then their anxiety and depression should diminish. Attaining a *positive mental state*, while undergoing pain management therapy, is a critical step toward reducing pain and suffering, and improving the overall quality of life of the patient—make sense?

The Mind/Body Relationship

Part of the patient experience is to educate them and give them a better understanding of how pain travels in the body. Please refer to my version of the **PITS Pain Diagram—Mind/Body Relationship** (see **APPENDIX B**). Basically, there are *four phases*:

- the first phase of *Activation* involves pain typically originating at the periphery of the body, whether it is on the skin, or in a muscle or joint, from some injury or painful medical condition. This typically starts from some source of injury, or from an infection, burn, or a surgical operation.

- The second phase is *Conduction* or travelling of the painful signals along the peripheral nerves in the arms, legs, trunk, and up-and-down along the central nerves in the spinal cord.

- The third phase of pain is called *Adjustment* and it relates to how the body dampens the pain signal, as it travels to the brain. Certain chemical substances like norepinephrine, serotonin, and endorphins, and others are secreted to help lessen the sensation of pain.

- The fourth phase is the brain *Experience* of the final pain sensation, which causes the actual sensory feeling of the pain and the emotional suffering components, that patients perceive.

The primary goal of the pain management team is to create relief strategies along the way that can *"block"* as many of these phases of pain as possible, to achieve the best overall result of reduced pain, and a better quality of life.

It is a daunting task to reach out to the millions of Americans who suffer from chronic pain, and to educate them on the benefits of the **PITS Program**. But I am committed to becoming one of the *new age* pain management voices in America, and to make the **P-I-T-S** educational pain management assessment and treatment philosophy available and affordable for everyone, to help solve the current opioid crisis and epidemic of pain in this country. There is *no nationally recognized universal educational pain program of this sort in this country yet!*

The **PITS Program** will help to support ongoing efforts from academic institutions, and existing pain management societies and experts, to address this national crisis. By getting the patients involved in their own pain assessments and pain treatment plans, chronic pain can be more successfully treated, like the disease that it is. I am going to do my best to see that the **Pain is the PITS Program** is elevated to one of the best educational practices, especially for the treatment of chronic and persistent pain, and to see that **P-I-T-S** is widely recognized as a universally accepted pain management guide. Along with this book, we will accomplish this through a variety of media outlets and platforms focusing on the internet website, as well as question-and-answer (Q&A) public meetings and seminars.

Initially, there will be the concept of virtual **PITS Pain Centers of America**, which will host pain management information and media content online on the **PITS Website**. Eventually, we might establish brick and mortar **PITS Pain Centers of America**, so pain sufferers can have direct access right in their own communities—like all the weight loss centers that currently exist. Integrative pain management will hopefully become part of the American lexicon, and not something one hides or shrinks away from, due to embarrassment.

Through time, **P-I-T-S** might provide lists of recommended pain care professionals who agree with the **P-I-T-S** *care philosophy* in cities and towns across America, for patient office consultation. We could offer 1-on-1 online telemedicine (**Tele-PITS**) consultation with a nurse or physician, group or individual therapy with a psychologist, or even gatherings with other pain patients to share their treatment stories. Patients could have access to **P-I-T-S** *recommended pain products* for sale, like TENS units, back braces, ice and heat packs, inversion tables and cervical traction devices, fish oils

and probiotics, and so forth, to help with the management of their pain. We are going to try to attempt this massive *grassroots effort* to see how many of America's painful lives we can change for the better.

It is going to be a two-way-street between the doctor and patient, each working *"50-50"* with the other. The doctor will provide their experience as the scientist, and their knowledge of evidence-based medicine, and their experience of what works and what does not work, when managing a particular chronic pain condition. The patient will be involved from the earliest assessment, and will develop knowledge about their pain condition, and the various options available to treat that condition. The patients ultimately determine if a particular treatment option is working or not, all based on their overall goals. Thus, this close working relationship between the pain management team and the patient is a critical component of the **PITS Program**. *There has to be a lot of patient-doctor communication and trust!*

Even though we will diagnose and treat pain like a disease state, pain itself is always subjective. This is unlike a neurosurgeon, for example, treating a patient with a brain tumor, where the care of this medical condition is primarily objective in nature. The neurosurgeon is going to be giving the patient the best options, given the known limits of brain surgery. The patient, although given a risk-and-benefit analysis, relies solely on the surgeon to provide a recommendation, based on statistics and historical outcomes in brain tumor management. So, unlike neurosurgery, pain management treatment will always involve a great deal of subjectivity. A pain management doctor must believe the patient's pain complaints, because unlike a brain tumor, the actual pain cannot be measured definitively. No doubt there is a known objective science behind pain causes and treatment, and this body of knowledge continues to grow rapidly, but when a patient says, *"It hurts,"* the doctor must give them the benefit of the doubt.

The patient's preference for treatment becomes an integral part of the process, where there are typically many avenues of care available, to achieve pain control and improve quality of life. It seems intuitive that pain management should be a patient's *"right"* and that everyone should be entitled to it. Unfortunately, for pain management, unlike the neurosurgical brain tumor example, successful pain treatment is often thought of as a privilege, and not taken as serious in everyday medical care. There are strong forces in this country, and around the world, which are trying to change this by pushing pain management as a right, and adding it to the patient's bill of rights. All of this remains to be seen as we go forward with our advancement of the Pain Medicine specialty.

The **PITS Program** is designed to assess and treat the many different types of pain, including acute pain, chronic non-cancer pain, and chronic cancer pain. We need to address pain in the very young and the very old. We need to address pain that exists after surgeries, chronic abdominal and pelvic pain, and even psychogenic pain. The various types of lower back pain, neck pain, headache pain, and face pain, all must be addressed. Other types of pain that **P-I-T-S** will treat are arthritic pain and the many different kinds of nerve pain, such as diabetic neuropathy, shingles pain, and complex regional pain syndrome (or reflex sympathetic dystrophy—RSD) pain. **P-I-T-S** will also be able to treat pain from tendinitis, bursitis, and fasciitis. There are several different pain mechanisms that patients need to be aware of in basic understandable terms. All of these different types of pain will be incorporated into the **P-I-T-S** *assessment and treatment protocol*, to help guide patients in looking for different ways to control their own pain. The **PITS Program** is truly simple and straightforward, and is ultimately a way for patients to finally address their disease, through a straightforward educational process of understanding expanded pain care options available to them—and how to incorporate the program into their daily lives.

In summary, below are the *basic steps* a patient can take in order to adopt the **PITS Program** in their daily lives, and thus reduce their acute and chronic pain burden:

- Patients first read the **Pain is the PITS Book** in order to get the big picture of modern-day pain management in America, and to develop a better understanding of their individual pain condition. They will be able to better understand the difference between assessment and treatment, have a clearer idea of the various pain management and

wellness strategies available, and better understand when to *go it alone* or *consult* with a medical or pain management team. The idea is to better identify certain pain conditions that may apply to them, and to then zero in on the possible treatment strategies, in order to improve overall comfort and function in life.

- Patients will be able to access their individual pain management program plan via the **PITS Book** or the **Pain is the PITS Program Website (painis-thepits.com)**, to then complete a baseline assessment and obtain their **PITS Score**. On the **PITS Website**, there will be sections featuring video and podcast presentations, and *Ask the Pain Expert* answers, which will help to further educate the patient. All of this pain knowledge will help them focus on weaker areas of their **PITS Score**.

- During certain times of the year, **PITS Meetings** will be held for all those patients who have signed up for the **Pain is the PITS** educational program and for the public at large, to have *Question & Answer sessions* where patients and pain experts and allied health professionals can meet face-to-face, so everyone can help each other through feedback from their own pain management experiences.

- As the **PITS Website** develops, patients will be able to access a network of pain management and wellness professionals in their community. These professionals, including the primary care physician, will comprise the pain management team—consisting of a physical therapist, chiropractor, psychologist, massage therapist, acupuncturist, neurologist, pain specialist and various surgeons, as needed.

- After getting the advice of their newly formed pain management and wellness team, and using the tools available on the **PITS Website**, the patient begins initial pain treatment protocols, and utilizes the **PITS Worksheets** to monitor progress and their personal experience (see **PITS Sample Worksheets** in APPENDIX C).

- Patients might eventually be able to access individual pain management specialists on the **PITS Website**, through web portals via telemedicine at an affordable cost, to ask questions and get more information about their individual pain problem(s). The overall goal is to always maximize your **PITS Score**.

"Less pain, more gain!"

Ultimately, each patient should begin to feel better as the weeks and months go by in the program. They will reach a reduced level of pain and improved quality of life, that they can live with comfortably, and maintain it through **P-I-T-S**.

The plan is to roll out the **PITS Program** on a regional, and then national basis, so that millions of pain sufferers can finally get a lasting relief plan they can incorporate in their daily life, to keep their pain burden to a minimum. Combining education with specific clinical pathways for its relief, the disease of *PAIN* can finally be brought out into the light, and treated like any other disease. Just think, when a patient is diagnosed with cancer, there are certain established treatment protocols that are employed, depending on the nature of the cancer, and individual patient factors. These cancer treatments have been adjusted and developed over time, and today there are many successes. With pain, the approach will be similar, where the pain team will document the pain condition, establish a course of action to treat and minimize that pain, and then evaluate results over time. As new research reveals new treatment options, these therapies can be incorporated into the **PITS Program**, and utilized when necessary.

Remember, the **PITS Program** *is a life program!* You do not just give up after a month or two. You do this kind of program for as long as you need for life, like a weight loss program for the disease of obesity. From my individual physician and pain sufferer point of view, I am sure this will make a big difference in helping to provide a better approach for pain care in America. Remember, chronic persistent pain is a disease!

CHAPTER 2

The Opioid Crisis in America

The *opioid crisis in America* had its potential start in the mid-1990s when semi-synthetic drugs like OxyContin were developed and prescribed as pain killers. This highly addictive medication certainly blocked the pain but did nothing to actually solve the pain issue. At that time, this level of pain care was usually reserved for cancer patients. This new pain medication, similar to the opium poppy, was being prescribed for all types of pain, and since the symptoms were often never fully addressed, the pain would often come back, and even worse sometimes.

According to the *Centers for Disease Control and Prevention (CDC)*, in 1996 doctors prescribed 670,000 oxycodone pills for pain relief. By 2002, doctors were prescribing more than 6 million pills per year, and by 2010, that number grew to almost 32 million pills per year. In 2002, more than 5,000 people in the U.S. died from opioid overdoses. By 2012, the sale of prescription opioids amounted to more than $11 Billion in the United States. In that same year more than 15,000 died from opioid overdoses. In 2017, more than 72,000 people died in the U.S. from drug overdoses of which two-thirds were attributed to opioids. Still the following year, 69,000 people died from both prescription and illicit-use heroin and fentanyl opioid overdoses. That was more than fatalities from auto accidents and gun violence combined! According to the *National Institute of Drug Abuse (NIDA)*, even though the U.S. accounts for only 5% of the global population, we consume more than 80% of oxycodone produced worldwide.

So, a main theme of this book is to discuss the opioid epidemic in America, and suggest a more integrative approach to pain management, which attempts to reduce the need for continuously escalating opioid prescriptions to control pain. The **PITS Program** *philosophy* of educational and clinical care can be the answer to improving the nation's pain management practices, without worsening the opioid crisis.

Over the last 20 years, the prevalence of chronic pain in America has been rising, and so has the healthcare cost of assessing and treating this increased level of chronic pain and suffering. Pain management professionals in this country were told 20 years ago that they were undertreating acute and chronic pain, and so the natural response was to increase opioid prescriptions, which by then had become easy to produce and readily available. Opioids were prescribed based on understood pain practice experiences through the years, and based on published literature, and expert opinion. Where in the past opioid prescriptions were mostly relegated for terminally ill patients, and with federal and state laws relaxed for physicians, opioids started being prescribed more frequently to treat acute and chronic *non-cancer pain* in the United States.

It bears mentioning at this point, without delving into a political commentary, that pharmaceutical companies were in a position to generate enormous profits, as the use of prescribed opioids became more widespread. It also bears mentioning that a significant part of the opioid crisis in America is due to abuses by patients and doctors, both in the writing of prescriptions and the illegal distribution of them, as well as sale of opioid narcotics without a medical prescription.

Around the year 2000, the *Joint Commission on the Accreditation of Healthcare Organizations (JCAHO)* set up new pain management standards for accredited facilities, which were focused mostly for hospitals and outpatient surgical centers. This gave rise to a national movement to recognize pain management as a crucial and legitimate medical protocol. Around this time, the concept of pain as the *fifth vital sign* was born, or what is commonly known as a patient's *pain score*—along with blood pressure, pulse, respiratory rate, and temperature. This was thought to help increase awareness for the right of patients to experience pain relief. This was supported by national pain organizations and the *Federation of State Medical Boards*, which reinforced the idea that physicians would not be prosecuted for prescribing opioid narcotics for legitimate medical purposes. Pharmaceutical companies that had developed opioid narcotic medications in the 1990s, such as OxyContin, began aggressive marketing campaigns assuring the medical community that the risks of addiction were small, and the benefits of better pain relief were great.

Thus, since approximately the year 2000, the medical community believed that the newly developed opioid formulations were highly effective and safe, and had minimal adverse effects when prescribed for legitimate patients in real pain. President Clinton had declared 2000–2010 the *Decade of Pain Control and Research in the United States*, drawing attention to the need for more pain research and the need for treating pain more aggressively, as the primary goals. By 2011, prescriptions for opioids had doubled, and with that, opioid analgesic-related deaths were responsible for more tragedies than suicide and motor vehicle accident deaths, as well as deaths from cocaine and heroin, combined. Also, at this same time, chronic pain as a disease state was affecting more Americans than diabetes and cancer combined—striking to say the least!

Now, as a response to all the chronic pain and all the opioids being prescribed, stakeholders started looking at the amount of opioid that patients were taking on a daily basis, as measured by **Morphine Milligram Equivalent (MME)** or **Morphine Equivalent Dose (MED)**—*MME is how other opioids compare to morphine in potency*—and its relation to death rates. For example, if a patient was on <100 MME per day, then the risk of a serious adverse event, like drug overdose and death, was a certain statistical percentage—but for >100 MME, there was a significant *"increased"* statistical risk to the patient. There were, of course, many other issues confounding the situation, like multiple scripts being written by different physicians, patient doctor shopping for more medications, patients mixing sedative-hypnotics medications with their opioids, and the constant problem of opioid drug diversion.

In 2011, the *Institute of Medicine (IOM)* was put to the task of identifying the extent of the pain management problem in America, and they came out with a report titled: *Relieving Pain in America: A Blueprint for Transforming Prevention, Care, Education, and Research*. The task force found that 116 million Americans had some level of pain lasting weeks-to-years and costing around 600 billion dollars per year for care, lost wages and workdays, and disability payments.

The IOM reported there were questions of the usefulness of long-term opioid use in terms of risk and benefit. They found a constant struggle between the balance of opioid pain relief and diversion and opioid abuse. In terms of science and research, the evidence suggests that short-term opioid use is beneficial, but those benefits decline over time as the pain relief aspect diminishes, and the chance of addiction increases. Plus, opioids are depressants by nature, and have been shown to depress various bodily functions, including our central nervous system, endocrine and gastrointestinal systems, our immune system, and in some patients make the even pain worse—a phenomenon called *opioid-induced hyperalgesia*—ouch!

Now, in response to the growing problem of opioid addiction, in March 2016, the Centers for Disease Control and Prevention (CDC) published the country's first ever opioid guideline for physicians. This 12-point guideline was intended to help physicians better evaluate the risk and benefits of opioid narcotics, in the big picture of pain management, and to consider alternative integrative care options going forward.

The CDC's new upper *"high"* opioid level is 90 MED for non-pain specialists and focuses on new patients starting out on opioid therapy. My **PITS Program**, again after 25-years of academic and clinical experience, sets an upper limit of 180 MME for *pain specialists* (+/− 25%) treating *legacy patients*—patients with a pre-existing history of chronic stable higher-dose usage for years. The idea is to allow new patients starting out on opioids, and legacy patients continuing with opioid treatment, a clearer understanding of what is considered low, moderate, and high levels of daily opioid usage, and the intendent risks at each level.

Initially the CDC focused on primary care physicians and not the pain specialists who have been dealing with patients on high dose opioids for years, if not decades. The CDC wants better communication with patients on the risk-to-benefit ratio of opioid use levels, and they want improved safety and alternative pain treatment options. They also want decreased risk associated with long-term opioid therapy, especially abuse, misuse, and addiction. Over the last few years, it seems that the new guidelines have influenced *all* physicians who prescribe. Most new pain patients starting on opioid therapy rarely go above 90 MME, and patients in general seem to have a better understanding of the issues surrounding long-term opioid therapy in today's society.

Moving forward, the key to using opioids in pain management will be:

- careful and complete patient evaluations
- not choosing opioids as first-line treatment
- conducting opioid abuse risk screening
- following up with patients and keep from continuously escalating opioid therapy
- conducting urine drug testing (UDT)
- checking the state prescription drug monitoring program (PDMP) for controlled substance prescriptions that patients receive

- establish exit plans for discontinuing opioid prescriptions
- zero or minimal use of benzodiazepine sedatives while on opioids

The **PITS Program** can help those who suffer from pain but want to avoid the vicious cycle of dependency and addiction from the use of opioids. It has been documented that even patients that follow the usage guidelines of an opioid prescription can become addicted—*no one is immune to the potential physical and emotional effects of different opioids.* The comprehensive approach of the **PITS Program** will quickly identify other pain management options before addiction can take hold. Also, communication through the future development of a **P-I-T-S** *Network* of pain management professionals and patients, will help pain sufferers reach out before the use of prescription drug therapy gets out of hand. Remember, as noted previously, the **PITS Program** is a life program to treat pain as a disease condition. You do not just give up after a month or two. This is a life changing event, like a surgical weight loss program for the disease of obesity.

Opioid and Narcotic Dosing Charts

Keeping in mind the current opioid crisis in America, while sensitive to the patient's pain treatment program, the **PITS Program** approach always attempts to avoid opioid dose escalations over time. For a comparison of typical dosage recommendations between the **PITS Program** and the CDC, I have created my version of a **PITS Opioid Narcotic Comparison Dosing Chart** (see **APPENDIX D**) for many different types of opioids. These types of dosing charts have existed for decades, developed through academic and clinical research, and patient care responses.

This opioid comparison dosing chart helps to demonstrate what is considered low-moderate-high risk ranges for different opioids, and provides a maximum recommended treatment guideline, considering the severity of a patient's pain condition and previous response to non-opioid therapies in the **P-I-T-S *treatment protocol***. In general, if a patient is considered a *low-risk candidate*, then they can have a higher dose of opioid for treatment, as needed. If a patient is considered a *high-risk candidate*, then they should not be on opioids at all, or they can have carefully monitored lower dose opioid levels, as needed.

This is only a guide, created out of my academic and clinical experience, not a hard-fast rule. Ultimately, levels of opioid therapy for individual patient care are left to the patient's specific pain treatment team, hopefully considering many of the factors I have outlined and discussed above. *Be careful!*

CHAPTER 3

The Proactive Approach

My experience and views on the subject of pain management in the United States comes after two and a half decades of training and hands-on clinical application, treating thousands of patients along the way. My **PITS Program** *philosophy* was developed throughout these years by caring for, not only the poor and indigent pain sufferers in a county hospital on Long Island, but also from caring for the more affluent pain sufferers in a multibillion-dollar private health network system. I quickly discovered that pain does not discriminate by religion, race, or financial condition. *Pain simply stinks, it is the PITS!*

Remember, the **P-I-T-S** *acronym* represents both assessment and treatment of pain. This is the simple genius of this educational program, where different pains need different options in the **PITS Program**. The program is designed to be tailored to the patient's needs and is *interactive* between the patient and their pain management team. There are many different pain care choices to consider, so my approach will help guide patients through the various options, all tailored toward improved wellness. The key is to be proactive in the program and to keep an open mind.

Some patients want medications to control their pain, and some patients do not. In general, there are anti-inflammatory pills, muscle relaxant pills, nerve agent pills, and opioid narcotic pills. Some patients do not mind injections, and others are afraid of needles. An injection can certainly help control pain—*patients just have to try it once and see*—and can help decrease

the need for opioid narcotic usage. Some patients are interested in physical therapy, and others are not. In those cases, some other complementary therapy regimen can be recommended, such as massage treatments, yoga, or possibly even acupuncture. Most people do not like the idea of surgery, and usually this option is reserved when nothing else will work. So, the **PITS Program** encourages exploring several different types of conservative options, and working your way toward a surgical option, when necessary. Patients usually know when they are close to needing a surgical procedure. *You see it on their face at some point* in their treatment course, if and when, the pain becomes unbearable.

On the point of narcotics, the misuse and abuse of opioid narcotics has become one of the leading healthcare problems in America. As previously mentioned, recent statistics point to this being a bigger problem than heroin, cocaine, and other illicit drugs combined. As of this writing, opioid narcotic usage has matched the use of marijuana in this country. It is no wonder why medical marijuana treatment indications, as well as recreational marijuana use, are increasing in this country, but not without its own pros-and-cons treatment issues.

America has been actively trying to address this narcotic problem as I write this book. Federal and State governments have cracked down on illegal drug shipments, and addicts are beginning to receive the help they so desperately need in drug rehabilitation centers. But a lot still needs to be done regarding the use of opioid narcotics and their ideal role in the treatment of pain.

Opioid and Depression Risk Screening

When a patient is considered a candidate for opioid prescribing, the approach that **P-I-T-S** takes is to individualize treatment doses based on that specific patient's pain situation—*one size DOES NOT fit all!* The accurate history of the patient's overall health issues and previous treatments is critical in determining the baseline for future pain management treatment options. Opioid levels, and frequency and duration of use, will be based on the patient's pain intensity situation, past narcotics prescriptions, and the prior failure of non-opioid treatment strategies. All patients being prescribed any opioid narcotic as part of their long-term **P-I-T-S** *treatment protocol* plan will be strongly encouraged to complete my version of an opioid risk assessment tool called the **PITS Opioid Risk Screening (PORS) Assessment** (see **APPENDIX E**)—or any other commonly used opioid risk screening tool.

Another issue that factors into the use of opioid narcotics as a treatment option in the **PITS Program**, is the patient's mental and emotional state, particularly regarding depression. If a patient is suffering from depression, then the use of opioid narcotics as part of the **P-I-T-S** *treatment protocol* plan needs to be carefully considered. In order to identify patients that could possibly be suffering from depression, each patient will be strongly encouraged to complete my version of a depression screening tool called the **PITS Depression Screening (PDS) Assessment** (see **APPENDIX F**)—or any other commonly used depression screening questionnaire.

Again, in general, if you are a *low-risk candidate* on assessment, then you can have a higher dose of opioid for treatment as needed. If you are a *high-risk candidate* on assessment, you should not be on opioids at all or you can have lower dose opioids levels as needed. This will provide an opioid use guideline and not a hard-fast rule. Opioid treatment will ultimately

be based on an individual patient's situation. Treating physicians and pain patients will always work together for the *optimal* opioid level, which is not always clear with the very many types of pain states and pain intensities that patients experience. As a general principal, when it comes to longer-term opioid use, physician and patient should seek the lowest effective dosing, with the least side effects, for the longest period of time—*without continuous dose escalation!*

Because of chronic pain and the growing opioid problem, the introduction of the **PITS Program** as an educational tool is excellent. Both doctors and patients will benefit with increased awareness of how to minimize the opioid epidemic moving forward, and how to expand the use of more integrative care options, for safer longer-term pain management. This book presents a **Clinical Pain Pathway** with **PITS Protocol Treatment** options, **Pain and Quality-of-Life Score**, **Opioid and Depression Screening**, **Narcotic Dosing Guidelines**, **Worksheets**, and much more. Collaborating with local medical communities all across the country, the **PITS Program** will educate pain sufferers on the benefits and dangers of opioids, help reduce the development of addiction to narcotics, find alternative sources of pain relief for people who experience chronic and persistent pain, reduce the amount of people addicted to prescription drugs, and help reduce healthcare costs throughout the country.

Always remember the *motto* of the **Pain is the PITS Program**:

"Feel better and live your life, because pain is the PITS!"

In my current clinical practice, when focusing on spine pain care initial evaluations, I always use the **P-I-T-S** *philosophy of care*. A lot of my patients through the years have said, *"Well Doctor I never thought of that,"* or *"That makes sense,"* or *"You have given me direction now so I can proceed more logically with my care,"* or *"Wow, you have made it so simple for me that now I can finally understand what all of my other doctors have been saying."*

This straightforward book and the media presentations on the **PITS Website (painisthepits.com)** will help millions of Americans, not just thousands, get access to this important educational material so they can start the *transformational comfort and function process*. Again, the key is to be proactive in the program with improving your overall pain and quality of life—you figure out where you have been, where you are now, and where you want to be in the future!

To help guide patients, I have developed a **P-I-T-S** *treatment protocol* with many treatment options for different pain conditions that affect most pain sufferers. In **CHAPTER 5**, the **PITS Treatments** chapter, I discuss specific causes of pain and list the typical **P-I-T-S** *treatment protocol* for each, along with many patient examples. My goal is to provide as many patients as possible with a real-life example of what their pain condition is, and how it can be addressed.

But it will always be up to the patient to adhere to the clinical pain relief pathway that is specifically developed for them. I will serve the role of pain management educator—your *pain coach* if you will. I will show you the possibilities toward improved comfort and a better quality of life, but individual patients must find comfort from a drive within themselves, a process that is as much physical as it is psychological—it really must be a proactive process.

In order to put their chronic pain into remission, patients are going to have to be self-motivated once they learn the program. Patients will realize that the maintenance of their own comfort and functional status will have to be on a priority basis, much like controlling and maintaining other disease states, like diabetes of high blood pressure. I will always provide you with educational guidance and I will always take your pain needs seriously. I will never say you are crazy, or it is all in your head, or there is nothing else to offer you for comfort, or you are just going to have to live with all the pain. *This kind of attitude is nonsense and counterproductive.* We are going to put the pain into a disease model, so that you will be offered assessment and treatment for life.

For any kind of pain, the **PITS Program** offers a direction of care—from head to toe, from migraines to bunions! So, I will always educate and motivate and offer direction for advancing your care options. *My gift in life is that I am an* **optimistic motivational educator**, *and I am going to continue to be passionate about passing the gift of my pain knowledge and experience on to as many people as I can, who are willing to listen to the message and improve their comfort and quality of life in the* **PITS Program**. My hope is that successful patients who learn the program will turn into what I call *critical patient thinkers*, and in turn, will spread the **PITS Program** *educational philosophy* to other pain sufferers going forward.

Through the years, many of my colleagues and patients have said, *"You should do this, you have a gift... this is real pain knowledge and a real easy program for pain patients to follow!"* So, I began to develop the **PITS Program** as an affordable educational program that pain sufferers can enter and follow. Our goal is to be proactive...to get the **P-I-T-S** *message of pain relief* to as many people as possible. We will do this with this book, through the videos and podcasts on the website, social media, and through many face-to-face **P-I-T-S** *Question-and-Answer Meetings* to be scheduled first on Long Island, then across America as the program continues to be popularized. This program will be a first of its kind, serving as a best practice universal guideline for personalized pain management, driven by the proactive interaction between patients and their pain management provider teams.

This program will help millions of pain sufferers achieve the best possible pain relief and quality of life possible. *Knowledge is power! Be proactive!*

CHAPTER 4

PITS Assessment: Pain and Quality-of-Life Score

The coordinated assessment of any pain condition is the first step toward achieving long-term pain relief. The patient must be honest about how they are feeling and what they have been through when a pain team is assessing their specific pain condition, and the pain team must use their experience and expertise—as well as other colleagues—to probe the intricacies of that pain condition in order to formulate the best plan of action moving forward with pain care.

Clinical Pathway for Pain Assessment and Treatment

One reason the **PITS Program** is successful is its simplicity. In a single page document, called the **PITS Clinical Pathway and Protocol for the Assessment and Treatment of Chronic Pain** (see **APPENDIX G**), the entire program of treatment of *ALL* chronic pain is outlined—and essentially for acute pain, since all chronic pain conditions first start out in an acute state. There are also similar, but more focused clinical guides for pain treatment of specific areas of the body, such as for chronic neck and back pain as seen on the **PITS Website**. The **PITS Program** is an educational guide to pain management in general, and offers a *multidisciplinary integrative clinical pathway* consisting of *four (4) steps*:

1. *Assessment of the pain.* Identifying the location and nature of the pain, taking a complete medical history of the patient, and identifying any psychological or social factors that might be present, are all part of a pain assessment. During this step, a comprehensive medical care evaluation is conducted involving a physical examination, examination of X-rays or other scans and images, and a diagnostic assessment. At the same time, a patient's baseline **PITS Pain and Quality-of-Life Score** (**PITS Score**) is first established.

2. *Development of a standardized plan.* This step includes building the pain management team and educating the patient about their pain condition. It involves identifying specific doctors, and other health professionals and specialists, which can help in the areas of anesthesiology, physical medicine and rehabilitation, neurology and psychiatry, spinal surgery, rheumatology, palliative care and oncology, internal medicine and family practice, pediatrics, OBGYN, or emergency room medicine, as necessary. After consulting with the newly formed pain management team, the patient is given various treatment options for their pain condition. At this point, the patient can be advised of the latest clinical studies or new treatment techniques, and the **PITS Patient Worksheets** are introduced.

3. *Implementation of pain treatment protocol.* This step of the pain treatment process involves the

P-I-T-S *treatment protocol* options, the core methodology of this pain relief strategy, and can be found in the next chapter. Remember, the *four categories* of treatment care are:

P is for Pills or medications, involving pharmacologic choices, whether they are anti-inflammatory medications of a non-steroidal or a steroidal nature, muscle relaxants, nerve pain agents, or opioid narcotic analgesics.

I is for Injections, which refers to interventional pain techniques, depending on the nature and severity of the pain. These can include epidural steroid injection (ESI) options, nerve blocks, joint injections, muscle or trigger point injections (TPIs), tendon injections, bursa injections, and so forth. Treatments can also include radiofrequency or burning pain relief procedures, and cryo-ablation or freezing pain relief procedures, if indicated. There are also diagnostic injection procedures, such as discography for certain spine conditions and CT scan myelograms for pinpointing the source of pain that might arise from spinal disc and spinal nerve problems.

T is for Therapy, which covers the four core types, including physical, psychological, sleep, and complementary therapy. Many patients first start out with the *physical* therapy category options, or all the non-pharmacological techniques, and include not only formal physical therapy (PT), but also chiropractic care and traction techniques, or occupational therapy (OT) techniques, as well as a home exercise program (HEP) and gym activities. We want patients to be as independent as possible with their activities of daily living (ADLs) using these basic approaches to physical care. There are also other advanced therapeutic techniques involving *physician care* as needed, including a physical medicine and rehabilitation (PM&R) doctor or a neuromuscular medicine and osteopathic (DO) manipulative doctor, especially when previous therapies are limited in their results.

S is for Surgery, or surgical intervention, if applicable. This treatment option is generally recommended after all other conservative options have been exhausted, but patients still remain in intractable pain. Surgery can entail a minimally invasive technique of the spine, joint, nerve, or tendon. It can entail a more invasive technique like spinal fusion for severe back pain or joint replacement for severe osteoarthritis joint pain. For certain abdominal and pelvic pain conditions, there is diagnostic laparoscopy or laparotomy surgical techniques, which are used when previous medical management is ineffective. There is also surgery to implant medical devices to control pain, as well, such as a spinal cord stimulator (SCS) or spinal narcotic pump therapy.

4. *Evaluation is the final step*. This final step is where the pain management team assesses the success of the customized treatment program determines if the patient's *goals* are being met—where patients are reaching an acceptable **PITS Pain and Quality-of-Life Score**. If additional treatment protocols are needed, then the treatment program will be adjusted and monitored for desired results. The key is close communication between the patient and pain management team, to ascertain which pain treatments are working and which are not—need to closely follow the pain *status* of the patient to maximize care. So, this critical step is a series of assessments and reassessments where the **PITS Score** is repeated to follow a patient's overall improvement.

Along with appropriate physician and nursing specialty care, another critical component is ***patient education***, which involves teaching patients to be *proactive*, by becoming aware of what their pain condition is, how to treat it, and how to minimize its flare-ups in the future. Assembling the proper pain management team is also vital, and the **PITS Program** can help you identify the proper medical personnel—through its anticipated community network of pain management providers—who agree with and support the **PITS Program** pain treatment philosophy.

Remember, the **PITS Assessment** is more than just the *physical diagnosis*. It also includes a *psychological evaluation* to assess anxiety and depression and allow for recommendations for cognitive-behavioral therapy as needed, in order to control the emotional component of the pain experience. It considers *sleep patterns*, and opens the door for *complementary therapies*, such as acupuncture, massage, yoga, essential oils, biofeedback, herbal medicines, and so forth. A patient's own understanding of the mind/body dynamic, with respect to the pain experience, is an important component of the pain relief process, and can lead to improved *social relationships*. The comprehensive evaluation of the patient's total condition—physical, psychological, and social—is what the **PITS Program** emphasizes, and represents the key overall pain management strategy, which helps promote greater wellness and faster healing.

PITS Pain and Quality-of-Life Score—PITS Score

The **PITS Program** focuses on evaluation and treatment of pain with the overriding goal of maximizing the patient's **PITS Pain and Quality-of-Life Score**. The **PITS Score** is the **"Holy Grail"** of the **PITS Program**!

Now, let us look at how the **PITS Score** is calculated. You can print the **PITS Score sheet** from **APPENDIX A** in the back of this book or download a copy from the **PITS Website (painisthepits.com)**. As a patient works through the categorical questions for each assessment section, it is important to have the best understanding of what the question is asking. There is no right or wrong answer for how much you agree or disagree with each of the categorical questions. Patients usually answer each question with the thought of a *weekly average* of *how they are generally feeling and what they are able to do in their daily lives*, when they fill out this assessment. The following paragraphs will help illustrate the focus point of each question, and help patients obtain the most accurate assessment of their pain condition as possible. Remember, better information *"in"* with the assessment portion of

the **PITS Program**, will result in better results *"out"* with the treatment portion of the program.

Remember the four **P-I-T-S Assessment Category sections**: **P-physical function**, **I-intensity of pain**, **T-thoughts and behaviors**, **S-social interactions**. Now there are three questions in each of these four sections, which add up to a total of 12 questions that form your **PITS Score**. Let us now explore these 12 questions in more depth.

Assessment Category Questions

P: *Physical Function*

1. You are able to work or take care of home and/or children?

The first section of the **PITS Score** is all about physical function, and the first subject you need to address when calculating your **PITS Score** is your *ability to work or take care of home and children*. This is part of the physical function section of the score, and it is very important. So, how do you answer this question?

When pain is controlled, and you are able to work full-time and take care of you children and do all the things you need to do around the house, that is great. But, if pain is keeping you from being fully functional, then that can be a problem. Are you missing work due to your pain? Are your children always nagging you because you cannot spend enough time with them because of your pain? Is your home always a mess because you cannot keep up with the housework?

If your answer to all three of those questions is yes, then that is obviously a low score. But, even if your answer to those questions is no, pain can still influence your ability to conduct these important functions.

The ability to deal with pain is different for everyone. Even if pain is not keeping you from doing these things, it could affect you in other ways.

Keep this in mind when you enter your score.

2. You are able to do some exercise?

The second subject in this section you need to address when calculating your **PITS Score** is your *ability to do some exercise*. So, how do you answer this question?

Doing exercise is a critical part of staying functional and keeping your pain from getting worse. Are you lying around on the couch all day because of your pain? Are you not going to the gym? Are you not following the home exercise program that your physical therapist recommended for you? This can be a problem.

It is important for everyone to exercise, but it is especially important for the chronic pain sufferer because of the need to stay fit and functional. The tricky part is that many pain sufferers feel increased pain when they exercise and think this is bad. The key is finding the right balance to get enough exercise without aggravating your pain condition.

For those who do not exercise regularly in the first place, this subject still applies, because it is an important part of pain management.

Keep this in mind when you enter your score.

3. You are able to do activities of daily living?

The third subject you need to address when calculating your **PITS Score** is your *ability to do activities of daily living*. What do I mean by this?

Activities of daily living include moving around your house, getting up and down the stairs, going to the bathroom and showering, cooking and cleaning, getting out to the store, and other tasks. If pain keeps you from doing these things, then that can be a problem.

The lowest score here would be for patients who are truly disabled and need assistance to perform these activities of daily living. But pain can affect anyone's ability to perform these activities on a regular basis. Being truly disabled is one thing, but varying degrees of pain can lead to varying degrees of disability—and affect each patient differently when performing these activities of daily living.

Keep this in mind when you enter your score.

I: *Intensity of Pain*

4. Your pain score levels are acceptable?

The second section of the **PITS Score** is all about intensity of pain, and the first subject in this section addresses the most basic—and most subjective—subject: *To what extent is your level of pain acceptable?* How do you answer this question?

Of course, this is the one question that every pain patient recognizes as the traditional pain score, the 0–10 scale. Although it is only one component of the **PITS Pain and Quality-of-Life Score**, it is a very important one.

One patient's acceptable level of pain might be very different for another. This speaks to the very subjective nature of rating pain that cannot be truly measured.

The key to answering this question is recognizing that you are not being asked to rate your level of pain. The key word here is *acceptable*. Chronic pain cannot be cured—but it needs to be managed. And your pain management treatment is based on the acceptable level of pain that you can live with day-to-day.

Keep this in mind when you enter your score.

5. Your duration of pain relief is adequate?

The second subject in this section when calculating your **PITS Score**, addresses the importance of understanding not only if your level of pain is acceptable, but also, how you feel about the *current duration of your pain relief*. What do I mean by this?

Once an acceptable level of pain relief has been reached—and this is different for every individual patient—it is important then to maintain this level of relief on a 24-hour basis.

There are many strategies for patients to prolong their duration of pain relief, and these are individualized based on the patient's pain condition, what has worked for them in the past, what has not worked, and what their preferences are for treatment, such as adding another medication, having an injection, or even considering surgery.

So, if you have found a successful treatment that gives you an acceptable level of pain, but only for a short while, which is a problem. The longer your pain relief lasts, the better your quality of life will be.

Keep this in mind when you enter your score.

6. Your treatment side effects are tolerable?

The third subject of this section of the **PITS Score** considers any *unwanted side effects of your current pain relief treatment*. Are these side effects tolerable? What do I mean by this?

If you are taking pain medication that makes you nauseous or dizzy, then that is not good. Many patients cannot take certain pain medication for this reason. They may opt for injections, but there are possible side effects there as well—especially with steroid injections and potential softening of tissue and bone demineralization effects, and blood sugar spikes in diabetics. Even physical therapy and chiropractic care can have side effects in the form of excessive treatment soreness and worsening pain, and this can be discouraging for patients.

There can be potential side effects to any pain management treatment. The real question is whether the benefit of the pain relief outweighs the negative side effects from that particular treatment.

Keep this in mind when you enter your score.

T: *Thoughts and Behaviors*

7. You are suffering from anxiety or depression?

The third section of the **PITS Score** is all about thoughts and behaviors, and the first subject in this section is critical. To what extent *is your level of anxiety and depression controlled?* It is perfectly normal for chronic pain sufferers to feel anxious and depressed, but that does not mean it cannot be controlled. So, what do I mean by this?

Uncontrolled pain can certainly lead to increased levels of anxiousness and depression. This is human nature. But what a lot of people overlook is that increased anxiety and depression in and of itself can lead to increased pain levels in many patients. Pain and anxiety transmission both follow a lot of the same nerve pathways in the brain. This is the basic mind/body relationship that has been recognized for a long time in medical care.

In addition to increasing your pain levels, uncontrolled anxiety and depression can also make it harder for you to focus on the things you need to do in order to combat your pain.

Keep this in mind when you enter your score.

8. You are getting restful sleep?

The second subject in this section of the **PITS Score** addresses the importance of restful sleep. Do you think you are *getting enough restful sleep?* What do I mean by this?

Restful sleep—also known as restorative sleep—is important for anybody. But it is especially important for the chronic pain sufferer. You need to get a restful sleep, so you are not waking up chronically fatigued all the time—thus making your pain worse.

What patients may not understand is that during REM sleep, which stands for *rapid eye movement* sleep, our bodies are repairing and rejuvenating. There is plenty of science and research behind the importance of getting a good night's sleep.

The typical range for most people is 6 to 8 hours of sleep. But do not forget we are talking about restful sleep.

Keep this in mind when you enter your score.

9. Your overall energy level is OK?

The third subject in this section of the **PITS Score** is about your energy level. How do you know if *your energy level is okay?*

Everybody needs to maintain a certain energy level to live life to its fullest, but it is especially important for chronic pain sufferers, for whom chronic pain can easily drain these energy levels and thus depress their quality of life.

What is worse, low energy levels make it harder for pain sufferers to focus on the things they need to do to combat their pain and get on with their daily tasks, not only at work but at home.

Keep this in mind when you enter your score.

S: *Social Interactions*

10. You are getting out with family and friends?

The fourth and final section of the **PITS Score** is all about social interactions, and the first subject in this section speaks to how much your pain might be preventing you from *getting out with family and friends.* What exactly do I mean by this?

Chronic pain affects many aspects of your quality of life. When it keeps you from enjoying time with your family and friends, this can be a problem. Social interactions are important for anybody, but especially for chronic pain sufferers, who feel isolated because of their chronic pain.

This isolation can lead to increased anxiety and depression, which can lead to increased pain. Furthermore, being around family and friends can provide the support you need to help with your pain management treatments.

Keep this in mind when you enter your score.

11. You are able to travel or do a hobby?

The second subject in this section of the **PITS Score** includes the idea of being *able to travel or do a hobby.* To what extent does your pain prevent you from doing these things? And why is it important?

If chronic pain keeps you from traveling in your car or on a plane, then this affects your quality of life on many levels. Not only might it keep you from traveling for vacation, but it can also affect your getting around day-to-day—like going to work or driving your kids to school. In addition to the practical limitations this can cause, it also leads to increased anxiety and depression, which leads to increased pain.

Likewise, if chronic pain is keeping you from enjoying your favorite hobbies, this can also discourage you and impact your quality of life.

Keep this in mind when you enter your score.

12. You have enough insurance coverage for pain care?

Remember, the fourth and final section of the **PITS Score** is all about social interactions, but the final subject in this section goes beyond just social. Do you have money resources or *have enough insurance coverage for pain care*—a socio-economic question? On the surface, this is a basic dollars and cents question, but it requires more than just a yes or no answer.

Economic stress can be a problem for anybody, but it is especially important for a chronic pain sufferer who might not have enough money or insurance coverage for their complete pain care.

The question is what is enough? You may have basic coverage for medications, but not for advanced treatments like injections, massage therapy or acupuncture. There are more and more nutritional supplements on the market that can help speed healing and control chronic pain—but these can be very expensive.

Not having these options within reach can cause anxiety and depression—again, leading to an increase in pain.

Keep this in mind when you enter your score.

So, these are the critical 12 categorical assessment questions that can instantly give patients a snapshot of their care progress. Remember, there is no right or wrong answer for how much you agree or disagree with each of the categorical questions. When you fill out this assessment, just answer each question on the basis of how you feel in *general* and how you are doing with your activities on *average* for the week, not just how you feel in the moment or in one given day.

PITS Score Summary

One of the most essential elements of the **Pain is the PITS Program** is the repetitive assessment and reassessments that are necessary, which gives a patient not only greater awareness and knowledge of their specific pain condition and how controlled their symptoms are, but also leads to greater awareness of the various remedies available to treat those ongoing symptoms. It is recommended that these assessments be conducted on a weekly basis, or monthly basis, to see where a patient stands with their overall program progress. This critical information provides the pain care team with the *big picture* of the desired level of comfort and functional status—the desired **PITS Score**—that is trying to be achieved by an individual patient!

Each of the twelve questions highlighted previously are answered on a scale of 0–10, where 0 is for ***totally DISAGREE*** and 10 is for ***totally AGREE***. So, with a total of twelve questions, a patient's maximum perfect score equals 120 ($10 \times 12 = 120$).

The following chart depicts the degree of pain control and quality of life that the patient experiences. The lower the score, the less control the patient has over their pain and overall quality of life. Likewise, the higher the score, the more control a patient has over their pain and quality of life:

PITS Score Ratings	
Excellent	101–120
Very Good	81–100
Good	61–80
Fair	41–60
Poor	21–40
Very Poor	0–20

The goal is to get your **PITS Score** to an acceptable level to *YOU*, the individual patient. One patient's score of 90 may be another patient's level of 50, where both patients are satisfied. Ideally, focusing on areas of the body that are experiencing the most discomfort, and going through the various **PITS Program** treatment options that are available, will help get the **PITS Score** above 100!

One benefit of the **PITS Program** is for the patient to identify persistent pain issues on a timely basis and take corrective action quickly. It is important to remember that the **PITS Score** levels are not a competition—they merely identify a patient's *individual* comfort level for pain tolerance. One patient's

tolerance for pain could be vastly different than another's. So, the trend is the higher the **PITS Score**, the better a patient is generally doing. Sometimes a pain condition may regress, but the patient can identify the regression quickly, and make immediate adjustments in their treatment options. Life happens, the weather changes, an old injury is re-aggravated—all of these things can bring the onset of a recurrent or new pain condition. The **PITS Program** allows patients to make timely adjustments and stay positive—*this is the key!*

To *summarize*, the four major phases of the **PITS Program** pain management **Clinical Pathway** are:

- Assessment
- Plan
- Implementation
- Evaluation

The ***Assessment*** portion of the program is triggered when a patient experiences a new or persistent pain sensation. Once the subjective pain is felt, a physical medical care evaluation should be scheduled. This type of examination may include the patient's medical history, the physical exam itself, possible radiology X-ray and MRI studies, and a diagnostic evaluation of the patient's pain condition.

Following this initial step, a customized ***Plan*** for acute or chronic pain care is then developed, using the **Pain is the PITS Program** guidance and the various medical professionals involved with the patient's case. These professionals can include internists, anesthesiologists, neurologists, vascular specialists, orthopedic surgeons, oncologists, physiatrists (rehab physicians), and rheumatologists—patients are often referred to more than one specialty area of care.

Along with the development of the clinical course of care, the patient educational component will be equally important to the success of the overall program. If a patient can be taught to understand his or her pain problem(s) in a simple **P-I-T-S** *framework*, and how the treatment plan(s) will work to relieve the pain symptoms, then they will already be well on the way to improving their **PITS Pain and Quality-of-Life Score**. In all the years that I have practiced pain medicine, I have come to believe that ***knowledge is comfort***. In most cases, the more knowledge a patient has, the more pain relief potential they can experience. *It is really amazing!*

In the ***Implementation*** portion, the four (4) major areas of integrative pain treatment to be started, again as necessary, are: ***Pills***, ***Injections***, ***Therapy***, and ***Surgery***. There are many subsets within each of these treatment areas, with a focus on integrative multi-modal pain care. Keep in mind, medications and injections will break the pain cycle, and allow patients to better rehabilitate. Then, therapy choices will help stretch, strengthen, and condition patients, so they can decrease recurrent pain in the future. Surgical options are usually a last resort and are reserved for patients that remain in intractable pain despite aggressive medical and interventional care, or in patients who experience worsening and/or persistent neurologic symptoms.

The **PITS Program** works most effectively when multiple treatments work in concert with one another.

So, psychiatric and psychological treatment is utilized when needed, restorative sleep tactics to help improve restful sleep are considered as necessary, and the use of supplemental complementary techniques such as yoga or massage therapy or acupuncture are encouraged in patients who want to explore these options.

The ***Evaluation*** portion, which is the continuous reassessment phase, is key to improving physical functioning, increasing energy levels, controlling anxiety and depression, and improving social interactions. Patient awareness of their **PITS Score**, and knowledge of their overall condition and treatment plan, is a core theme of the **PITS Program**. Making the necessary lifestyle changes, for the ultimate quest for a better life with less pain, is the key!

After all, the ***motto*** of the **Pain is the PITS Program** is: **"Feel better and live your life, because pain is the PITS!"** *Sound familiar?*

CHAPTER 5

PITS Treatments

There is an epidemic of pain in the United States which has led to increase opioid prescribing, along with an advancing opioid addiction crisis issue, and all of these factors have left us with a lot of unanswered questions surrounding future treatment options. How much of this pain management care is making a difference in a patient's life? What does the science and research say about long-term opioid use for chronic pain? What are the costs of long-term pain care? Do we have a unified approach that patients can understand and follow to maximize their comfort and quality of life? The **Pain is the PITS Program** is meant to be both educational and therapeutic and can help address many of these issues and concerns.

This section of the book will discuss an important aspect of the **PITS Program—the Patient Worksheets**, a sample of which is found in **Appendix C**. You can print them from the glossary section of the book or download them from the **PITS Website: www.pain-isthepits.com**.

The **Patient Worksheets** are a key tool in *identifying, measuring, and treating a patient's pain condition*. These worksheets include the all-important **PITS Score Sheet** (also shown in **Appendix A**). The **Patient Worksheets** consists of five (5) separate pages as listed below:

Page 1—**Patient Information** (with Medical History)

Page 2—**PITS Score Sheet** (the Assessment Tool)

Page 3—**PITS Treatment Protocol**

Page 4—**PITS Treatment Timeline**

Page 5—**Patient Notes & Questions**

The **Patient Worksheets** can be completed for each body region where the patient feels pain, if necessary, and a **PITS Score Sheet** can be used for each separate pain condition within that body region if a patient desires. There are six (6) major body regions that the **PITS Program** identifies as general areas in which patients experience pain. They are:

- Neck and Back
- Head and Face
- Arm and Hand
- Leg and Foot
- Abdominal and Pelvic
- Chest

Other general pain conditions and painful subject areas that the **PITS Program** addresses are **Cancer-related pain**, **Acute pain** from injury or surgery, **Arthritic pain**, the common **Emergency Room pain** issues, **OBGYN and Pediatric pain**, and lingering **Post-Surgical Pain Syndromes**. Once the general region of the body is identified, where the actual pain condition presents and the specific pain diagnosis is determined, then the **Patient Worksheets** are very important to allow the patient and the patient's pain care team to create a personalized **P-I-T-S** *Assessment and Treatment Program*, based on the severity of the pain and quality-of-life issues.

The *first page* of the **PITS Patient Worksheets** lists the patient's basic information, including contact information and medical history. This page is also where the patient identifies the region of the body where they are experiencing pain and list the medications they are taking for pain and non-pain issues. There is a section where the patient can list specific pain problems and their respective diagnosis, and a section to list allergies, such as certain dyes, antibiotics, or latex products. There is a section to list the primary pain management specialist involved in the patient's treatment, and other medical professionals involved in the patient's overall care. Other medical conditions should be listed, including previous heart trouble, high blood pressure, emphysema or asthma, sleep apnea, kidney problems, thyroid problems, liver or hepatitis issues, stomach ulcer or gastritis issues, and abdominal pain or endometriosis history. Does the patient exhibit skin rashes, do they have a bleeding disorder, or is there any history of cancer, seizures or stroke? A complete medical history is vital in order to arrive at an optimum pain management strategy. The last thing a pain management specialist wants to do is to treat the patient's pain condition in one area of the body only to cause another problem in a different body region.

The **second page** of the **PITS Patient Worksheets** is the **Pain and Quality-of-Life Score Sheet** or the PITS Score, previously seen in **Appendix A**, and discussed in **CHAPTER 3**. It is important to obtain a baseline measurement of the patient's initial pain condition, so pain management strategies can be modified as needed.

On **page three** of the **PITS Patient Worksheets**, the active **P-I-T-S** *treatment protocol* is listed based on the fundamental tenets of the **PITS Program**. Patients are encouraged to become actively involved in their pain relief treatment, which includes self-examination and regular consultation with the pain management team. It is recommended that patients regularly visit the **PITS Website** for the educational videos and podcasts that are relevant to their pain condition. Patients are also encouraged to attend the periodic educational **PITS Meetings** for question-and-answer sessions, which will be held throughout each year, for interactive learning from physician-to-patient and from patient-to-patient. These meetings have been piloted and have had positive feedback.

On **page four** of the **PITS Patient Worksheets** is the **PITS Program Treatment Timeline** (see **APPENDIX H**), which helps the patient monitor improvements in their pain condition, and measure these improvements against certain milestone markers. The idea is to move a patient from an acute pain management care scenario, into a less serious chronic pain management longer-term program if necessary—*remember, nearly all chronic pain first starts out as acute pain*. The goal is always to see the patient's pain condition improving, and if it is not, to make necessary adjustments in the pain treatment protocols accordingly. The degree of the patient's involvement in his or her pain management program will dictate how quickly adjustments can be made.

On **page five** of the **PITS Patient Worksheets** is a section for **Patient Notes & Questions**, where patients can make notes and reminders to themselves, and list any questions and concerns that they may have with their future pain care. These issues can be addressed in ongoing evaluations and treatments with their pain management team, or at a future **PITS** *Question & Answer Meeting* with the general public.

Now, we will get into more detail of the various pain treatment options, as highlighted by the **P-I-T-S** *acronym*: **P-pills**, **I-injections**, **T-therapy** and **S-surgery**. The following treatment suggestions are not intended to be a complete list, but rather, examples of the types of options in each of the *four sections* of care available to a pain sufferer:

Pills—When over-the-counter (OTC) medications stop working and a visit to the doctor or nurse practitioner is needed, then prescription medications are introduced. In terms of treatment options under the pill or medication category, there are many different choices, including anti-inflammatory medications, muscle relaxants, nerve pain agents, and opioid narcotics. Opioids are recommended only to be prescribed short-term for a severe acute pain state, or considered longer-term for a more lingering severe chronic pain state, as a last resort depending on an individual patient's clinical course.

Under *anti-inflammatory medications*, there are two major groups: nonsteroidal anti-inflammatory drugs (NSAIDs) and steroids. In terms of NSAIDs, examples include Motrin (ibuprofen) or Advil (ibuprofen), Aleve (naproxen), Mobic (meloxicam), Celebrex (celecoxib), and many other nonsteroidal medications. Under the steroidal section, the most common are Prednisone and the Medrol Dosepak (methylprednisolone).

Muscle relaxants are the next kind of pill category. Examples include Flexeril (cyclobenzaprine), Zanaflex (tizanidine), Robaxin (methocarbamol), Baclofen (lioresal), Skelaxin (metaxalone), and other types of muscle relaxants. The **PITS Program** does not favor the use of Soma (carisoprodol), because this drug is more of a barbiturate sleep medication with muscle relaxant-like activity, and has the potential to be habit forming, like opioids.

Nerve pain agents include Neurontin (gabapentin), Lyrica (pregabalin), Lidoderm Patch (transcutaneous lidocaine), Cymbalta (duloxetine), Elavil (amitriptyline), Pamelor (nortriptyline), and other nerve pain agents.

Finally, as a carefully weighted option in the pill category, there are *opioid narcotics*, both short-acting and long-acting types. For short-acting opioids, there is codeine or tramadol (Ultram), hydrocodone (Vicodin), oxycodone (Percocet), and tapentadol (Nucynta). There is also, hydromorphone (Dilaudid), morphine (MSIR), and others. For long-acting opioids, we have OxyContin (oxycodone), MS Contin (morphine), Nucynta extended-release (tapentadol), Duragesic Patch (transcutaneous fentanyl), Butrans Patch (transcutaneous buprenorphine), and others. When using opioid therapy in general, it is important to note that a significant side effect of prolonged opioid use is constipation. It is important that patients are moving their bowels at least once every two days, and if not, to consider constipation treatment medication. The **PITS Program** utilizes my version of a stepwise protocol called the **PITS Treatment of Opioid-Induced Constipation** sheet (see **APPENDIX I**).

This summarizes the pill (medication) protocol choices, based on the patient's pain problem, and any other medical problems or allergies that may exist. A large part of medication therapy under the **PITS Program**, is to monitor dosage levels and frequency,

and document pain relief results quickly and accurately. When adjustments to medications are necessary, they can be made with the medical professional's guidance, in a timely fashion, and reduce the possibility of any setbacks in the patient's pain management program.

Injections—The next section in the **P-I-T-S treatment protocol** is injection therapy. There are many types of injections that can be utilized based on the specific pain issue and the patient's medical history. The selection of which injection is most appropriate depends on several factors.

An example of an injection is an *epidural steroid injection (ESI)*, which is used to treat an inflamed *"pinched* nerve," typically due to a bulging or herniated spinal disc. Without getting too technical, different ESI approaches depend on where the inflammation is located in the spine. There are ESI injections that are targeted for cervical (neck), thoracic (mid-back), lumbar (low back), or caudal (lumbosacral or tailbone area) locations. Epidural injections can also be of a transforaminal (neural foramen side-of-the spine) approach, to target one or more specific nerve root areas along the spine.

Another category of injections are the *nerve blocks*, which include peripheral nerve blocks and sympathetic nerve blocks. Peripheral nerve blocks could include facet nerve blocks that control pain to the spinal facet joints along each side of the spine, the greater occipital nerve in the back of the head, intercostal nerves around the ribs, or the median nerve in the wrist. For sympathetic nerves, there are the stellate ganglion block in the neck for someone typically experiencing upper extremity sympathetic pain, the lumbar sympathetic block for diagnosing and treating different leg pain conditions, or other sympathetic blocks.

In another category of injections, there are *joints* that could be injected if they develop pain and inflammation, such as cervical, thoracic, or lumbar facet joints in the spine. There is the sacroiliac joint giving buttock, hip, and back pain. There are shoulder, hip, knee, and other synovial joints that can be injected especially for osteoarthritis inflammatory pain.

Another category in the injection protocol is *trigger point injections (TPIs)* for painful muscle spasms, or Botox injections for chronic migraines and for intractable muscle spasm pain. There are *tendon injections*, such as biceps tendon or tennis elbow injections. There are *bursa injections* in the shoulder or hip or other areas. There are *fascia injections*, such as plantar fasciitis in the feet. This summarizes injection therapy options under the **P-I-T-S** *treatment protocol*. Under the **PITS Program**, timely adjustments are encouraged based on patient feedback and lifestyle preferences.

Therapy—This section of the **P-I-T-S** *treatment protocol* includes four general categories of therapy, and considered the core approaches, including *physical, psychological care, sleep strategies*, and *complementary care techniques*.

First off, most professionally provided therapy choices consist of physical therapy and chiropractic care and traction, with a large segment of that care focused on back and neck issues. There are special chiropractic tables for decompression to safely stretch and realign the spine. There is also an inversion table that patients can use on their own, 10–20 minutes at a time at the beginning and end of the day, using their own body weight to decompress the spine.

A lot of therapy techniques are designed to increase flexibility, strength, and endurance, so patients can maintain their comfort and functional status as they live their lives. There are also occupational therapy techniques. One of the best ways for patients to learn self-improvement strategies is to stay in shape—right? So, exercise in moderation can be a good injury prevention tool, which can help reduce recurrent episodes of a painful injury. Joining a gym or performing a regular home exercise routine (HEP), is a recommended pain management strategy, and a part of the therapy protocol of the **PITS Program**. Another aspect of therapy is maintaining a proper nutritional diet—a body properly fueled will heal faster than a body poorly nourished.

Often, pills and injections are the precursors to therapy, where the pain condition is lessened by *breaking the pain cycle* enough—then patients can better perform physical and chiropractic therapy, and their home exercise program (HEP), all done in an effort to help decrease recurrent pain moving forward. Sometimes the pain condition persists, even after pills and/or injections, and the patient is required to participate in physician-directed therapy care. Often these are patients who suffer from chronic persistent neuromuscular pain and impairment—victims of stroke, traumatic brain injury (TBI) and spinal cord injury (SCI), multiple sclerosis, Parkinson's disease, and so forth. These patients may need neuromuscular medicine experts, such an osteopathic physician expert, or a physical medicine and rehabilitation (PM&R) doctor—also known as a physiatrist.

Secondly, in terms of psychiatric and psychological therapy care, it is important to control anxiety and depression and other conditions. In terms of anxiety, Xanax (alprazolam), and Klonopin (clonazepam) are commonly used, hopefully for only short periods, because of their potential for habituation and negative drug interactions—especially when used in conjunction with opioid narcotics. In terms of depression, Zoloft (sertraline), Effexor (venlafaxine), Cymbalta (duloxetine), Wellbutrin (bupropion), or other anti-depressive medication are used. Also in this category, cognitive-behavioral therapy (CBT) is important for changing thought patterns and using distraction and other strategies to help control painful sensations, especially for post-traumatic stress disorders (PTSD), and other kinds of conditions.

Thirdly, in terms of restorative sleep therapy strategies, restful sleep is an important factor in relieving chronic pain symptoms. This is done with lifestyle changes and supplements, and actual prescription medications, as needed. Lifestyle changes include, not drinking caffeine at night, making sure the bedroom is quiet and cool, not doing a lot of vigorous exercise right before sleep, and so forth. In the supplement category, we can consider chamomile tea, melatonin, valerian root, or other supplements. In the prescription medication category, there are short-term FDA-approved sleep drugs, such as Ambien (zolpidem) and Lunesta (eszopiclone), or longer-term sleep-inducing drugs used *off-label*, like trazodone (Desyrel) or Elavil (amitriptyline).

Fourth and finally, there are a wide range of complementary therapy techniques to help promote wellness and healing. Therapies to be considered include acupuncture, massage, yoga, Pilates, Reiki, hypnosis, herbal therapy, essential oils, magnets, and low-level laser therapy. Millions of chronic pain sufferers look to complementary care options to support their primary conventional care options—prescription medications, physical therapy, injections, and the need for surgery. Adopting an *integrative pain care approach* is an essential theme of the **PITS Program**.

Surgery—The final section in the **P-I-T-S** *treatment protocol* is the surgery option, which should be utilized when all other treatment protocols were not successful or were not possible. *Minimally invasive surgical techniques* are preferred, if a patient's condition fits this criterion, and are increasingly available now with advances in physician training techniques and advancing technology options. For the most part, the least invasive surgical techniques offer the shortest possible recovery time and less intense postoperative pain. There are now minimally invasive surgery (MIS) techniques, such as MIS decompression spine surgery, joint arthroscopy, nerve release in the carpal tunnel, Achilles tendon repair, and other rupture injuries. More invasive surgical procedures include, multilevel laminectomy and discectomy choices, for persistent back and neck pain, and many other types of procedures.

Today *total joint replacement* of the shoulder, hip, knee, or other joints is more common and less invasive as in past years. This type of surgery is performed frequently and successfully in many patients.

Regarding abdominal and pelvic pain, *diagnostic laparoscopy and laparotomy* are frequently needed both diagnostically and therapeutically. For hernia pain in the groin and abdomen, hernia repair surgical procedures are frequently performed endoscopically by a general surgeon.

Moving forward, new techniques are being developed for *minimally invasive implantable devices* to treat different pain conditions. In the spinal area, there is the spinal cord stimulator (SCS) for using electric current to typically treat persistent back pain, and the implantable spinal pump device, known as an intrathecal infusion device-IID, for pinpoint delivery of spinal narcotics and other medications directly into a patient's spinal fluid—for treatment of persistent cancer pain when indicated, for example.

The *most invasive surgeries* are usually reserved for patients who develop intractable pain, whether due to a severe acute injury, or due to years and years of chronic persistent pain that becomes intractable at some point. Spinal decompression and fusion with hardware instrumentation is often recommended in very difficult pain management cases related to the cervical, thoracic, and lumbar regions of the spine—especially if patients develop severe degeneration and spinal instability. These spinal fusion cases to repair an advanced degenerative spine are the most invasive of surgeries, and generally require the longest recovery period.

In reviewing the **P-I-T-S** *treatment protocol*, there is an important pain care treatment priority that patients will frequently have to keep in mind. Contrary to popular thought, *getting the pills right* is not the top priority for individual pain management programs. This is one of the reasons for opioid prescribing levels and why opioid narcotic addiction is so prevalent in the United States today.

The **PITS Treatment Priority Table** (see **Appendix J**) establishes the order of priority for the **P-I-T-S** *treatment protocol* and is at the core of the **P-I-T-S** *wellness philosophy*. The recommended **P-I-T-S** *treatment priorities* are listed below:

- *Mind and Body Therapy*. This is the *top priority*. This means doing everything possible, including making important lifestyle changes to promote individual wellness, prior to pursuing *aggressive pill therapy*, or other treatment options. This priority includes addressing sleep issues, starting a home exercise or physical therapy program, pursuing psychological therapy with a group or one-on-one guidance, considering yoga or Pilates, attempting massage or acupuncture therapy, and other potential therapy approaches.

- *Pill Therapy*. This is the second priority, getting the medications right, for those patients who need them in the short run, or for longer-term treatment.

- *Injection Therapy*. This is the third priority, and

often utilized to break a patient's pain cycle and speed up healing, when therapy and medications are not offering enough relief.

- *Surgical Therapy.* This is the last priority, baring a true emergency situation, and utilized when a patient needs a physical or mechanical fix if they remain in intractable pain despite medications, injections, and therapy.

Since the overall goal of the **PITS Program** is to maximize the **PITS Pain and Quality-of-Life Score**, it is imperative that patients remain functional at work and continue to be a homemaker where applicable. Patients need to start and maintain an exercise routine to keep their pain at bay, increase their energy levels, and have improved mood and sleep habits. Patients need to keep learning that mental and emotional health is a crucial element of any pain management program, and they need to maintain control of anxiety and depression, or this can lead to exacerbations of pain. Also, it is important that patients have improved social interactions with family and friends, so they do not feel isolated. As important, and should not be overlooked, is a patient's need for adequate insurance coverage for continued pain care options, so they can explore not only conventional care of pills-injections-therapy-surgery, but also, consider complementary care options of massage-acupuncture-yoga-supplements. All of these care points are constantly encouraged by remembering the **PITS Program** *Motto*:

"Feel better and live your life, because pain is the PITS!"

Remember, chronic pain is a disease, make no mistake about it, with known permanent pathologic changes in the nervous system now well recognized in this country by physicians and insurance companies and the government. It is a very real problem affecting millions of Americans, and their families. It has physical, emotional, and social components that affect pain and quality of life. Although we cannot measure pain, per se—*it is what the patient says it is*—we can measure, in a sense, other aspects of the patient's life like their functional status, their disability level, what they are doing in their life in terms of interests and socialization, and even their dependence on others. Pain in this sense is very real, and again, it is treated in a disease-model fashion. Chronic persistent pain takes on a *bio-psycho-social* disease model of care, unlike most other medical problems that are just biological in nature—it is indeed a multidimensional model of disease management.

Remember, the **PITS Sample Worksheets** are there for patients to use as an ongoing guide to keep developing their individual pain assessment and treatment program with their expert pain team. This book is not a static technical medical text where, *"Here is the information, good luck."* Rather, it is a real living, breathing, and understandable proactive educational program, with realistic tangible assessment and treatment relief results!

All the elements of the **PITS Program** are now in place, which are only tools, and not effective if they are not utilized. The program is designed to be an individualized approach to pain management with active participation by the pain sufferer. Through the use of this book—and the educational website—a long-term wellness solution to reduce acute and chronic pain is offered. ***You are now on your way to improving your pain and quality of life forever!***

CHAPTER 6

PITS Treatment Protocol for Specific Types of Pain

As we develop different **P-I-T-S** *treatment protocol* care scenarios for many of the different pain conditions that cause patient suffering, it is important to first outline the different categories of pain that form patient diagnoses. The **PITS Diagnostic Categories of Pain** sheet (see **APPENDIX K**) outlines the six different types of pain conditions or processes. The **PITS Program** addresses these different types of pain in the body, and many pain states typically have more than one cause of pain, making it a bit more complex and challenging. The following is a list of the *six major pain types*:

- **Biomechanical**—a *nociceptive* pain cause—like spinal discs and joints.

- **Soft Tissue**—another *nociceptive* pain cause—like skin and muscles.

- **Inflammatory**—an *inflammation-related* pain cause—like osteoarthritis and pancreatitis.

- **Neuropathic**—a *peripheral or central nerve* pain cause—like diabetic neuropathy and spinal cord injury.

- **Dysfunctional**—an *undetermined* pain cause—like migraines and fibromyalgia.

- **Psychogenic**—a *psychiatric-related* pain cause—like anxiety and depression-related disorders.

Remember, each cause of pain does not live in a bubble. There is a lot of overlap among all the different pains and their various mechanisms that cause us to hurt, and many patients unfortunately have multiple pain diagnoses. As patients start to build their tailored **Pain is the PITS Program**, there is a treatment priority order of care that helps focus on the most essential components first, in accordance with the **PITS Program** *philosophy* of treatment. Then, the patient works their way up as needed with additional treatment priorities, based on their comfort and quality of life goals, or previously determined **PITS Score** level.

When patients and their pain team decide to consider opioid narcotic therapy as a choice of medication, especially if other non-opioid medications fail to offer enough relief, then a **PITS Opioid Risk Screening (PORS) Assessment** is obtained (see **APPENDIX E**)—or any other opioid risk questionnaire can be utilized. This will help match a level of opioid usage that is most appropriate based on multiple patient evaluation factors and the specific clinical pain situation. Also, if patients are suspected of suffering from an element of depression, it will be important to obtain a **PITS Depression Screening (PDS) Assessment** (see **APPENDIX F**)—or any other depression questionnaire can be utilized to factor in a level of depression as a risk factor when opioid narcotic levels and duration of opioid therapy are considered.

PITS Treatment Protocol for Specific Pain Conditions that bring Patients to seek Professional Diagnostic and Therapeutic Care

Low Back Pain

SUMMARY: Low back (lumbar) pain is the number one leading cause of pain in America that drives thousands of patients every month to see their primary care physician and urgent care centers. Only the common cold beats low back pain out as a reason for an office visit. Billions of dollars each year are spent in America on caring for low back pain, and it is the leading cause for disability in middle-aged adults. It is estimated that 80% of adults will experience an acute low back pain incident, and that 25% percent of all chronic persistent pain in America fits the category of low back pain.

There can be many different causes of low back pain, thus the initial complaint of excessive pain should start the *clinical pain management pathway* with an initial evaluation assessment with a medical doctor or appropriate specialist. If you have low back pain that is lingering, and you cannot manage on your own, then an initial evaluation from your doctor would typically include:

- Going through a history of how the pain began and the nature of the pain. Is the pain sharp like a knife, dull like a toothache, or hot and burning like a stove? What does the pain feel like at its highest and lowest intensity, what makes it feel better and feel worse, and are there any other associated symptoms, like numbness and tingling? What other circumstances could be contributing to the pain, whether it is another physical condition, a psychological issue, or a social factor in the patient's life?

- Then a physical examination would be performed, focusing on the neuromuscular system and other related body systems, depending on the location of the pain, to help discover different *pain generators* in the back.

- Then your doctor would take a close look at any kind of studies or X-rays you may have had or need, such as plain films or regular black-and-white X-rays, CT scans, MRIs, EMG/NCS for nerve-related pain, and the like, to help confirm a source(s) of pain.

- Then your doctor would formulate an assessment and diagnosis of what type or types of back pain you are experiencing, whether from muscles, joints, spinal discs, and so forth, and then develop an appropriate treatment plan.

- After the assessment phase of the clinical pathway, you would start the **P-I-T-S** *treatment protocol* implementation.

- After a cycle or two of pain care options—pills, injections, therapy, and surgery if needed—you should reach a point where your pain and quality-of-life goals are being met and you are satisfied with your progress and overall care.

There are several causes of **acute low back pain**:

- *A muscle strain* with periodic or continuous muscle spasm-like symptoms.

- A *ligament sprain* from injury to different spinal ligament segments.

- It could be of a fascia or other soft tissue nature, causing *fasciitis*.

- A *bulging or herniated disc* leading to back and leg symptoms, or from one bone in the low back slipping in front of, or in back of the other, called *listhesis*.

- *Facet* pain, which are spine joints in the low back on each side that support structure and motion, which can get inflamed and degenerated from an injury.

- A flare of *sacroiliitis* or inflammation in the sacroiliac joints, which are low back-pelvic joints just above each buttock.

- *Discogenic* pain from a slip-and-fall, which is pain that arises from an injury in a disc itself. The spinal discs have nerve endings, and they can be irritated and be a source of low back pain.

- *Spinal stenosis* is a narrowing of the spine that typically happens slowly through a chronic process over decades. With acute injury, however, inflammation and compression in the spine can be due to a pre-existing stenosis condition.

Teasing out the acute cause of pain or suspected causes can lead us to a definitive plan of treatment. Fortunately, acute low back pain conditions usually settle down and healing occurs within weeks or a few months with conservative treatment. ***If low back pain extends beyond six months, then it becomes a chronic pain condition.*** Therefore, I will discuss each of the common types of low back pain causes, first from an initial acute phase, and then from a chronic phase perspective if pain persists. Remember, *all chronic back pain first starts out as acute back pain.*

The **Pain is the PITS Program** will hopefully try to help standardize an educational guideline plan to treat different painful conditions, for whatever specialty of medicine that is involved, and for all the pain patients of America who could benefit from this knowledge.

There are lots of different doctor specialties to help patients with low back pain, including:

- Interventional anesthesiology

- Physical medicine and rehabilitation (or physiatry)

- Neurology or psychiatry

- Spinal surgeons (both Orthopedic and Neurosurgery)

- Rheumatologists

- Palliative care and oncology doctors (if you have end-of-life or cancer-related back pain)

- Internal medicine doctors and family care practice doctors and pediatric doctors, as well as OBGYN physicians, are all considered primary care doctors, and the vast majority of patients in the United States have their initial back pain evaluation and treatment care with this huge group of doctors.

- Many patients are also seen initially in *urgent care centers*, and in a true emergency pain situation there are always emergency room physicians available for assessment and triage of potential life-threatening back pain symptoms—from an abdominal aortic aneurysm, for example.

The next section will deal with the specific initial presentation of acute and chronic adult myofascial-muscle spasm low back pain, as well as other causes of adult low back pain. We will put aside back pain in children for now, we will assume that the cause of back pain is not cancer related, and we will assume that acute trauma with fractures of the spine is not the cause of low back pain. The discussion will center on *six different causes of low back pain*, the most common conditions seen in clinical practice, that may or may not involve leg pain, and how the **P-I-T-S** *treatment protocol* can be applied in each instance.

Specific Low Back Pain Conditions

1. Lumbar Myofascial Pain Syndrome (MPS)

The first type of low back pain is acute and chronic Lumbar Myofascial Pain Syndrome. Implementing the **P-I-T-S** *treatment protocol*, the first course of action for the treatment of low back pain which is muscular or spasm-like in nature, is to recommend certain **Pills** or medications. Most medications to treat this condition will be of a nonsteroidal anti-inflammatory and acetaminophen nature, or a short course of oral steroids. Also, certain muscle relaxants can be added for the muscle spasm symptoms, but one must be careful of the potential side effect of too much sedation off-setting the positive benefit of the muscle-relaxing effect. Only for severe pain, should patients consider a short course of short-acting opioid narcotic analgesics. In time, with rest and limited activity, some physical therapy with modalities (heat, ice, stim, and ultrasound), or chiropractic care and traction if the pain lingers for weeks, will the initial pain resolve, and full healing will occur.

Once the pill regimen has been tried, but proven only partially effective, then trigger point **Injections** (TPIs) can be considered. This is a local anesthetic injection, typically alone or in combination with other substances—steroids, vitamins, tissue spread enhancers—which is injected through the skin directly into a muscle spasm to try and *"break it"*—through the muscle-relaxing action of the local anesthetic. Injections are commonly used along with physical **Therapy**—the third section of the **P-I-T-S** *treatment protocol*—in conjunction with more ice, heat, massage therapy, and stretching, to try to lessen the spasms, so they are not as incapacitating. Trigger point injections can be helpful, and they can be repeated weekly or monthly for a short while, as needed.

If these injections are temporarily successful but persistent spasms still exist, then some patients proceed toward Botox (onabotulinum toxin type A) injections to break the spasm condition in hope of achieving longer-term relief. Botox is denatured botulinum toxin that is injected safely as a chemical, working at the neuromuscular junction in muscle and nerve sites, to relax the spasms for up to three months and sometimes longer. Local anesthetic injections for trigger points typically offer relief that last for days or weeks, but Botox injections can have relief duration for many months at a time. Botox injections are the most aggressive conservative treatment for persistent myofascial pain, but also the most expensive. Check with your insurance carrier to see if your health plan covers this type of treatment.

Also, as a part of the therapy treatment protocol, patients can consider psychological and restful sleep therapy options, as well as complementary therapy care options. For example, if a patient did have a mood disorder from acute pain, the increased anxiety and depression needs to be addressed. The treating physician may start a short course of antianxiety or antidepressant medication or talk therapy in this case.

Patients must be sure that they are getting as much restorative sleep as possible so that they are not fatigued. It generally follows that the more fatigue a patient feels during the day, the more pain they will experience. Finally, within the therapy category, complementary treatment techniques incorporating multidisciplinary pain control strategies may be considered, such as acupuncture, massage, yoga, essential oils, low-level laser therapy, biofeedback, herbal medicine, and so forth.

The final **P-I-T-S** *treatment protocol* section, **Surgery**, is not common for myofascial release, unless there was entrapment of critical nerves or other structures where a surgeon would need to release the restricting muscle.

As mentioned previously, there are other types of low back pain that could be helped with this treatment regimen, which include acute back *sprains and strains*. These are the most common reasons for low back pain and are generally self-limited. Hopefully with medications, injections and physical therapy, patients can get back to their normal home activities and work status.

After the treatment protocols have been followed—assessment, plan, and implementation—the next phase is evaluation. This is the period when the patient reassesses their pain condition after treatment and measures it against the pain goals they had previously set for themselves. As basic goals, patients need to stay functional and resume as much productivity as possible. They need to improve their comfort in general and have better control of the pain itself, with little or no side effects of the treatment. The evaluation phase is designed to measure changes in the pain condition, hopefully seeing improvement, and maximizing ones **PITS Score**. If the myofascial condition becomes intractable, surgery might be the final option.

Now if myofascial pain were to persist beyond six months, this would be considered a **chronic low back pain** condition. Keep in mind that myofascial pain can coexist with other causes of persistent low back pain, such as a disc problem, stenosis, or facet joint or sacroiliac joint issue. Remember, there are multiple pain generators in the lumbar spine that can persist after acute injury, which can subsequently lead to a chronic pain syndrome. If myofascial pain persists, then a primary physician or pain specialist will want to tease out other primary spinal pain reasons that may be feeding into a secondary cause of persistent spasm.

For chronic myofascial low back muscle spasm pain lasting more than 6 months, treatment is going to be along a continuum of the same options that were used for acute pain, utilizing anti-inflammatories or muscle relaxants as needed, and periodic trigger point injections, but for an extended period of time for periodic moderate-to-severe pain flares.

Other possible therapies for myofascial pain are the use of an inversion table, for self-traction home care, or formal chiropractic-directed decompression table treatment in an outpatient office setting. These will aide in stretching out the spine and muscles, and more importantly, patients should begin to develop a home exercise program (HEP) regimen centered around stretching and strengthening muscles to help decrease recurrent spasm pain.

Some patients will need to seek more specialized physician care through a neuromuscular medicine expert or osteopathic medical professional, or a physical medicine and rehabilitation (PM&R) expert. These physicians often provide short and longer-term care in a comprehensive program to optimize a patient's functional status, like the use of osteopathic manipulative therapy (OMT). It is important to remember that earlier treatment protocols, such as trigger point injections, can be used throughout the treatment process, and in many instances will complement physical therapy options, as patients continue to rehabilitate in their pain care program. Myofascial pain is often under diagnosed and under-appreciated as a severe cause of persistent low back pain.

PATIENT EXAMPLE: A 25-year-old male was otherwise well until he slipped down a flight of steps at his house and suffered an acute low back pain episode. The pain was mostly restricted to his low back without any radiating symptoms into his legs. He applied some ice to his low back and did some stretching and took a dose of Motrin. His pain persisted for several days. He did his normal activities and he had complete resolution of the original discomfort, without seeking medical advice, in about a week's time. He stopped taking his Motrin. He stopped applying heat and ice and got back to his normal activity, thereafter.

This is the most straightforward example of acute sprain and strain. Had he had a persistent myofascial muscle spasm type pain in his back after a week, he may have sought medical treatment, and again, if on physical examination was found to have a palpable knot in his back, he may have been a candidate for a trigger point injection (TPI) with a local anesthetic injection like lidocaine or bupivacaine (Marcaine). If he needed TPIs and his pain resolved, then it would have been both pills and injections that helped him.

Now, if he had pain that persisted for a month, his physician may have put him in physical therapy, to have a therapist use heat, ice, ultrasound, and stimulation to try to break the spasm with stretching and a home exercise program for conditioning and strengthening. All of this may have been necessary if his pain persisted for a month or two, again, with eventual resolution of symptoms—where he would have been through pills, injections, and therapy. Again, there is no true surgical indication for chronic low back pain of a myofascial pain nature.

2. Lumbar Radiculopathy

The second type of low back pain is Lumbar Radiculopathy or sciatica, classically from a bulging or herniated spinal disc. Many patients present with acute sciatica symptoms for different reasons, but most of the pain incidents are related to an injury of some sort. These injuries occur from accidents on the job or motor vehicle accidents, from slip-and-falls or recreational sports, from lifting a heavy object, or from a simple body movement that causes an injury, such as sneezing or even from getting in and out of a car. Lumbar discs can be very fragile at times, and with the right twisting motion or traumatic forces, spinal discs can crack, fissure, bulge, herniate, or even have a whole piece come off—causing acute low back and radiating leg symptoms. If lumbar radiculopathy symptoms continue for more than six months, then it is considered a chronic condition.

Like any pain condition discussed in this book, lumbar radiculopathy patients enter the clinical pathway for pain management with a pain complaint, and then they schedule a consultation with a medical professional as needed. The evaluating team will develop a history, perform a physical examination, review imaging studies (X-rays/MRI) or other tests (EMGs), and finally make a diagnostic assessment and develop a plan for pain care.

Upon completion of the initial assessment and establishment of a plan, the treatment plan is then implemented. It is imperative that the medical team and the patient find the right medical professional to treat sciatica pain. Typically, medical doctors will start implementing a plan of anti-inflammatory medication and physical therapy. With acute sciatica pain, many patients will experience some relief within weeks-to-months, even if they do nothing. However, many more patients can experience relief much sooner by following the **P-I-T-S** *treatment protocol*.

With a herniated and inflamed disc, the herniated disc piece contacts and inflames a spinal nerve(s) in the back, and this results in nerve pain that typically shoots down the leg. Compression and inflammation of spinal tissues and nerves is the pathologic disease process. Thus, a patient should be treated first with anti-inflammatory drug **Pills**, such as OTC (over-the-counter) Motrin/Aleve or prescription NSAID, and even oral steroids if necessary. Often an oral steroid, such as the Medrol Dosepak, will be prescribed for six days with tapering doses in order to offer relief by breaking the acute inflammation cycle caused by the herniated disc. If there is an associated muscle spasm in the back, doctors can add a muscle relaxant to help relief tightness, like Flexeril or Baclofen, for example.

If there is severe acute pain, often a short course of short-acting opioid narcotics may be prescribed, like tramadol or Percocet, for example, but typically after the initial round of non-narcotic medications has been tried. Hopefully, with rest for no more than a day or two, the patient will be capable of performing normal activities and the pain will start to resolve. Early on, if persistent pain necessitates a course of physical therapy or chiropractic care with traction, then this course of action will be to optimize a patient's range-of-motion and flexibility and to improve strength and conditioning, ultimately to help decrease recurrent pain moving forward.

Chiropractic care may be used in certain acute pain situations, but if the patient has a large, herniated disc, then sometimes chiropractic manipulation can make the problem worse. That decision is up to the discretion of the patient and the chiropractic physician. If it is their judgment that the disc herniation needs to have an **Injection** to further reduce the pain, then an epidural steroid injection (ESI) can be considered, especially if the pain condition has persisted for a month or two. In addition, if the patient still has high pain scores and cannot return to work or is not able to do normal activities, then interventional pain management is indicated sooner than later.

A board-certified pain-trained interventional anesthesiologist, physiatrist, or neurologist physician mostly performs epidural steroid injections. If there is inflammation in the epidural space around nerves, then an epidural steroid injection under fluoroscopic X-ray guidance can be performed on an outpatient basis—in an office, surgical center, or outpatient hospital care setting. Delivering a very powerful depot particulate steroid directly to the inflamed area to treat spinal inflammation, as well as to help stabilize the spinal nerve pain impulses, is the key to this very safe minimally invasive procedure. As a rule, all patients will have had an MRI imaging study or CT scan prior to performing an ESI, to better define the inflamed compressed disc area(s) and allow for pinpoint accuracy of the planned steroid injection. Many times, the lower three discs (L3-4, L4-5, and L5-S1 levels) are the culprit because of the body's susceptibility for increase pressure in these areas.

If a herniated disc was discovered at the L4-5 level on a lumbar MRI, then an epidural steroid injection could be performed at that level in an outpatient setting under X-ray guidance to better target the area for procedural accuracy and safety. Epidural steroid injections are powerful—thus, a patient should receive no more than three injections within a six-month period to avoid excessive demineralization of bone and softening of tissue. Also, the frequency of injections beyond this recommendation could suppress the body's adrenal glands, important hormone glands above each kidney, which are natural producers of our body's own steroids. Keeping within this injection window will allow bone, tissue, and the adrenal glands to fully recover before any future injections are contemplated.

If after one or two injections, there is no appreciable relief, then a third injection is typically not performed. If anti-inflammatory injectable steroid medication is not enough to break the pain cycle, that indicates a more mechanical pathology, and not an *inflammatory* pathology that is persisting, such as ongoing *mechanical* nerve compression. It is not unusual for pain patients to complain that injections have not worked, and this is an indication that there is a more physical issue that now needs to be addressed. But it is important to try injection therapy first, to rule out a spinal inflammation issue. It is when there is persistent pain after injection therapy is performed, that pain management professionals would then look to an ongoing neurologic compromise of nerves. Patients would present with persistent numbness or weakness of the legs or feet, at which point a surgical consultation may be necessary with a spine surgeon, to consider possible decompression surgery to lessen the risk of patients suffering permanent nerve damage and disability.

Prior to choosing any surgical option, and in conjunction with medication and injections to break the pain cycle, the **P-I-T-S *treatment protocol*** emphasizes **Therapy** choices to rehabilitate patients. Physical therapy optimization for strengthening and conditioning, and psychiatric and psychological therapy as needed for a patient's mental health state, are critical elements of care. A lot of ongoing acute and chronic pain symptoms can wreak havoc on a patient's *"psyche."* Avoiding excessive anxiety and depression is very important to the overall success of the program. Also, making sure that the patient is getting as much restorative sleep as possible is important, so that sleep disruption does not exacerbate pain itself and destroy a patient's mood. Finally, patients may consider other therapeutic techniques to complete the multidisciplinary therapy care options. These other complementary techniques can include yoga and Pilates, acupuncture and massage, Reiki and meditation, biofeedback, herbal medicines and essential oils, and many other therapies.

Now continuing with the **P-I-T-S *treatment protocol***, if pills, injections, and therapy are unable to get pain under control, then a **Surgical** consultation is the next step. With a large, herniated disc, maybe a minimally invasive discectomy or a laminectomy—the removal of tissue or bone to decompress the spine—may be the answer. Typically, a straightforward herniated disc does not require a spinal fusion. A spinal fusion option is usually reserved for patients who suffer with multi-level degenerative compressive problems or spondylolisthesis, involving one vertebral body slipping over another in the spine, leading to *spinal instability*. This type of procedure often requires the placement of hardware or spinal instrumentation to correct the problem.

If any surgery is necessary, then the risk and benefits of such a procedure would be discussed with the patient, and a decision made as to whether the surgical plan should proceed. In general, surgical options are considered only if patients remain in intractable pain despite aggressive medical and interventional pain management treatment, or the patient experiences ongoing or progressive neurologic deficits. Also, the surgical option must be scheduled to fit into the patient's lifestyle—family life, job, school, seasonality, and so forth—in order to minimize the stress to the patient and accelerate the patient's return to a more normal life.

The success of the **PITS Program** depends upon patient awareness and willingness to re-evaluate their pain condition on a regular basis, in concert with the **P-I-T-S *treatment protocol***. The patient must always reassess their condition while keeping their personal pain condition goals in focus. This is the key for the patient to *maximize* their **PITS Score**.

In general, the patient's goals should include improved comfort, return to function and productivity, and that the **P-I-T-S *treatment protocol*** has minimal side effects. The patient wants to ensure that they are controlling anxiety and depression and improving their social interactions. Statistically, even for acute herniated disc problems, sixty percent of patients experience relief within the first month by using conservative care techniques, and ninety percent of patients improve after two or three months. With more persistent pain symptoms, patients move along a program protocol that would lead pain treatment into a subacute phase between three to six months, and into a chronic lumbar radiculopathy phase beyond six months.

PATIENT EXAMPLE #1: A 49-year-old female with a job in retail had a slip-and-fall at work and experienced acute radicular pain in her leg with numbness and tingling. She went to her employer's physician, who diagnosed her with lumbar radiculopathy—sciatica. At the start of her Workers Compensation (WC) treatment guideline of spine care, she was given a course of anti-inflammatory medication with the Medrol Dosepak, and the muscle relaxant cyclobenzaprine.

After approximately seven days her pain condition persisted, and the doctor placed her in a physical therapy program for six weeks. During the physical therapy program, the patient experienced partial improvement. Her back pain subsided, but she still had persistent leg pain. Eventually, the doctor prescribed a lumbar MRI imaging study, after the six weeks of conservative therapy, which revealed a herniated disc at the L5-S1 disc level compressing a spinal nerve root.

She was then referred to interventional pain management for consideration of an epidural steroid injection (ESI) to treat spinal inflammation from the disc disruption and the nerve impingement. She had two injections a month apart, after WC authorization between each injection, without excessive steroid side effects—hot red face, weight gain, blood sugar elevation, stomach upset, vaginal spotting, or leg muscle cramps—and this resolved 90% of her leg pain. She had improved functionality and needed less pain medication thereafter, and never needed to consult with a spine surgeon. She did not suffer acute anxiety or depression during her treatment course. With the help of the analgesic sleep aide Tylenol PM, she did have restorative sleep during this period. She did not consider complementary techniques, like acupuncture or massage or yoga.

She returned to the employer's physician for evaluation and was deemed clear for return of work full duty. She did well thereafter, without recurrent pain. Had this patient not resolved her symptoms after multiple pills, up to three ESIs, and several courses of therapy, then she would have been referred to a surgeon to determine if she was a candidate for discectomy—removal of the disc component that was contacting the spinal nerve—known as *spinal decompression*. If she needed a discectomy, then after a short course of rehabilitation after this very successful surgical procedure, she would have obtained clearance to return back to work at that point in her pain care program.

If she had unfortunately failed to get relief with surgery, and her pain persisted into a six-month period and up to 1-year of healing, she would have been considered a chronic pain patient at that point and instructed to follow the extended **P-I-T-S** *treatment protocol* plan for chronic persistent low back pain of a lumbar radicular nature.

Pain and disability are common with work-related injuries, especially in cases where pain lingers for a while. Statistically, very few patients return to work if they have been out for more than twelve months with

unresolved pain complaints. So, it is critical that all acute pain patients, especially work-related patients, move through the treatment options in a timely fashion to optimize recovery and return to an appropriate work schedule as soon as possible.

PATIENT EXAMPLE #2: A 27-year-old male recreational runner had finished a 5K race up and down hills in his hometown. He had warmed up pretty well before the race, but shortly after the run he felt tightening in his back and pain down his leg. It was centered in his right buttock muscle area.

He took some Advil after the race. It helped somewhat, but again he had that one area of spasm in his buttock area that persisted. It felt like a *"big knot"* and it was very bothersome to him. He never experienced type of pain in the past and felt that he could have sciatica. Heat, ice, and stretching did not resolve this knot and the periodic pain he felt down his right hamstring.

His girlfriend thought that he may have some type of myofascial muscle-related pain. She had a history of this type of pain in her neck and had seen a pain specialist and received a trigger point local anesthetic injection to break her neck spasm. He felt this might also help him, so he saw a physiatrist who specialized in muscular care, and the physician recommended a myofascial trigger point injection in the right piriformis muscle.

Two days after receiving this type of injection in the piriformis muscle in the buttock under X-ray guidance from a local interventional pain care provider, much of the runner's acute spasm had resolved and he achieved an improved level of comfort. However, after about two weeks the pain returned at about half of the original intensity. He returned to his pain specialist, who repeated the piriformis trigger point injection. Again, he experienced approximately two weeks of relief, but this time he started physical therapy with modality treatment of heat, ice, and TENS unit—transcutaneous electrical nerve stimulation—therapy. This course of action resulted in a further reduction of pain down to approximately 25% of the original level.

He resumed his recreational running activities a month later. During the subsequent few months most of his pain resolved, including any pain down his leg. It turned out that the piriformis muscle was irritating the *sciatic nerve* just below it, resulting in the periodic radiating sciatica leg symptoms. Now, had this patient's pain level persisted despite multiple local anesthetic trigger point injections and physical therapy, and the sciatica symptoms became worse, then an MRI followed by an epidural steroid injection—if a lumbar disc problem was discovered—could then be considered for longer-term relief. In the case of myofascial pain syndrome in the spine/buttock muscles, there are no surgical options. But with persistent sciatica from a spinal disc disruption, there are typically surgery options available as needed. In this case example, the patient did well with conservative treatment.

In these first two acute and chronic low back and sciatica pain scenarios it was important to get early assessment so that care could be started and continued in a timely and progressive manner. It has been proven that when severe acute pain is controlled quickly, then chronic pain is less likely to set in and persist due to permanent changes in the central nervous system. This is an unfortunate, but all-to-common process known as *sensitization*.

With the **P-I-T-S** *treatment protocol*, pills and injections are important to break the pain cycle and to allow for rehabilitation to begin with optimal therapy, whether in the form of physical therapy or chiropractic care or both, to strengthen and condition muscles in order to decrease the recurrence of pain moving forward. Surgery is always a last choice when intractable pain continues, despite medical and interventional pain management, or if there is ongoing or progressive neurologic compromise—severe sensory loss, worsening weakness, loss of reflexes or bowel-bladder-sexual function loss.

PATIENT EXAMPLE #3: A 32-year-old female was otherwise well until playing competitive tennis with her tennis partner. One hour after her match, she started having low back pain with some radiating symptoms through her right buttock and into her leg. She went home and rested, took an Advil anti-inflammatory medication, but the pain seemed to persist. The pain was bothersome to her, so she rested for a week laying off her tennis and other activities.

The pain persisted with some numbness into her right leg. She went to a nearby walk-in urgent medical care facility, and the staff physician on duty diagnosed her with sciatica symptoms. She was prescribed the drug Mobic—meloxicam, a nonsteroidal anti-inflammatory medication—for a week, and she was advised to rest a few more days. She was also prescribed the muscle relaxant Baclofen, for some spasms she was experiencing. Her symptoms worsened over the next 2 weeks and she returned to her regular internist for reevaluation. She was prescribed a two month-long program of physical therapy (PT) to see if this could break her pain cycle, as a conservative medical management measure. Over the course of her PT treatment her condition improved, but her symptoms were not completely resolved, and she was still not able to resume full physical activity. She returned to her internist who ordered an MRI imaging study of the lumbar low back spine to rule out the possibility of a spinal disc derangement—bulging or herniated disc that could be resulting in a *spinal nerve impingement*.

The MRI indeed revealed a herniated disc at the L4-5 disc level, and realizing the patient had no progressive neurologic numbness or weakness, she was able to avoid an immediate spinal surgeon consultation. Thus, she was referred to an interventional pain management specialist who felt she was an excellent candidate for *cortisone* injection therapy.

She proceeded with two epidural steroid injections (ESIs) to relieve her spinal inflammatory pain, and ultimately, she returned to her usual level of activity after achieving significant relief. Epidural steroid injections are powerful, and therefore, no more than three injections are advisable within a six-month period had her pain persisted—practitioners typically do not need more than three ESIs to fully treat the spinal inflammation, and they do not want to soften tissue and weaken bone where the steroid is injected. Fortunately, the patient experienced significant relief with two epidural steroid injections a month apart, and along with her medications and a short course of therapy, she was fully restored to normal pain-free activities.

In the foregoing patient example, had the patient failed to improve after the medications, therapy, and two or three epidural steroid injections, then she would have been a candidate for a surgical spine consultation pursuant to the **P-I-T-S** *treatment protocol*.

With her progression of pain and neurologic symptoms, and with her sciatica worsening where she could barely walk, she would have sought a surgical opinion for a discectomy and/or laminectomy. This is a minimally invasive procedure to remove a piece of disc and bone that is compressing a spinal nerve. In the hands of a trained spine surgeon, this is common surgery with relatively low surgical risk, and would give her a chance at a long-term cure outcome.

In a more advanced scenario, had this patient progressed with intractable pain after the first surgical decompression, then a reoperation consideration for a spinal fusion could have been determined if indicated, otherwise the patient would have been a candidate for a spinal cord stimulator (SCS) trial, a specialized type of stimulation wire therapy of the spinal cord. This trial modality uses mild electrical impulses to treat the area of the spine that is responsible for the ongoing back and leg pain. If after the trial week this form of treatment demonstrates some relief from the pain condition, and her sleep and activities have improved, she may be a candidate for implantation of permanent epidural leads or a surgical paddle and a longer-term pulse generator under the skin.

If all these protocols had been exhausted, and her pain persisted, then she could be a candidate for longer-term oral narcotic therapy or a spinal narcotic injection trial candidate and consideration of a morphine pump implantation for control of ongoing intractable pain symptoms. Fortunately, these two options are less likely scenarios.

Remember, if the patient had undergone the discectomy and again experienced recurrent pain, after consulting with her original surgeon or obtaining a second opinion, she could have been a re-operative candidate. If she ever developed *spinal instability*, then she would be a spinal fusion candidate typically with spinal hardware stabilization placement.

In reality, it turned out that this particular patient experienced recurring pain six months after her discectomy and she needed a spinal fusion to help stabilize her spine. She received a two-level spinal hardware stabilization, and after six months of healing returned to most of her pre-injury activities, barring the competitive tennis part. In the end, she was disappointed that she needed a spinal fusion, but was satisfied with the ultimate result. In conclusion, this is an example of lumbar radiculopathy moving from possible medical pain management resolution to interventional pain management resolution of symptoms, and then finally moving toward a surgical resolution.

In summary, when it comes to lumbar radiculopathy, it is important to begin pain treatment options in a timely fashion in order to break the pain cycle as soon as possible. Patients should realize that following the **P-I-T-S** *treatment protocol* allows them to fully rehabilitate and get back to their jobs, family, and daily activities as quickly as possible. Remember, the first option of the **P-I-T-S** *treatment protocol* is **Pills**, and in this case consisted of non-steroidal anti-inflammatory medications. The next option of treatment when pain persists are **Injections**, and in this scenario would necessitate lumbar epidural steroid injections, typically offering weeks-to-months of relief. These are strong steroid minimally invasive injection procedures, performed under a fluoroscopic X-ray, mostly on an outpatient basis. It is usually recommended that some form of **Therapy** begin in conjunction with the initial protocol of the **PITS Program**. Therapy can include physical therapy, chiropractic manipulation, traction, or just re-establishing a home exercise and gym program. Patients are encouraged to maximize flexibility, biomechanics, posture, strength, and conditioning, all to keep debilitating pain in *remission*. Sometimes patients seek the help of a rehabilitation physician, osteopathic manipulative physician, or a neuromuscular medicine expert.

Realize that if patients are not candidates for injectable steroids, such as patients who cannot stop anti-coagulation blood thinners like Plavix or Coumadin, then oral steroids are the next best choice like the Medrol Dosepak (methylprednisolone) to treat inflammation. In addition, if patients have a lot of back spasms with their herniated disc, then muscle relaxants can be used for a short course or for long periods of time while they rehabilitate. Some patients maintain a hypnotic sleep effect when taking muscle relaxants that have sedative effects, like Flexeril, Baclofen, and Zanaflex, and this often helps with restorative sleep. Also, if patients have persistent nerve pain sensations, then they can have a nerve pain agent to slow down the pain, like Neurontin and Lyrica, or a drug like Elavil. Centrally-acting analgesics can help with back and nerve pain, like the mild opioid Ultram or Ultracet. With more persistent or severe cases of pain, the use of stronger opioid narcotics, either short-acting or long-acting, can be trialed for a period of time until patients are fully rehabilitated. If this opioid treatment scenario is needed, it is important to have a patient risk-versus-benefit discussion, and to be cognizant of the morphine milligram equivalents (MMEs) being used, to help minimize opioid complications.

Remember, when the first three **P-I-T-S** *treatment protocol* choices—pills, injections, and therapy—have not substantially relieved the pain condition, then **Surgery** is the final option to consider. If patients have never had a surgical consultation, and their pain might ultimately be controlled with surgical decompression, then these patients should seek a surgical consultation. The surgical option can range from minimally invasive to more invasive surgeries. Discectomy, foraminotomy, laminectomy, all the way up to spinal fusion in the most severe cases, are surgical are potential options. Some patients who have already had surgery and are not deemed candidates for further surgery, can consider the implantable devices for persistent lumbar radiculopathy, such as the spinal cord stimulator or spinal morphine pump. *Never give up—always stay hopeful!*

3. Lumbar Spinal Stenosis

The third type of low back pain is Lumbar Spinal Stenosis. This progressive painful condition develops as people age, where painful symptoms usually start in their fifties and sixties. Patients will typically experience persistent pain in their back and in their legs, especially with prolonged walking.

When patients feel pain in their legs from spinal stenosis, this condition is called *neurogenic claudication*. This is different than *vascular claudication*, which is due to a blood flow problem, which can also cause patients to have pain in their legs. Spinal stenosis is a physical problem in the spine where narrowing of spinal tissue and structures leads to mechanical and inflammatory painful symptoms. The word *stenosis* means narrowing.

When a structure in the spine is progressively narrowing, the spinal nerves start to become impinged and irritated. This can be caused by a hypertrophied ligament issue, a disc derangement problem, calcifications or osteophytes, facet joint arthrosis, or congenital stenosis—born with a narrowed spinal canal. Any narrowing of structures related to the spinal cord (central) or spinal nerve roots (foraminal) can cause intense pain and inflammation known as spinal stenosis.

In keeping with the **P-I-T-S** *treatment protocol* for chronic lumbar spinal stenosis beyond six months or more, there are pills or medications, injections, therapies, and surgical options that the patient and their pain care providers should consider.

For **Pills** or medications, anti-inflammatory drugs, such as non-steroidal or oral steroids, may be considered if there are flares of severe pain. With spasmatic symptoms, muscle relaxants can be added to the pain management strategy. For persistent nerve pain, centrally-acting analgesics, such as Tylenol or the mild opioid tramadol, can be considered. For severe pain, stronger opioid narcotics, both short-acting and long-acting, can be dosed on a short or long-term basis depending on the patient's clinical situation and preference. For spinal stenosis, all the pill categories apply for care.

For **Injection** categories, epidural steroid injections (ESIs) are warranted to treat spinal inflammation from spinal stenosis to break the pain cycle, especially if nerve impingement is discovered on imaging studies. If patients have accompanying back spasm pain with spinal stenosis, then trigger point local anesthetic injections to relieve persistent spasms may help.

When it comes to **Therapy**, all categories apply for low back pain with spinal stenosis. For physical care options, there are chiropractic care, traction, physical therapy, home exercise, gym, and direct physician care. For all the other multidisciplinary therapies of care, including psychological care, restful sleep, and complementary care techniques, there are many choices and approaches to consider.

For **Surgery**, there are minimally invasive techniques, with devices placed outside the spinal canal between what are called spinous processes to distract a stenotic area, and more invasive options, as needed. Spinal decompression that involves a laminectomy or fusion option is very successful for spinal stenosis, especially if patients have intractable pain or worsening neurologic compromise. A highly trained spine surgeon can perform this surgery on many levels of severe stenosis and can even offer *reconstructive* spine surgery, if necessary. Again, patients will have a thorough risk-and-benefit discussion with their spine surgeon, especially if their quality of life is deteriorating, before proceeding with major surgery.

PATIENT EXAMPLE #1: A 60-year-old male was otherwise well until he woke up one day from bed with a *"sore"* back. This pain persisted for weeks despite taking OTC (over-the-counter) anti-inflammatory medication. Many months later, he felt some numbness in his legs when walking, but without any neurologic compromise of bowel and bladder function or weakness in the legs. Six months later, he noticed swelling in his ankles, especially when he felt severe numbness in the tops of his legs with prolonged walking.

He sought medical attention with his primary physician, who suggested some physical therapy and a stronger medication. The patient was not a big medication person in general, so he felt that maybe some physical therapy could help him. He did a course of two months of strengthening and conditioning, but he only felt worse. He still had trouble walking and still experienced periods of numbness in his legs.

His back did not hurt as much at this point, but he still had persistent leg symptoms with activity. He noticed that arching his back forward offered some relief, especially when he was food shopping at the local market and leaning on the shopping cart. He returned to his primary care physician with ongoing pain, and a CT-scan imaging study was ordered.

The CT-scan revealed moderate-to-marked lumbar spinal stenosis at the L3-4 level. He was referred to a spine surgeon at this point who offered a decompression and fusion option, but first recommended an interventional pain management consult, for the patient to consider injection therapy. After consulting with the pain specialist, he underwent two lumbar epidural steroid injections (ESIs), under fluoroscopy X-ray guidance, in an outpatient office setting. The injections were two weeks apart.

His overall pain condition was 50% better after these injections, without steroid side effects of a hot red face, excessive weight gain, mood irritation, stomach upset, or leg muscle cramps. He felt that he did not need to return to the surgeon at this point. He got back to his normal activity and only took Tylenol infrequently for what he attributed to *pain of normal aging.* Had the pain not resolved, or had it worsened, then a surgical decompression option could have been pursued moving forward with spine care, as seen in the next patient example.

PATIENT EXAMPLE #2: A 66-year-old female, with a history of multilevel marked lumbar spinal stenosis, had a deteriorating condition over the last five years as she tried to stay active. She had tried many different NSAIDs or non-steroidal anti-Inflammatory drugs, several types of physical therapy and yoga therapy, and multiple epidural steroid injections (ESIs), all of which failed to give her lasting relief. In the beginning, the ESIs lasted for six months, but lately they only provided relief for a few weeks.

She had a friend who had talked to a spine surgeon about a similar condition, and that friend eventually ended up with a lumbar fusion with resultant relief. The patient struggled with the surgery decision because of her busy schedule, but eventually asked her internist for a recommendation to a spine surgeon, in order to get a better understanding of her surgical options.

A month later, she met with a neurosurgeon who felt that spinal surgery would be a good option to break her intractable pain cycle. The surgeon and patient had a risk-and-benefit discussion about the possibility of doing a lumbar decompression fusion surgery. The patient eventually opted for this course of action, after getting no relief from another month of physical therapy, and underwent a two-level lumbar fusion with instrumentation at the local hospital.

She responded well postoperatively, as was expected, and left the hospital three days after surgery. Two weeks later she had a follow-up visit with her surgeon, and X-rays were taken that confirmed the fusion hardware was in the proper position and alignment. Three months later she was back to her daily activities, and at six months after a follow-up lumbar CT scan revealed a solid fusion, was at full unrestricted activity enjoying her life again.

Assume for a moment that this patient had lumbar fusion and did well for many years, but had recurrent pain thereafter, and was deemed not to be a surgical reoperation candidate. In that case, she could be a candidate for the spinal cord stimulation (SCS) lead trial modality, especially if she had recurrent persistent back and leg pain.

If she had failed a spinal cord stimulation trial, and still suffered with severe pain symptoms, then she could consider a trial of long-term opioid narcotic therapy, if this was agreeable to her. However, if she failed a high-dose oral narcotic therapy attempt, because of insufficient relief or excessive side effects, then she could be a candidate for the spinal morphine narcotic test trial.

If for any reason all the advanced implantable modalities failed, then she would have fallen back on other aspects of the **Pain is the PITS Program** with its multidisciplinary integrative treatment approaches. These would include mind-body complementary therapy trials, and many other options, for the ongoing pursuit of an acceptable **PITS Score**.

4. Lumbar Facet Pain Syndrome

The fourth type of low back pain is Lumbar Facet Pain Syndrome. This is a condition of inflammation and degeneration of the lumbar spinal facet joints. These are paired vertebral joints, much like synovial knee and hip joints, which can wear-and-tear and break down over time, with normal repetitive twisting and bending of the low back. They are another common source of pain in the lower back. When patients are experiencing hyperextension with lateral bending back pain and have palpable pain over the *sides* of their spine typically above the waist, they can be suspect for facet pain syndrome. Imaging, such as plain X-ray, CT scan, or MRI studies, which reveal facet hypertrophy and arthrosis of these joints, can confirm advanced disease.

Relating to the **P-I-T-S** *treatment protocol*, anti-inflammatory medications or **Pills** apply as an initial option, considering OTC (over-the-counter) or prescription strength choices. If the facets give the

patient muscle spasms, then a muscle relaxant can be prescribed. Facet pain is a type of joint pain which does not involve a true nerve problem issue, so nerve pain agents are not typically used for this condition. As needed, short-acting opioid narcotic analgesics can be offered for persistent moderate-to-severe low back pain of a facet origin.

Injection therapy options are therapeutic joint steroid injections or diagnostic facet nerve local anesthetic blocks. These two interventional pain management approaches are performed under fluoroscopic X-ray in an outpatient setting. Typically, the steroid is directed directly into one or more joints either on one side or both sides of the spine in order to break the pain cycle by reducing inflammation. If steroidal injection directly in the joint gives prolonged periods of relief, then this option can be repeated—up to three injections in a six-month period as needed. The key is not to put too much steroid in a concentrated area too often, or the patient runs the risk of deteriorating joints, softening bone, and weakening tissue. If these injections are spaced appropriately—typically two months apart for medical necessity—this allows this injection therapy to be safe and therapeutically effective for patients.

Many interventional pain doctors may prefer to do a diagnostic facet nerve injection with local anesthetic outside of the joint to *block* the nerve supply that controls pain, as an initial first step. If this diagnostic facet nerve injection is successful with a certain amount of relief and duration, then patients may choose to undergo a radiofrequency (RF) burning of the facet nerves for longer-term relief of facet joint back pain. Typically, this methodology can result in relief for three-to-six months duration or possibly longer, before the facet nerves *regrow* and pain returns.

When discussing **Therapy** options for facet pain syndrome, all the basic therapy categories apply—physical therapy, chiropractic care, traction, home exercise, gym, and direct physician care, as needed. The main goal is always to optimize the patient's flexibility, biomechanics, strengthening, and so forth, in order to decrease recurrent pain to a tolerable level. In addition, all the psychological pain tolerance approaches, restful sleep strategies, and complementary therapeutic techniques may apply based on the individual patient's needs.

The **Surgery** option for pain relief in treating this condition, known as isolated facetectomy or removal of part or all of the joint area, is aggressive and not common as an isolated surgical technique to decompress the spine. Facetectomy is usually done along with other surgical decompressions of the lamina, another bony area in the back of the spine, and the spinal discs—or in conjunction with spinal fusion.

PATIENT EXAMPLE #1: A 28-year-old male who was partying at his friend's house, fell down ten steps in the house, and sustained an acute low back pain episode. His friend drove him to the hospital where X-rays were negative for any kind of fracture or dislocation. He had a lot of soreness and pain with lateral bending and hyperextension of his back and was given two different medications in the emergency room—a muscle relaxant and an anti-inflammatory medication.

He was told to rest and then follow up with his internist if pain persisted. He was not better in two weeks, and when he followed up with his internist, he was prescribed a course of physical therapy. The patient did a full 6 weeks of physical therapy, three times a week, with instruction in an ongoing home exercise program (HEP). His moderate-to-severe pain slowly resolved over the subsequent two months, and he was back to his usual walking and climbing stairs. He continued to do well thereafter, without recurrent pain.

PATIENT EXAMPLE #2: A 38-year-old male salesperson was involved in an automobile accident on the expressway and suffered an injury to his low back area. His lawyer referred him to an orthopedic spine specialist, who after a thorough history and physical exam evaluation, along with an MRI of the lumbar spine, diagnosed the patient with a bulging disc and multiple levels of moderate facet joint degeneration.

The orthopedist prescribed medication and physical therapy as the first steps toward recovery. The medications only made him sick, and after eight weeks, even the physical therapy failed to produce any positive results. Despite having a bulging disc on the MRI, he

was not experiencing any sciatica-like symptoms with shooting pain in his legs. His pain remained localized in the back area over the lateral facet joint area sides of the spine.

The orthopedist discussed the use of injections to try and relieve the pain, and the patient was referred to an anesthesiology interventional pain specialist to consider facet joint steroid injections to treat the persistent low back pain. After two sets of facet steroid injections two months apart, the relief was short term, lasting for only one month in duration. The injections indeed reduced the pain level by 80%, and without steroid side effects of a hot red face, excessive weight gain, mood irritation, stomach upset, or leg muscle cramps, but the relief just did not last.

At that point, the interventional pain specialist recommended the minimally invasive procedure of radiofrequency lesioning (RFL) or burning of facet nerves for longer-term pain relief—also known as radiofrequency ablation (RFA). This intervention was anticipated to block the facet nerve transmission, and thus stop the painful facet joint sensations, for months or longer. The patient subsequently had the outpatient procedure performed on the right-sided facet joints, under fluoroscopic X-ray guidance and IV-sedation at a local surgical center, and felt great a few days later. He felt sore initially for a day from the procedural discomfort itself, but the post-procedure pain settled down quickly after icing the area. He chose to have the same procedure for his similar left-sided facet pain 2 weeks later, and again he did very well.

He returned to the original orthopedist who cleared him to return to full activities with no restrictions. In this case, the patient's quality of life, work status, and recreational activities were fully restored with the help of medical and interventional pain management, while avoiding the surgical option.

5. Sacroiliac Joint (SIJ) Dysfunction and Sacroiliitis

The fifth type of low back pain is Sacroiliac Joint Dysfunction (mechanical pain) and painful Sacroiliitis (inflammatory pain). Essentially, the sacroiliac joints (SIJs) connect the back of the pelvis to the lower spine, so there is a left and right SIJ. Much like the paired facet joints, the sacroiliac joints can get inflamed, and can become degenerated and dysfunctional. Using our **P-I-T-S** *treatment protocol* options, sacroiliac joint pain is first approached with nonsteroidal anti-inflammatory medications or **Pills**, especially for treating sacroiliitis. If there is spasm component, then using a muscle relaxant can help break the spasm-related pain. Since this type of joint pain is not typically a nerve pain problem, anti-neuropathic medication, like Neurontin (gabapentin), is not usually prescribed.

Centrally-acting analgesics apply as options, like Tylenol or the mild opioid tramadol, as needed. For severe cases, stronger opioid narcotics can be prescribed, both of a short-acting and long-acting nature. Typically, opioid treatment begins with short-acting narcotics, like Percocet or Vicodin, but again if patients require multiple doses a day to control symptoms, then a long-acting narcotic may be warranted for a short while.

As a side note, some patients on prolonged narcotics will develop a sense of tolerance to opioids, and will need other aspects of the **PITS Program** to regain the lost comfort. In this case, a well-constructed integrative approach to the management of chronic pain is the preferred approach, as opposed to the historical approach of prescribing more and more opioids. Sometimes, if patients become tolerant to one kind of narcotic, physicians can perform what is called an opioid rotation, or switching to an equivalent analgesic dose of a different opioid narcotic. By switching to a different narcotic, patients can often recapture control over their pain.

In terms of **Injection** therapy, sacroiliac joints can be injected with a steroid as an interventional technique, typically repeated two months later, if necessary, to obtain a measure of prolonged relief. If that relief is short lived, then radiofrequency lesion or burning of the joint can be performed, much like for the facet joint RFL procedure, for the aim of achieving longer-lasting relief. Remember, the sacroiliac joints are paired joints on each side of the lower spine below the waist connecting the sacrum to the ilium with ligament attachments, so some patients opt for a complementary care technique called *prolotherapy*. Prolotherapy involves injecting certain irritants, like high-sugar solutions, into the sacroiliac ligament to try to promote healing and tightening of the joint, in an attempt to make it less dysfunctional.

As for **Therapy** options, physical therapy and care therapy techniques are very important to get patients to a more comfortable spot and keep them functional. As previously mentioned, most pain management teams prefer to exhaust all conservative pain treatment protocols before choosing a surgical option. This is sound pain management practice, provided that the patient is not suffering with an excessive quality-of-life issue, and they are continuing to move forward with their pain treatment protocol. There are also lots of complementary techniques that can be offered, such as yoga, acupuncture, massage, biofeedback, herbal therapy, essential oils, and so forth.

Surgery options for sacroiliac joint pain are limited and used when the joint is fractured and unstable, usually in severe trauma situations, or from a process of severe inflammatory degeneration over years. If chronic sacroiliac joint pain becomes progressively intractable from severe arthritic joint degeneration or sacroiliac joint dysfunction, then a minimally invasive surgery (MIS) titanium joint fixation procedure can be performed, by an orthopedist trained to provide this type of operation, to stabilize the joint area and provide lasting pain relief.

PATIENT EXAMPLE: A 50-year-old male who had a previous lumbar fusion five years ago started developing low back and buttock pain after twisting and turning while repairing his automobile in the driveway. He had persistent pain despite applying ice and had taken a muscle relaxant which he had in his medicine cabinet.

He felt a little bit better for a day or two, but the same pain returned. It was mostly over his right low back and buttock area. He was worried about his previous fusion repair and returned to his original surgeon. After examination and X-rays of the lumbar spine, he was diagnosed with sacroiliac joint pain over the lower part of his spine and buttock below his lumbar fusion scar.

He was instructed to do a month of physical therapy, which included stretching, heat, ice, TENS unit and other modalities, but his pain was not appreciably better. He was eventually deemed to be a sacroiliac joint steroid injection candidate by his physical therapist, and was referred to an interventional pain specialist, who agreed with the recommendation after consultation.

The patient had the joint injection performed under fluoroscopic X-ray guidance in an outpatient setting and did well without side effects. There was a 75% reduction in overall pain symptoms within the first week after the procedure. The patient subsequently came off his medications and got back to his normal activity. Now, if the sacroiliac injection resulted only in short-term relief, then the patient would have been eligible for radiofrequency (RF) ablation of sacroiliac joint nerves, for an attempt at longer-term relief and better rehabilitation moving forward.

6. Lumbar Degenerative Disc Disease (DDD)

The sixth type of low back pain is **Lumbar Degenerative Disc Disease**. Lumbar degenerative disc disease (DDD) pain typically happens as aging occurs and the spinal discs lose their water content hydration, and start to decrease in height. This can unfortunately result in progressive chronic pain symptoms. Active patients in their thirties and forties seem to be affected the most with this condition.

The lower three lumbar discs take most of the pressure (pounds per square inch=PSI) and this puts them at risk of deteriorating. Patients who are active with sports or have strenuous jobs with a lot of bending and twisting, or who suffer back injuries early in life, are at increased risk of speeding up the degenerative disc process. Most patients with lumbar degenerative discs complain about non-radiating *mechanical* low back pain—axial in nature and in the center of the spine—usually from sitting for extended periods of time. Sitting increases pressure on the lower discs more than standing, and often it is hard for patients with this condition to find a comfortable position.

Using the **P-I-T-S** *treatment protocol*, treatment for this condition usually starts with nonsteroidal anti-inflammatory medications or **Pills**, or plain Tylenol. If there are associated spasms, then a muscle

relaxant is added. For more moderate-to-severe pain, a short-acting opioid narcotic can be prescribed while other pain management options are evaluated.

As far as **Injection** pain options, some patients find relief from lumbar epidural steroid injections, especially if degenerative discs start to compress spinal nerves. Some patients with persistent discogenic pain will undergo diagnostic multilevel lumbar discography to better define the actual disc level(s) that are causing the pain. Lumbar discography involves pressurizing discs with contrast material to determine the disc pathology and to see how the patient responds with their pain symptoms. With certain painful discs, and depending on insurance coverage, intradiscal electrothermal therapy (IDET) can be offered as a minimally invasive outpatient procedure, which uses heat to safely burn discogenic nerves for an attempt at relief.

Along **Therapy** lines, patients will be encouraged to keep their core muscles in shape, either in physical therapy or with a home exercise program. The key core muscle groups are the lumbar paraspinous, buttocks, hamstrings, and abdominal muscles. Many patients attempt yoga or Pilates, as well, to stay flexible and core strong.

In severe pain cases, patients seek consultation with a spine surgeon to consider lumbar spinal fusion as a **Surgery** option, for decompressing and stabilizing multilevel degenerative disc disease. Surgical spinal disc replacement procedures are also an option for certain patients.

PATIENT EXAMPLE: A 40-year-old firefighter who had been battling blazes for twenty years, started to develop an increasing low back pain ache that was slowing down his normally busy days at the firehouse. Despite Motrin and a few days of rest, the low back pain increased, especially sitting around at the firehouse.

He asked his internist about doing some physical therapy, and after six weeks of strengthening and conditioning, he felt 80% improved. He resumed his active firefighting duties, but intense back pain returned, so he went to the local hospital emergency room for evaluation. After a physical examination and completion of a lumbar MRI study, he was diagnosed with marked degenerative disc disease at the L4-5 and L5-S1 disc levels. A neurosurgeon on call came to see the patient and prescribed Percocet and a steroid Medrol Dosepak for discharge home.

The patient was given instructions to follow up with the neurosurgeon in two weeks if his condition did not improve. When he returned to the surgeon his pain had only slightly improved. It was recommended that the patient have a diagnostic lumbar discogram test, which involved injecting pressurized contrast material into spinal discs to determine the levels of provoked pain, to better determine which lumbar discs were the most painful and which discs could be repaired with surgery if necessary.

The patient was referred to an interventional pain specialist who explained the risk and benefit of discography. The pain specialist explained that it was a test that was meant to be painful in order to find the affected discs, but it was the best way to provide accurate information for the surgeon. Pain medication is often administered after this type of provocative painful procedure.

The patient agreed to the diagnostic discogram, which revealed that only the L5-S1 disc appeared to be affected, and not the L4-5 or L3-4 discs, as originally thought. When the patient returned to his spine surgeon, he was offered a single-level lumbar spinal fusion with instrumentation to control his painful symptoms. The patient did not want to have the disc fusion surgery as recommended, but rather, wanted to try interim measures in the hope of avoiding the surgical procedure altogether.

The surgeon mentioned that a lumbar epidural steroid injection (ESI) might offer temporary relief, and so the patient returned to his pain specialist for the injection. The patient had a L5-S1 level epidural steroid injection that gave him 2 weeks of 50% relief and no side effects. The patient was offered a second injection but was now interested in a longer-term fix for his condition, and eventually returned to his surgeon to proceed with the spinal fusion.

Immediately after the surgery, and three months later into the rehabilitation process, the patient realized he was feeling much better, and had basically returned to full normal activity after 6 months. He was pleased that he had made the right choices in the pain management process. He had failed medical pain management, then failed interventional pain management, and finally ended up with a successful surgical pain management option.

So, these are some of the common types of acute and chronic low back pain conditions, accounting for nearly a quarter of all the chronic pain that exists in the United States. Never give up on the trying to get your desirable level of comfort and functional activity goals as you move through the assessment and treatment process. Sometimes the pain goes away in a few days, or a few weeks, or a few months, or a few years, or maybe never, but 100% pain relief is not always achievable with certain chronic low back situations—right? Rather, controlling the pain at an acceptable level is more reasonable for many patients, where your focus on optimizing your **PITS Score** through time is the real key to meaningful relief and a better quality of life!

I trust this chapter will serve as an educational platform, with different patient examples of pain care scenarios, so that patients can see where their own pain *"fits in."* I have created a separate chapter at the end of this one, called **PITS Educational Pearls of Pain Care Wisdom**; and at the end of the book there is an extensive **PITS Glossary of Pain Terms** section for added information on specific topics, like pain conditions, medications, procedures, and so forth. Remember not to skip these important sections of the book, because they are vitally important as reinforcers of the overall pain knowledge that will help ensure your success in the **PITS Program**!

Neck Pain

SUMMARY: When is the last time you heard, "This is a real pain in the neck"? All of the various types of **neck (cervical) pain** account for one of the top five most common pain problems in America. Most of the physical mechanical and inflammatory problems that lead to acute and chronic low back (lumbar) pain symptoms, also affect the neck structures. A lot of the same spinal structures in the lumbar spine exist up in the cervical spine in the neck. Thus, it stands to reason that patients can develop cervical pain symptoms in a similar way as lumbar symptoms—through normal aging, injuries at work, motor vehicle accidents, through competitive and recreational sports, slip and falls, and so forth. Cervical spasms, herniated discs, spinal stenosis narrowing, facet joint arthritis and inflammation, and degenerative cervical disc disease are the common painful conditions in the cervical spine area.

When patients seek medical advice from their physicians and pain management specialists regarding their cervical pain complaints, it is the initial complaint of *PAIN* that starts the clinical pain management pathway with an initial evaluation assessment. Similar for low back problems, the primary care physician (PCP) or pain specialist will:

- Take a complete history of the pain condition—when did it start, how does it feel, what pain level is it rated, what makes it better/worse, are there any associated factors, what treatments have been tried so far, and so forth.

- Conduct a physical examination with particular attention paid to the musculoskeletal and neurological systems.

- Review radiology studies and other tests, if completed or available.

- Make an assessment with a diagnosis of the suspected pain type(s).

- Formulate an initial plan for pain management care moving forward.

After the assessment and plan phases of the clinical pathway comes the **P-I-T-S** *treatment protocol* implementation. After a cycle or two of pain care options, patients move to the evaluation part of the clinical pathway. This is the critical determination as to whether the patient's pain and quality-of-life goals are being met. Cervical spasms, radiculopathy from nerve irritation, spinal stenosis, and degenerative joint and disc conditions are all treated in a similar fashion as lumbar spinal pain conditions—considering **Pills** or medications, **Injections**, **Therapy** (physical, psychological, sleep strategies, and complementary therapies), and **Surgery**—as the four sections of the **P-I-T-S** *treatment protocol* options.

All of the **P-I-T-S** *treatment protocol* options apply to acute and chronic painful cervical conditions. There are the same basic medication or **Pill** choices—anti-inflammatories, muscle relaxants, nerve pain agents, and opioid narcotics—which can be tailored to a patient's particular clinical situation and preference. The pain management plan takes into consideration the expertise of the pain care team, and the scientific evidence and research currently available, in terms of what works and what does not work. It is a balanced treatment approach that follows a multidisciplinary pain management plan. Often the use of different medications for various types of pain gives the patient a *multi-modal* treatment approach focusing on using smaller amounts of different medications rather than a large amount of one medication. This strategy may result in better pain relief and less side effects for the patient.

Injection options, depending on the main cause of pain, would be cervical trigger point local anesthetic injections for spasms, epidural steroid injections (ESIs) for herniated discs and spinal stenosis to treat spinal inflammatory pain, and facet joint and facet nerve injections to treat facet joint degenerative pain and inflammation.

All the **Therapy** categories apply, including physical options like chiropractic care, gentle traction, physical therapy, home exercise, gym, and specialized physician care if needed. Many chiropractors are cautious when manipulating the sensitive structures in the neck, so it is usually gentle chiropractic care in the neck area when patients pursue this option. Psychological care and sleep strategies are other important therapy types, as well as complementary therapy approaches like acupuncture, massage, yoga, and other techniques as needed.

Surgery, from minimally invasive to more invasive care, is offered as needed, to round out all the **P-I-T-S** *treatment protocol* options. Through new technology and research, surgical approaches to alleviate pain, particularly spinal fusion surgery, have advanced greatly. This is especially true for anterior cervical discectomy and fusion (ACDF), where this is commonly performed through an anterior (front) neck approach (rather than from the back of the neck), where patients typically make a much faster and less painful recovery.

With expert spinal surgical care, many patients leave the hospital on the same day or the next day to heal at home over the ensuing months. The surgical incision is typically hidden in a patient's natural neck creases and heals well.

Specific Neck Pain Conditions

Cervical Myofascial Pain Syndrome of the neck is treated conservatively, with medications or **Pills**—anti-inflammatory and muscle relaxants—trigger point **Injections**, various hands-on **Therapy** approaches, and without the need for **Surgery** release techniques for typical myofascial spasms, in general.

Cervical **Herniated Discs**, **Cervical Spinal Stenosis**, and **Cervical Degenerative Disc Disease**—similar to low back herniated discs, stenosis, and degenerative discs—are treated with the anti-inflammatory medications or **Pills**, muscle relaxants, nerve pain agents, centrally-acting analgesics, and opioid narcotics, as needed. Epidural steroid **Injections** can be used to treat spinal inflammatory pain and are safe minimally invasive outpatient procedures. Of course, trigger points can be done if there are persistent associated neck spasms. The integrative **Therapy** approaches for cervical herniated discs and spinal stenosis all apply. As far as **Surgery** being considered, operations are typically restricted for patients who develop or experience persistent or worsening neurologic compromise, or for ongoing intractable pain and spinal instability.

Lastly, we have **Cervical Facet Joints** that can become irritated and degenerated, much like lumbar facet joints. These are paired joints on each side of the cervical spine to help with stability and movement. Anti-inflammatory medications or **Pills**, muscle relaxants, centrally-acting agents like Tylenol, and opioid narcotic medications apply. Facet joint and facet nerve **Injections** apply. If we are doing facet joints or facet nerve blocks, then following up with radiofrequency lesioning—a technique using heat to control pain by *"deadening"* nerves—may offer longer-term relief of facet neck pain. Whereas steroids alone may last weeks to a month perhaps, radiofrequency pain relief may last three-to-six months, or longer. All of the **Therapy** options apply to facet pain treatment. **Surgery** is not common for just facets alone, but in severe cases of advanced degeneration and subsequent spinal impingement, this option can be considered, typically along with a spinal fusion.

So, these are some of the chronic neck pain etiologies and their **P-I-T-S** *treatment protocol* options of care. The neck pain patient examples that follow will be almost similar to the low back patient examples, as lot of the *spinal pain generators* are similar in the back and neck. Discs that can cause pain, joints that can become painful, and muscles that can spasm are the typical pain generators in the neck that can lead to chronic persistent painful conditions.

1. Cervical Myofascial Pain Syndrome Patient Example

A 35-year-old male was working as a carpenter when he was hurt on the job sustaining a neck injury, when a wooden board slipped off scaffolding above him and landed on his neck. He went to the emergency room where he was found not to have any fractures, but had reversal of his normal cervical lordosis on X-ray. He did have bruising in the back of his neck with some muscle spasm on physical examination. He was given anti-inflammatory medications and an ice pack and was told by his workers' compensation doctor to take a couple of weeks off to rest, use ice and heat, and do some gentle stretching. He was given a prescription for physical therapy to try, as well, to loosen up some of his ongoing spasm.

He experienced persistent pain however, and after another physical examination and a negative MRI for herniated disc, was found to have active trigger point myofascial knots on both sides of his neck at about the C7 spinal level. It was suggested that he consider a trigger point injection (TPI) with local anesthetic to try to break his spasm pain cycle.

The patient then sought consultation with a neurologist, but had negative EMG and nerve conduction studies, to determine if there was *nerve damage* from his injury. He still experienced some residual spasms, so he decided to undergo local anesthetic trigger point injections, as suggested earlier. This provided him with

50% relief overall of his neck pain for 2 weeks with improved functionality and less need for medication usage. The patient was then offered a Botox injection for longer-term relief of his spasm, which he felt was too aggressive for him. He did not feel comfortable with the idea of *Botox*, although considered very safe and effective injection option, when indicated.

At this point, the neurologist suggested another month of physical therapy, with modalities, and a home exercise program (HEP), which helped tremendously in relieving his residual spasm. He was able to return to work and resume full physical activities shortly thereafter, and felt that he finally had his quality of life back.

2. Cervical Radiculopathy Patient Example

A 49-year-old female mother of three was vacationing with her children at Disney World. She was exiting one of the rides when she felt a *"crick"* in her neck. She had been on a flume ride with a precipitous drop at the end of the ride and had been aggressively waving her arms back and forth with her children. About 30 minutes after exiting the ride she began to experience numbness in her left hand. It felt like her thumb had fallen asleep.

The condition improved slightly during the day, but returned later that night, when they were out to dinner. She took some Advil anti-inflammatory medication which helped for a bit. When she eventually returned home after her vacation, the numbness came back and persisted for weeks. She went to her medical doctor who felt she may have had a pinched nerve in her neck, and was subsequently sent for an MRI imaging study. The MRI study showed two herniated discs, one at the C6-7 disc level and one at the C7-T1 disc level, and were believed to be the cause of her ongoing pain and neurologic symptoms. At this point, she was referred to a pain specialist.

The patient, who was conservative by nature, was given the option of an epidural steroid injection (ESI). She wanted to take some time to do some research on this recommendation. She consulted with one of her friends who had a similar injection and was reassured that it was safe and well tolerated. Just to be sure, she went online and found information on this type of injection,

and realized that it was probably like having an *epidural* for a baby. She understood that it involved using a needle that could be placed into the epidural space, under X-ray guidance, through which a steroid could then be administered, to treat *spinal inflammation* directly at its source.

After consulting with her pain management doctor again, and after her questions were answered, she underwent an outpatient epidural steroid injection under X-ray guidance. The first injection offered her a 50% percent reduction in pain within one week, without any side effects. She then wanted to start physical therapy, so she got a prescription for six weeks, to strengthen the cervical area and to help decrease recurrent pain. Thankfully, a lot of her symptoms had resolved after the therapy was completed, and she slowly got back to her normal activities.

Had her pain persisted, she could have been offered a repeat epidural steroid injection, to decrease even more spinal inflammation, and achieve a longer period of relief. The patient understood that up to three epidural steroid injections in a six-month period was safe. If, even after epidural steroid injections and medications and more physical therapy the pain persisted, then she would have been referred to a spine surgeon in keeping with **P-I-T-S *treatment protocol***.

If she wanted to pursue complementary care techniques, then she could have chosen acupuncture, massage, yoga, biofeedback, essential oil therapy, and many other available options. Now, if the numbness started leading to weakness, in other words, there was evidence of progressive neurologic compromise, then she would have been a more serious surgical candidate.

Realize, that some patients can experience elements of residual pain, even after a successful spine surgery. For example, after an anterior cervical discectomy and fusion (ACDF), other issues can arise such as epidural fibrosis scarring, or a new disc herniation. If this were the unfortunate case for this current patient, and she still had persistent pain even a year after surgery, then she could be a candidate for re-operation or a spinal cord stimulation (SCS) lead modality trial to relieve ongoing discomfort. If she was not a re-operation candidate, then she could certainly consider spinal cord stimulation testing with a pain specialist. If this SCS trial was successful, then she could go on to longer-term implantation of the pulse generator and permanent spinal cord stimulation lead wires, which she could adjust as needed through time, to maintain comfort and quality of life moving forward. There are different companies in the U.S. that specialize in SCS neuromodulation devices, so it is up to the pain specialist and individual patient as to what system is ultimately chosen.

3. Cervical Spinal Stenosis Patient Example

A 70-year-old man was noticing persistent pain in the base of neck while pursuing his gardening hobby. He was proud of his garden, but it required a lot of maintenance care, and now he felt like he was starting to pay the price with all his ongoing neck pain. The dull achy pain continued despite Tylenol, and he could not take Motrin because of a gastric bleed history.

His primary physician gave him a prescription of tramadol (Ultram) and put him in physical therapy, for what was thought to be cervical strain and sprain, due to his gardening activity. When the symptoms worsened, and the patient started feeling numbness in his right hand, he was then referred to a pain specialist, who promptly ordered a cervical MRI imaging study to rule out spinal derangements that might be amenable to future interventional pain management.

The MRI revealed multilevel moderate-to-severe spinal stenosis at the C4-5, C5-6, and C6-7 levels, but no herniated discs. The patient was then offered an epidural steroid injection (ESI) to decrease spinal inflammatory pain, and allow improved activity. He had undergone a total of three epidural injections, over the next four months, which were successful in controlling the numbness symptoms he had experienced earlier. He was maintained on a low dose of Neurontin (gabapentin) for keeping the numbness at tolerable levels, and slowly resumed his gardening. He never had to see a spine surgeon or pursue any other complementary techniques to treat his symptoms.

4. Cervical Facet Pain Syndrome Patient Example

A 42-year-old male was involved in an automobile accident that resulted in a whiplash injury, causing him neck pain. He had gone to the emergency room where X-rays were negative for fracture or dislocation. He was sent for MRI imaging studies that showed no disc herniation and no arthritic problem.

The patient had initially presented to the ER with spasms in his neck, and had been prescribed anti-inflammatory medication and muscle relaxants. The patient also tried narcotics, but they made him *"sick to his stomach."* He eventually saw a pain specialist, and was diagnosed with cervical facet pain syndrome, from a whiplash injury. It was recommended he undergo a minimally invasive, multilevel cervical facet medial nerve branch diagnostic injection, to determine if his cervical facet joints could be the source his persistent neck pain.

This pain was also giving him headache-like symptoms. He was told by his pain management specialist that if this diagnostic local anesthetic injection provided significant relief, he could then be a candidate for a radiofrequency lesioning (RFL) procedure for longer-term care of his painful facet joints. He underwent the diagnostic block successfully, and then the radiofrequency ablation procedure a week later, in a comfortable outpatient setting. The combination offered him 50% relief overall. His persistent headaches were also improved with the procedure. He slowly recovered further, over the next month, and was able to come off his medications. He was able to resume full normal activities, shortly thereafter.

5. Cervical Degenerative Disc Disease Patient Example

A 75-year-old female executive, who frequently traveled between the United States and Europe, awoke one morning in her London hotel room with severe neck pain and spasm. She remembers being on her cell phone for a two-hour-long conference call the day before, with her head *"bent"* all that time.

She took some ibuprofen which helped for a couple hours. She had a massage at the hotel, but this seemed to make the pain worse. She felt a burning sensation at the base of her head that spread out between her shoulder blades. When she arrived back in the U.S., she visited her primary care physician, who sent her for X-rays of her cervical spine.

The X-rays showed greater than 50% decreased disc height of the C6-7 disc. The pain persisted for the following month, and was disturbing her sleep and quality of life, especially with her hectic travel schedule. She was eventually referred to an interventional pain specialist, who ordered an MRI in consideration of injection therapy. The specialist prescribed Lyrica (pregabalin), to help treat some of the direct nerve pain, and offered an epidural steroid injection to treat spinal inflammatory pain, after the MRI revealed multilevel degenerative disc disease (DDD), the worst of which was at the C6-7 level. The Lyrica helped somewhat with nighttime pain and sleep, but the days were still full of bothersome symptoms of neck stiffness and pain.

She eventually had an epidural steroid injection, but with no relief at all. When she returned to her internist, she was referred to an orthopedic spine surgeon to see if a surgical option could help alleviate her ongoing pain at this point. She was informed by the spine surgeon of the risks and rewards of this surgery for a woman of her age, and at the same time, did not want to be forced into retirement due to persistent pain.

The surgeon offered her a C6-7 spinal decompression and fusion procedure with hardware placement, which would require one month off from her job, for expected healing. She chose to have the surgery in the Spring, because that was a good time for her to take a break from work, to have plenty of time to recuperate. She indeed had an anterior cervical discectomy and fusion (ACDF) procedure, and after a month, excitedly returned to her job. She experienced 80% pain relief two months after her surgery, and 90% relief overall, after six months. This was quite satisfying to her, and she resumed full activity, not only at work, but also with her personal life.

So, these are some of the common types of acute and chronic neck pain conditions, accounting for one of the top five overall pain conditions in the United States. Following the **P-I-T-S *treatment protocol***, patients are educated as to their relief options, involved in their pain management decisions, and taught how to monitor their progress. Their very participation in the **PITS Program** helps the patient reduce stress and relieve the anxiety, that persistent pain can often cause, and puts them on the path to reducing pain to a tolerable level and improving activity.

I trust this chapter will serve as an educational platform, with different patient examples of pain care scenarios, so that patients can see where their own pain *"fits in."* I have created a separate chapter at the end of this one, called **PITS Educational Pearls of Pain Care Wisdom**; and at the end of the book there is an extensive **PITS Glossary of Pain Terms** section for added information on specific topics, like pain conditions, medications, procedures, and so forth. Remember not to skip these important sections of the book, because they are vitally important as reinforcers of the overall pain knowledge that will help ensure your success in the **PITS Program**!

Headaches

SUMMARY: Headaches are the second most common pain reason why patients seek relief from their primary care physicians, or neurologists. Migraines, especially when not controlled well, can be very debilitating to the millions of Americans suffering from this difficult condition. Cluster headaches, although not as common as migraine and tension-type headaches, can make patients feel like the world is coming to an end. The pain of a cluster headache can become extremely intense, and often needs emergency room care to get it under control. Tension-type headaches are like the *stress headaches* of everyday busy life, but still, can be quite bothersome.

All headache types start out acutely, but depending on the frequency and duration of symptoms, these headaches can often lead to chronic recurrent painful conditions. Acute and chronic headaches cost the country billions of dollars each year in healthcare expenditures, lost productivity, lost workdays, and disability. It is important to note that *primary* headaches—migraine, tension-type, and cluster—are different than *secondary* headaches which are caused by conditions like concussion, aneurysm, abscess, and tumor. This focus of this chapter will be on primary headache types.

When patients seek medical advice for bothersome headache symptoms, it is this initial complaint of *PAIN*, that starts the clinical pain management pathway with an initial evaluation assessment. Just like for back and neck pain, the primary care physician, neurologist, or pain specialist will take a complete history of the patient's headache symptoms. When it comes to headaches, a carefully detailed specifically-directed history will provide the most important information on what type(s) of headache the patient is suffering from. It is often what the patient describes, typically as the worst symptoms, which leads to the specific headache diagnosis.

Next along the pathway, comes a directed neurological physical exam, which is often *normal* for headache patients, believe it or not. If there is any major concern about possible abnormal pathology in the brain, then a brain CT scan or MRI will be ordered, to rule out secondary headache causes, like aneurysm, infection, or tumor. An assessment with a diagnosis will be made, and finally, a plan of treatment will be formulated, to start controlling the headache symptoms.

After the *assessment* and *plan* phases of the clinical pathway, comes the **P-I-T-S *treatment protocol*** implementation phase. After a cycle or two of headache pain care *implementation* treatment options—**Pills**, **Injections**, **Therapy**, and **Surgery**, if ever needed—the patient moves to the *evaluation* part of the clinical pathway. This is the critical determination as to whether the patient's pain and quality-of-life goals are being met, and basically, how their pain treatment plan is working and how their **PITS Score** is improving.

Specific Headache Conditions

1. Migraine Headaches

As far as **migraine headaches** are concerned, some of the latest scientific research is that patients are born with a *"migraine brain"*—which is a central neurologic condition, relating to genetic hyperexcitability in the brain, which can be activated at any point in a patient's life. Migraines are a classic example of a dysfunctional or undetermined type of pain, and there are different variations of migraines. Most migraine sufferers are female, there is a strong genetic link among families, and fortunately, most migraines become less intense or

go away after menopause.

Migraine attacks have a vascular and neuropathic nature to them, and have many *trigger events*, that can lead to activation of various painful symptoms. Certain muscle spasms around the head and neck can trigger migraines. Certain foods, not enough sleep, and hormonal changes during a menstrual cycle, can all trigger migraines. Even changes in the weather and barometric pressure, and life's stressful moments, can trigger a migraine attack.

So, the number one way to treat migraines is to have patients embrace a proactive lifestyle-modification approach to keep migraines from starting in the first place. Patients need to remember in their own personal experience, by typically keeping a pain diary, what they are doing in the minutes or hours before a migraine presents:

- are they ingesting wine or sulfite-containing foods, or cheeses?

- is there excessive stress in their work, or home life?

- does the patient have poor sleep habits?

- are there certain activities that give them spasm pain, which can then trigger a migraine?

When the patient is more aware of their individual situation, there are preventative and prophylactic approaches that can be pursued, to prevent migraines from starting and escalating. Once patients have an acute episodic migraine attack, short acting analgesics like Motrin, Tylenol, a triptan or ergotamine, can break the headache cycle. However, migraines typically have 4–72 hours duration of moderate-to-severe, pulsating, unilateral—but sometimes bilateral—quality pain, aggravated by physical activity, and associated with nausea and/or vomiting, and hearing and sight sensitivity. In prolonged severe cases, a short-acting opioid medication may be required.

At any time, if patients start to *transform* what are just episodic migraine attacks into chronic migraine headaches, with fifteen or more attacks per month, that last four hours or more, then the patient needs an around-the-clock baseline prophylactic analgesia with medications that keep headaches at bay—Topamax, Elavil, or a beta blocker like Inderal.

Botox injections every three months around the face, head, and neck, as a prophylactic chronic migraine prevention tool, is an FDA-approved effective therapy, especially if patients cannot use oral prophylactic medications. Also, new *gene-related* prophylactic migraine medications like Aimovig, Emgality, and others, and electric stimulation devices for migraine prophylaxis, are now FDA-approved in America. There is a lot of ongoing research in this area.

Unfortunately, many chronic migraine patients often suffer from *medication overuse headache (MOH)* syndrome, sleep disorders, and mood disorders. For example, patients are at risk of worsening migraine symptoms if they are taking prolonged or excessive amounts of an opioid, triptan, ergot, simple analgesics like Motrin, Aleve, or Tylenol, or combination analgesic, like Fioricet. Patients need to keep in mind that taking more and more medication can make migraines more difficult to treat. Most severe migraine patient sufferers are treated by migraine neurology specialists, and follow a multidisciplinary pain management approach, for best outcome results.

Patient education and motivation, and following the **P-I-T-S** *treatment protocol*, will be the keys to longer-term success. Remember, when it comes to treating migraines over an extended period of time, until they start to ease up and become less frequent which they often do later in life after menopause, the treatment course is indeed a *marathon* and not a *sprint*.

PATIENT EXAMPLE: A 30-year-old female had suffered intermittent migraine headaches in childhood, which became worse after her pregnancy. She started developing headaches at a frequency of eighteen attacks per month. She was under the care of a neurologist and was taking some Motrin and Tylenol occasionally. These medications were ineffective, and when she returned to her neurologist, she was prescribed Imitrex, to be used as an abortive migraine medicine.

She tried this for a period of time with some relief, but again many months later, she started having persistent headaches. Her neurologist put her on the prophylactic long-acting analgesic Topamax. She was titrated up on Topamax as her baseline medication over a two-month period, and started having fewer recurrent episodes. She made certain lifestyle changes, like avoiding migraine triggers with her diet choices, getting more sleep in general, and trying to get back to a more normal routine daily schedule.

The patient avoided any excessive activity, and was soon able to resume a more productive life, at home and at her work. She did not have migraines with auras. She knew about the risk of taking excessive opioid narcotics, or any other short-acting excessive analgesics, which could lead to rebound headaches. She sought out nutritional counselling, and improved on a long-term basis with Topamax, and with short acting anti-inflammatories for breakthrough pain, thereafter.

If the patient's migraines had persisted despite prophylactic migraine medication and abortive medication, and she developed chronic migraine pathology—15 or more attacks per month each lasting 4 hours or more—then she would be a candidate for FDA-approved Botox injections. Only in intractable migraine cases would a patient ever progress toward a surgical option consultation. These situations could include myofascial entrapment of frontal and ocular nerves, temporal area myofascial spasm with nerve entrapment, or any occipital muscle nerve triggers, which could be precipitating her migraines. Surgical migraine procedures are not common, but again, there is evidence that for certain intractable migraine patients with neuromuscular entrapment, they may be beneficial as a last resort.

2. Tension-Type Headaches

A **tension-type headache** is by far the most common type of primary headache that afflicts patients, and is usually self-limited. Most people have had a tension-type headache from time-to-time, and like migraine headaches, can have different triggers. Tension-type headaches are typically not severe in nature, are not localized or throbbing, and are not made worse with activity. It goes to reason, not a lot of patients are rushing off to their medical doctor for this type of pain.

Tension-type headaches can last from 30 minutes to several days, have a pressure tightening bilateral feeling, and are not associated with nausea or vomiting, or sight and hearing disturbance. By excluding other types of primary and secondary headaches, most often physicians conclude that their patient is suffering from a tension-type headache.

When episodic headaches are triggered by muscle spasms in the head and neck area, then simple analgesics, like Motrin, Aleve, and Tylenol, and combination analgesics containing caffeine, can be enough to break the pain cycle. If chronic tension-type headaches prevail, then using a prophylactic medication agent, like Elavil (amitriptyline) or Effexor (venlafaxine), may provide relief. Lifestyle modifications are going to be the key in keeping these headaches at bay, and these can include stress management techniques, exercise, stretching, and improving restorative sleep. Most patients do not feel disabled by tension-type headache, and most of these headaches lessen in occurrence, as we age.

PATIENT EXAMPLE: A 50-year-old female librarian was reportedly putting some books on a bookshelf in her local library, when she felt some tightness in her temporal head regions. She had some persistent pain at home later that night, and took four Advils. This helped somewhat, but she continued to have headache symptoms that were bothersome to her. She did not have any neurologic symptoms, and never had any history of migraine attacks. She did feel that she was under a lot of stress at home. That evening her headache persisted, so she took two ES Tylenol. She experienced some relief by morning, and steady improvement over the next few days. Within a week, her headache symptoms were completely resolved. She was back to her full activity and was happier at home, after straightening out her stressful home situation.

This is typical of a tension type headache, again, the most common occurring type of headache that patients experience. Now, if this tension headache had persisted, she could have been placed on a nonsteroidal anti-inflammatory medication. If she was found to have muscular trigger points on examination, and were thought to contributing to her headaches, then she would be a candidate for trigger point injections (TPIs) of local anesthetic, in an attempt to break the spasm-related triggers. If the local anesthetic trigger

points were indeed effective, but short lived, then she would have been a candidate for Botox injection consideration, for longer-term relief of her myofascial muscular spasms.

3. Cluster Headaches

Cluster headaches are the third type of primary headache, and consistently the worst pain intensity headache that a patient can experience. This type of headache affects men more than women, unlike migraine, and is typically seasonal, occurring more frequently in the spring and fall. It is a severe localized pain that is unilateral behind one eye, or the other, that can occur many times a day, lasting up to one hour at a time. These cluster attacks can last for a few months and then go into remission for years. Cluster headaches are vascular and neurogenic in nature, and also have triggers, like alcohol intake.

During these excruciating attacks of pain, patients can be agitated, violent, and even threaten suicide. Treatment consists of 100% oxygen in an emergency room in conjunction with lidocaine-soaked nasal cotton applicators that can block nerves—the sphenopalatine nerve plexus—in the back of the nasal passages, to break the pain cycle. Triptan and ergotamine medications are also frequently used to abort severe pain. For intractable cluster headaches, slow IV histamine infusion can be effective. Prophylactic medications include drugs like Zanaflex (tizanidine) and Doxepin (desipramine), among others.

PATIENT EXAMPLE: A 42-year-old male who had been suffering seasonal cluster headaches for four years but otherwise healthy, had experienced an acute episode of pain in the fall when he was bringing his child to college. He took Motrin and Tylenol with some relief. When he returned home, he had persistent headache pain behind his left eye. He felt like banging her head against the wall to relieve the severe symptoms.

His wife ended up taking him to the nearest emergency room, where the emergency room doctor promptly confirmed a cluster-like headache attack. The patient was offered 100% oxygen therapy, and after ten minutes into the therapy, most of his symptoms had resolved. He was put on Doxepin (desipramine) as a prophylactic medication, and his usual course of clusters had resolved within a month. He resumed his normal activities, and without recurrent headaches for years.

As a reinforcement, below is a summary of the **P-I-T-S *treatment protocol*** for headaches:

Pills—Advil, Tylenol, or Motrin to ease headache pain, at least short term. If and headache pain persists, the patient should consult with their primary care physician or neurologist, for prescription medication choices. If pain is excruciating, and ongoing outpatient medications offered no relief, then the patient should consider an emergency room visit.

Injections—Botox (onobotulinum toxin A) injections, for chronic migraine prophylactic therapy, are FDA-approved and are effective, and minimally invasive as an interventional pain management strategy. Five units of Botox are injected, in each of thirty-one specific spots, around the frontal (front) region of the face, the temporal (side) region, the occipital (back) region of the head, the cervical (neck) region, and in the trapezius (top of the shoulder) region. Botox injections, if successful and tolerated without excessive side effects, can be given every three months as a maintenance therapy without causing an immunologic problem for a patient. The risk and benefits of this type of procedure are discussed between physician and patient when considering Botox injections, as with any interventional pain procedure. Patients may be a little sore afterward, but Botox injection is a very well tolerated procedure, much like receiving a small-needle trigger point injection with a local anesthetic for other spasm-related bodily pains.

Therapy—Therapy for all three of the common headaches can involve manual, cognitive-behavioral approaches, and taking complementary herbal supplements—like butterbur and feverfew—as preventative therapy. Chiropractic care, to release cervical subluxations and muscle triggers of a mechanical nature, can be helpful. Physical therapy for flexibility, strengthening and conditioning, to keep spasms in remission, can also be quite helpful.

Surgery—Only in rare cases will a surgical option be considered for the relief of headaches. For certain entrapment-related nerve and muscle intractable migraine headaches, patients may seek a surgical option, where specialized surgeons release nerves and muscles around the head to ease theses neuromuscular triggers. Again, surgical techniques are reserved for intractable pain, when previous aggressive medical and interventional injection techniques have failed. Surgical procedures on cranial muscles are rare. One of the triggers for migraines can come from within the nose, where trigeminal nerves can become irritated. In this case a turbinectomy, or decompression of the turbinates, can be performed to remove this trigger irritation source.

So, the realistic treatment option expectations of pills, injections, therapy, and surgery should always be discussed, between patient and pain care provider, in open communication with any complicated headache situation, and patients need to understand that lifestyle modification strategies are always the most important and effective strategies for long-term treatment success.

I trust this chapter will serve as an educational platform, with different patient examples of pain care scenarios, so that patients can see where their own pain *"fits in."* I have created a separate chapter at the end of this one, called **PITS Educational Pearls of Pain Care Wisdom**; and at the end of the book there is an extensive **PITS Glossary of Pain Terms** section for added information on specific topics, like pain conditions, medications, procedures, and so forth. Remember not to skip these important sections of the book, because they are vitally important as reinforcers of the overall pain knowledge that will help ensure your success in the **PITS Program**!

Arthritis

SUMMARY: Painful **arthritis** conditions are one of the top five pain reasons why patients seek medical help. Arthritis affects millions of Americans and is one of the leading reasons for disability in this country. **Osteoarthritis (OA)** is progressive inflammation and degeneration of cartilage and joints, through normal wear and tear aging, or results from accelerated degeneration secondary to injury. Osteoarthritis affects many joints in the body, but especially the weight-bearing joints, such as the hips and knees. Hands and shoulders are also commonly affected. It is the progressive inflammation and pain that leads to internal joint derangement and destruction, and all of this pathology starts to inhibit a patient's quality of life, through lack of strength, range-of-motion, and mobility. **Rheumatoid arthritis (RA)** is an autoimmune medical-type of arthritis, which can be very destructive to joints if not treated, and can affect other bodily organs. There are many specific FDA-approved rheumatologic drugs that can treat the symptoms of RA and slow the progression of joint degeneration. Whereas, osteoarthritis can be managed by different physicians, like internists, orthopedists, and so forth, a rheumatologist specialist typically manages rheumatoid arthritis, especially when patients need IV-infusion medication treatment.

When patients seek medical advice from their physicians and other allied healthcare providers concerning arthritis-type pain complaints, it is this initial complaint of *PAIN*, that starts the clinical pain management pathway. Just like for back or headache problems, the primary physician—or orthopedist, rheumatologist, or pain specialist—will take a complete history of the pain, and then conduct a directed physical examination with particular attention to the musculoskeletal system. Any needed tests or studies are then ordered and reviewed, if not already completed—X-rays, CT scan, MRI, blood work, bone density and so forth—in order to make an assessment and diagnosis. The final step is to formulate a pain management care plan.

Once the pain management plan is implemented with one or two cycles of **P-I-T-S** *treatment protocol*

options, the patient is always re-evaluated to measure whether the patient's pain condition has improved or worsened; in other words, are the patient's quality-of-life goals being met, and is the **PITS Score** improving.

Recurrent acute arthritis flares of joint pain involve an inflammatory mechanism of pain and swelling, which can then lead to biomechanical mechanisms of pain, where physical joint destruction unfortunately takes place. It is these chronic pathologic changes in joints that eventually persist, and lead to the chronic arthritic pain state that many of us suffer with, typically on a daily basis.

The accelerated cycle of recurrent acute flares of inflammation, which cause pain through the physical destruction of the joints, can come from normal wear-and-tear aging or from post-traumatic and post-surgical arthritic joint changes due to previous injury or surgery. An acute episode of arthritic pain is typically short lived, but chronic daily arthritis pain can persist for a lifetime, as many of us already realize.

Specific Arthritis Conditions

1. Osteoarthritis (OA)

As far as **osteoarthritis** is concerned, if the patient experiences mild-to-moderate pain symptoms and follows the suggested **P-I-T-S** *treatment protocol*, the patient will start with a course of non-steroidal anti-inflammatory medications or **Pills**, such as Motrin, Aleve, and other prescription anti-inflammatory choices. For severe inflammation cases, short courses of oral steroids are often used, like the Medrol Dosepak or prednisone. If osteoarthritis is associated with muscle spasms around joints, then muscle relaxants can also be used, like Flexeril or Robaxin. Centrally-acting analgesics like acetaminophen (Tylenol) and the mild opioid tramadol (Ultram), and stronger opioid narcotics like Vicodin or Percocet, are often considered for severe degenerative pain.

Injection therapy will usually involve trigger point injections for joint-related spasms or the use of lubricating viscosupplementation medication, like the rooster comb or chicken cartilage shots, injected directly into the affected joint(s) to help stimulate motion and help the patient maintain normal activity maximum possible range of motion. If inflamed joints get out of control, then patients will often come to a physician for joint injections with local anesthetic and steroids. Degenerative joints can get severely inflamed from time to time, and if a course of injectable steroids can help deliver periods of relief for many months, then this can help patients break the pain cycle, rehabilitate better, and have a better quality of life. Just remember, only so much steroid can be injected into joints through time, or the steroid itself can damage joints and soft tissue.

In the **Therapy** category, patients are encouraged to maintain an active lifestyle where the key to maintaining mobility is summed up in the saying, *"Motion is the lotion."* Patients should protect their joints through a strengthening routine, such as cycling. Usually, physical therapy is followed by a home exercise program or a gym-exercise program for maintenance therapy. Additionally, patients can seek physician assessment help, such as physical medicine and rehabilitation or neuromuscular medicine osteopathic expertise. Patients also seek out an orthopedist or rheumatologist as needed for various joint pains. Many patients with complex arthritic issues will often choose this physician level of consultation to explore more comprehensive therapeutic strategies. Chronic oral steroid use is discouraged because this can lead to accelerated bone destruction and may worsen osteoporosis.

If patients are candidates for minimally invasive procedures, such as arthroscopy, before a joint replacement, then often patients will go for arthroscopies of knees, hips, and shoulders to *"clean up"* the joint and experience some level of pain relief. Only in the most severe cases of a bone-on-bone scenario will patients seek a **Surgery** opinion and have complete joint replacements.

Currently, shoulders, hips, and knees and even ankles can have total joint replacements for successful long-term care in selected patients. In the past, total ankle replacements were not perfected but now patients are undergoing ankle replacements quite successfully. This is true specifically in cases of advanced osteoarthritis and joint derangement, and when ankle fusion is not desirable. Full joint replacement is reserved for patients who have intractable pain despite aggressive medical and previous interventional pain management.

The **P-I-T-S** *treatment protocol* is available to treat acute or chronic arthritic pain, and as with other pain conditions, can be successfully complemented with other care strategies. These will include cognitive-behavioral therapy, yoga, and herbal supplements, and other choices.

PATIENT EXAMPLE: A 69-year-old male having enjoyed an active lifestyle through his 40s and 50s, developed some right knee pain after excessive gardening. He had noticed some swelling of his knee and took some Advil but the pain persisted. He tried some rest and some normal activities for several days, but because he was feeling a clicking in his knee, he went to his primary care physician who ordered X-rays. The X-rays showed no fracture or dislocation, but there were moderate degenerative changes noted.

It was explained that he was having bothersome arthritic joint changes and to consider some supplements such as glucosamine and chondroitin. He tried this approach, and after about two months, experienced about 25% relief. The patient tried to resume his gardening activities, but this re-aggravated his knee.

He decided to go to a local orthopedist who ordered an MRI imaging study, which showed an advancing degree of osteoarthritis spurring in his knee. He was given a course of physical therapy for strengthening and conditioning and this helped for a short while, but again, did not fully resolve the issue.

After a return visit to the orthopedist, it was suggested that the patient might be a candidate for viscosupplement injections, such as Synvisc or Supartz. His orthopedist explained the risk-and-benefit of the series of injections and the patient decided to proceed. The patient had three ultrasound-guided right knee joint injections over a period of three weeks, and experienced a dramatic 90% improvement in his pain condition. He was able to resume his activities, and did well thereafter, very satisfied with his care.

Advancing this scenario, had the patient not sought the injection treatments, and his osteoarthritis had progressed, then he might have been a surgical candidate for arthroscopy or total joint replacement at some point—like a bone-on-bone scenario. Perhaps a minimally invasive arthroscopy procedure could be considered to give him some temporary relief, but full knee replacement—the most aggressive surgical treatment in the **P-I-T-S** *treatment protocol*—would have been his only option for lasting pain relief and improved functional status.

2. Rheumatoid Arthritis (RA)

Rheumatoid arthritis follows a similar **P-I-T-S** *treatment protocol* as osteoarthritis, with some different medication choices available—such as injections and intravenous infusions of medication which are often required when severe rheumatoid arthritis symptoms flare.

In terms of **Pills** or medications, nonsteroidal anti-inflammatory, such as Motrin, Advil, Aleve, Celebrex, and so forth, and oral steroid like prednisone medication choices, are used as primary initial therapy to suppress the inflammatory flares and other symptoms that arise from this debilitating autoimmune and progressive disease.

There is a category of rheumatoid arthritis treatment drugs, known as disease-modifying anti-rheumatologic drugs (DMARDs), which are critically important and frequently started for patients to slow down disease progression. The autoimmune pathologic process is the key difference between osteoarthritis and rheumatoid arthritis. DMARDs include Remicade (Infliximab) and Humira (adalimumab) and are administered through IV infusion every 6–8 weeks, depending on the rheumatologist and patient response.

Without getting too technical, these DMARDs work as tumor necrosis factor (TNF) category agents and are the first line of treatment at certain receptor sites in the body. If patients do not respond appropriately with first line agents, then a second line IV-infusion medication, like Orencia (abatacept), a biologic-category agent, can be attempted to suppress T-cell immune activity. Research has shown that T-cells in our body play a primary role in starting the chain of events that lead to inflammation, pain, and destruction

in RA, so the goal of IV-infusion treatment is to put the rheumatoid arthritis symptoms into remission.

If moderate-to-severe pain continues, despite the primary medical treatment attempts for RA, then additional analgesics, like short-acting opioid narcotics, can be considered to help break the pain cycle and improve the quality of life for the patient.

As for **Injection** treatment options, certain patients may benefit from direct intra-articular joint injections of local anesthetic and steroid like Kenalog or Depo-Medrol, to treat severe pain and inflammation. These joint injections are typically performed no more than every 3–6 months—to optimize relief and minimize potential joint damage from the steroid itself through time.

The **Therapy** category for RA is identical to that of osteoarthritis and involves all option aspects—chiropractic care, physical therapy, stretching, home exercise-gym, and doctor-related care. Joints in general, need to maintain as much range-of-motion as possible, and strengthening and conditioning is the best practice to keep patients flexible and mobile.

Lastly, **Surgery** options are reserved for patients who remain with intractable joint pain, despite aggressive medical and interventional pain management plans, and range from minimally invasive arthroscopy to total joint replacement programs. Patients usually know when they need the surgical option because they are no longer *able to move!*

PATIENT EXAMPLE: A 62-year-old female who had rheumatoid arthritis for years, was following a conservative course of treatment. She had no severe pain symptoms and bony destruction of her hands. She started developing some pain after doing the dishes one day, which persisted even after taking Tylenol and Advil.

She had no active rheumatologist following her and was never on any rheumatoid arthritis intravenous medication protocols to keep her rheumatoid arthritis from destroying her body's normal tissues. She went to her internist, and after blood work came back with high rheumatoid factors, her physician had promptly referred her to a rheumatologist for a specialized evaluation.

After a full workup, her rheumatologist recommended a course of intravenous medications which consisted of Remicade IV-infusion therapy. She was then put on Orencia infusion therapy, which helped her hand symptoms, and put her disease into remission. She followed this treatment protocol with periodic infusions as her rheumatoid arthritis worsened, but had reasonable control of usual pain symptoms using periodic doses of Ultram. She preferred not to be on any stronger medications.

With some short courses of oral prednisone through the years, she was able to manage her rheumatoid arthritis pain comfortably. Had this patient needed a joint injection, she would have been referred to a sports medicine physician or interventional pain specialist to discuss this risk-and-benefit option. If she needed an orthopedic surgeon consultation for advanced joint destruction replacement, then again, she would have considered this option if she remained in intractable pain.

Arthritis in any form is one of the most debilitating pain conditions experienced by any patient. Arthritis is not curable, and therefore the pain can never be eliminated, but it can be managed successfully by following the **P-I-T-S** *treatment protocol*.

I trust this chapter will serve as an educational platform, with different patient examples of pain care scenarios, so that patients can see where their own pain *"fits in."* I have created a separate chapter at the end of this one, called **PITS Educational Pearls of Pain Care Wisdom**; and at the end of the book there is an extensive **PITS Glossary of Pain Terms** section for added information on specific topics, like pain conditions, medications, procedures, and so forth. Remember not to skip these important sections of the book, because they are vitally important as reinforcers of the overall pain knowledge that will help ensure your success in the **PITS Program**!

Face and Jaw Pain

SUMMARY: Trigeminal neuralgia and temporomandibular joint (TMJ) syndrome are two of the common causes of persistent chronic pain in the face and jaw region. **Face and jaw pain** complaints are one of the top five most common chronic pains in America. Trigeminal neuralgia is a type of neuropathic pain that can be quite disturbing to patients, and temporomandibular joint disease is a type of dysfunctional pain state that can be a constant reminder of chronic jaw pain.

Specific Face and Jaw Pain Conditions

1. Trigeminal Neuralgia

Trigeminal neuralgia is an irritation of a nerve in the brain that causes pain typically through the jaw and teeth and middle of the face. It can be triggered by touch to the skin or chewing foods, or other trigger mechanisms. It can be very debilitating to patients, especially due to the sharp, lancinating and shooting nature of the pain. Many trigeminal neuralgia patients with prolonged severe cases are referred to a neurologist for longer-term care.

Pill or medication treatment choices from the **P-I-T-S** *treatment protocol* include anti-neuropathic medications, such as Tegretol, Neurontin, Lyrica, Elavil, and others. Sometimes, anti-inflammatory medications, like Motrin and Aleve, can be effective. If the patient is experiencing jaw muscle spasms, then typical muscle relaxants, such as Zanaflex and Baclofen, can be used. The mild centrally-acting opioid analgesic tramadol can be used for trigeminal neuralgia, and stronger opioid narcotic analgesics for severe pain cases.

Injections that can be used are local anesthetic steroid injections placed around the nerve at the base of the head under fluoroscopic X-ray or CT-guided imaging. These injections are typically done by a pain specialist or a neurosurgeon. If the diagnostic/therapeutic injection is successful, then a chemical neurolysis with glycerin or phenol can be injected in a similar fashion at the base of the head under imaging, to try to give longer lasting relief by deadening the nerve. In other cases, Radiofrequency lesioning (burning) can be performed for longer-term pain control. This is proven minimally invasive method that can be performed under oral or IV sedation on an outpatient basis.

In terms of **Therapy** options, strengthening of the face muscles may be attempted, but success might be limited. Relaxation, stress-relieving strategies, and other complementary care approaches, such as acupuncture and essential oils, can help with symptom control.

In terms of **Surgery**, CyberKnife ionizing radiation beam technology, or Gamma Knife stereotactic radiosurgery approaches, can be offered to ablate the trigeminal nerve. A craniotomy at the base of the skull can be performed, where neurosurgeons can decompress the trigeminal nerve by using a Teflon spongy pledget or other fatty tissue, to pull the nerve away from its compressive vascular and bony skull structures. These different surgical techniques are often successful in offering selected patients longer-term relief of intractable pain from trigeminal neuralgia. Remember, the risk-and-benefit analysis of each procedural technique is subject to a discussion between the patient and their neurosurgeon before consenting and proceeding.

PATIENT EXAMPLE: A 39-year-old female started feeling numbness and burning pain in the right side of her cheek, in the absence of any specific history of trauma, infection, or illness. The pain was bothersome to her, and over several months became burning, sharp, and stabbing. It was worse when she chewed certain foods, or at times when she touched her face. The pain was located over the right side of her face, and the area was very sensitive in general.

She was concerned, so she made an appointment with her primary doctor. After taking a history and after a neurologic head exam, the doctor felt she may have a developed trigeminal neuralgia. She was given a course of Tegretol (carbamazepine) as an anti-neuropathic agent to help ease some of her pain. She was slowly titrated up on the Tegretol over a month, and this was successful in keeping her **PITS Score** low, on a fairly regular basis.

Had this patient's pain not been controlled with the oral medications, then she could have been referred to a neurosurgeon, who would have considered a procedure for longer-term relief of trigeminal neuralgia. This might have included a minimally invasive technique, such as a neuroablative chemical injection through the patient's cheek, or a CyberKnife treatment, or a microvascular decompression craniotomy procedure. Again, these are some of the neurosurgical procedures for longer-term relief of bothersome trigeminal neuralgia that fails ongoing care in the **P-I-T-S** *treatment protocol*.

2. Temporomandibular Joint (TMJ) Syndrome

Temporomandibular joint syndrome is dysfunctional type of pain and can have several causes. One of the most common causes of this type of pain is when people clench their teeth and develop myofascial spasms in the jaw and joint area. Another cause could be progressive arthritis in the TMJ, as seen in older patients. Still, another common cause for the development of painful TMJ symptoms is after an injury to the area, such as with a car accident or sports injuries, which cause trauma to the face and jaw. Many patients feel the pain at the junction of the jaw and skull, from opening and closing the mouth and chewing foods, which can be quite debilitating. Unfortunately, TMJ dysfunction is a common cause of facial pain. It is this severe irritation and impingement around and within the temporomandibular joint, which causes many patients to seek medical attention.

Regarding the **P-I-T-S** *treatment protocol* for TMJ treatment options, **Pills** or medications that are anti-inflammatory in nature, and centrally-acting analgesics, such as Tylenol, are often used to suppress symptoms. If the condition is accompanied by jaw spasm, then using a muscle relaxant can break the pain cycle, and help relax the temporomandibular joint to allow healing. Nerve pain agents are not typically used, but opioid narcotics can be used for severe cases. The use of opioid narcotic analgesics is only a fall back, should patients fail non-narcotics medications at first.

Injections of the temporomandibular joint with local anesthetic and steroid are sometimes necessary to relieve TMJ pain, and are typically performed by an oral maxillofacial surgeon, or a pain management expert. In terms of steroid injections, it is always important to space these treatments over a reasonable period—every 3–6 months as needed—to avoid bone and joint tissue damage which could affect the very function of the joint itself.

Conservative **Therapy** involving the use of a bite block, and strengthening of the jaw muscles, can be employed along other common approaches—psychiatric care, improving sleep patterns, and utilizing complementary techniques—to help in the overall pain management of temporomandibular joint pain syndrome.

In the worst-case scenario, patients will seek a **Surgery** opinion to see if they need an operative procedure on the joint to release pressure and reduce dysfunction, especially for severe intractable cases that fail more conservative measures. The need for surgical decompression is not a common course of treatment, but is available for those patients who continue to struggle with a poor quality of life.

PATIENT EXAMPLE: A 25-year-old female had a dental procedure done for a cavity. A week later she noticed some pain when opening her jaw on the right side. This worsened over the next two weeks and was associated with periods of jaw spasm. She returned to the dentist who felt that there was no problem with the cavity but she may have a case of temporomandibular joint irritation. She was given prescription-strength Motrin and Skelaxin muscle relaxant, but at the end of a week, her symptoms had not improved. She was told to try a bite block at night and try to relax as much as possible. She tried this for a month, but again had persistent pain.

She was referred to an osteopathic doctor who did some gentle manipulation of the temporomandibular joint to try to release some tension and irritation. This helped for a short while, but again, pain returned and was persistent. She was then referred to an oral maxillofacial surgeon who felt that she may have an inflammation flare in her joint. She was subsequently given an ultrasound-guided injection of local anesthetic and steroid into the joint at the surgeon's office. She tolerated this procedure well, and was surprised that a lot of pain was gone in just two days.

The patient was now able to resume normal activities by just taking over-the-counter Advil periodically. She was quite pleased with the overall results of her

care. Now, if the pain had not settled down even after **Pills**, **Injections**, and **Therapy**, she may have been a **Surgery** candidate for a *release* of the joint, which is the most aggressive treatment for temporomandibular joint pain.

I trust this chapter will serve as an educational platform, with different patient examples of pain care scenarios, so that patients can see where their own pain *"fits in."* I have created a separate chapter at the end of this one, called **PITS Educational Pearls of Pain Care Wisdom**; and at the end of the book there is an extensive **PITS Glossary of Pain Terms** section for added information on specific topics, like pain conditions, medications, procedures, and so forth. Remember not to skip these important sections of the book, because they are vitally important as reinforcers of the overall pain knowledge that will help ensure your success in the **PITS Program**!

Myofascial Pain Syndrome (MPS)

SUMMARY: In general, any skeletal muscle in the body can become inflamed or injured and result in acute and chronic pain and spasm. Many times, spasms are short-lived, because every so often when we *"pull a muscle"* the spasm pain eventually heals in a few days, weeks, or a month. This is typical of a neck or back muscle, or a groin or hamstring muscle. However, if pain and spasm persist for whatever reason for more than six months, then it becomes a more chronic condition, which is then referred to as **myofascial pain syndrome**. This is a pathologic process where muscles develop deep taut ischemic bands of irritated muscle and fascia and become what are known as active *trigger points*, where if you press on them, you can feel a characteristic intense sharp radiating pain.

Most patients develop trigger point myofascial pain in several areas of the body, including the neck and shoulder area, mid-back, low back, and in the buttock area over the piriformis muscle. The piriformis muscle, which is deep in the middle of the buttock area, lies over the sciatic nerve, so when this muscle is active with spasm, the pain can mimic that of sciatica—normally brought on by a bulging or herniated disc. If the piriformis muscle is chronically active with pain, then it is referred to as *piriformis syndrome*.

These myofascial pain conditions are primarily muscle problems, either as a direct result of muscle damage, or secondary to some other underlying irritant pathology. For example, if spinal nerves were irritated from spinal disc problems, and realizing that spinal nerves go to the muscles of the spine, then it goes to reason that the spinal muscles can reflexively spasm to guard the spine and prevent further injury. This scenario represents a secondary cause for muscle spasm. A primary cause would be the case if the spinal muscles were directly damaged by a traumatic injury or surgical procedure.

It turns out, myofascial spasm is very debilitating to patients, often under-diagnosed and treated, and can be a major source of disability. For millions of Americans, many acute spasm injuries from work-related incidents, motor vehicle accidents, slip-and-falls, sports activities, and so forth, continue to hurt beyond six months and become chronic pain problems.

For myofascial spasms, whether acute or chronic, patients can begin utilizing the **P-I-T-S** *treatment protocol* by starting with a course of anti-inflammatory **Pills** or medications, like Motrin, Aleve, Mobic, diclofenac and so forth, and a muscle relaxant, like Flexeril, Zanaflex, Baclofen, Robaxin, and so forth, to try and break the pain and spasm cycle. Centrally-acting analgesics, like Tylenol and the mild opioid Ultram, and stronger opioid narcotics, like Tylenol/codeine, Vicodin, Percocet, and so forth, are started if severe pain persists after this initial course of medications.

In terms of **Injection** treatment options, the mainstay for active myofascial trigger points are trigger point injections (TPIs). Trigger point injections are considered safe, minimally invasive, office-based injections of local anesthetic combined with any other active additive substance, such as a steroid, Sarapin (natural plant biologic substance), vitamin B12, and others.

In addition, Botox (onobotulinumtoxinA) injections are offered to patients who have persistent trigger point intractable pain, despite repeated local anesthetic injection attempts. Botox injections, which block the chemical substance acetylcholine in muscles, can offer three months or longer relief duration from persistent severe spasm pain. Although Botox is not FDA-approved for this type of pain treatment, some insurances do cover it. Otherwise, patients often will pay out-of-pocket for the injections because they find them so effective and beneficial in their overall pain management care.

Therapy is the mainstay of treatment for myofascial pain, especially for persistent acute spasms that may continue for up to three months, and for chronic myofascial pain spasm that persists beyond three months. With the help of physical therapy and a home exercise program (HEP), patients need to stay in the best shape possible with biomechanical and postural awareness and training, flexibility, strengthening, and endurance exercise, to keep myofascial pain in remission. An active exercise program should also include yoga, acupuncture, and massage therapy, to complement physical therapy programs. The main goal for patients suffering from this type of pain is to put active trigger points, which are areas with sharp shooting radiating pain when pressed, into an inactive state where muscles are now just sore when pressed and more manageable.

A home exercise program (HEP) is going to give patients the greatest hope for longer-term maintenance of relief from myofascial spasms. There will be flares of spasm from time-to-time, for sure, but when muscles are conditioned, these exacerbations of pain will typically be less intense and of shorter duration. In addition, chiropractic care is often attempted to break the spasm cycle through manipulation techniques in the office, or through manipulation-under-anesthesia (MUA) as an outpatient procedure at a surgical center. Finally, in terms of therapy options, physical medicine and rehabilitation specialists (physiatrists) and osteopathic neuromuscular medicine specialists can be consulted for long-term care in difficult cases of chronic spasm from spinal cord injury and stroke patients.

In terms of **Surgery** care options for the treatment of myofascial pain syndrome, primary surgical release of intractable spasms is reserved for nerve structures which are entrapped by inflamed and scarred myofascial tissue. There is a small percent of piriformis pain syndrome patients, where the piriformis muscle in the buttock entraps the sciatic nerve. If pills, injections, and therapy cannot release a piriformis muscle spasm, then specialized surgeons can do an exploratory surgical technique where they separate the sciatic nerve from the piriformis muscle entrapment to relieve the pain. These procedures are rarely performed. They are reserved for intractable pain patients who have muscle spasm that is entrapping a nerve, and other conservative **P-I-T-S** *treatment protocol* options have failed.

Rounding out the **P-I-T-S** *treatment protocol* therapy options are all of the other available multi-disciplinary approaches and techniques that can offer relief such as stress management strategies, and cognitive-behavioral therapy. Other important factors are the ability to achieve restorative sleep, so patients are not waking up fatigued. Lack of functional sleep can exacerbate spasm and magnify any pain condition.

PATIENT EXAMPLE: A 45-year-old male was taking out the garbage one day and he felt a pulling sensation in his low back. He had some back spasms an hour later and applied ice and took Tylenol. This helped for a short while, but the spasms came back even more severe the next day.

He made an appointment to see his internist, who after a history and examination palpated an active trigger point in his left lumbar paraspinous muscle. He was given a short course of the muscle relaxant Flexeril, and the anti-inflammatory Naprosyn, but the Flexeril made him too sleepy. Because of his persistent spasms, his doctor wrote him a prescription for six weeks of physical therapy, 3 times per week. The physical therapist used the modalities of heat, ice, and stimulation, as well as, ultrasound and a TENS unit, to break the spasm initially.

After one week with this approach, the patient started strengthening exercises and stretching exercises. He was eventually instructed on a home exercise program (HEP). This course of therapy helped tremendously, after one month he still had some residual pain, but this resolved through time.

Had this severe recurrent trigger point spasm pain persisted, he could have been referred to a pain specialist for a trigger point injection of local anesthetic to try to break the spasm. If the pain persisted, a Botox injection could have been considered.

I trust this chapter will serve as an educational platform, with a patient example of a pain care scenario, so that patients can see where their own pain *"fits in."* I have created a separate chapter at the end of this one, called **PITS Educational Pearls of Pain Care Wisdom**; and at the end of the book there is an extensive **PITS Glossary of Pain Terms** section for added information on specific topics, like pain conditions, medications, procedures, and so forth. Remember not to skip these important sections of the book, because they are vitally important as reinforcers of the overall pain knowledge that will help ensure your success in the **PITS Program**!

Fibromyalgia

SUMMARY: Fibromyalgia is a chronic soft tissue pain that is felt throughout the body but mainly in the head and neck area, upper and lower torso, and the extremities. It is characterized as a dysfunctional type of pain, like migraines, and especially affects women who experience anxiety and high stress, suffered from a severe infection, or suffered a severe traumatic event.

With persistent symptoms beyond three months, patients can develop a chronic *fibromyalgia pain syndrome*. This syndrome is diagnosed solely on the patient history of pain complaints and was recently recognized by the American College of Rheumatology as new diagnostic criteria for fibromyalgia. The diagnosis is made after a host of diagnostic patient history questions aimed at determining what is called a widespread pain index (WPI) and a symptom severity score (SS Score).

Fibromyalgia pain affects the whole body with widespread pain and severe tender spots that can exist in areas of the neck and shoulder, torso and buttocks, and arms and legs. It is not specific to spasms like myofascial pain syndrome but can be considered along that kind of continuum of soft tissue pain disorders. Fibromyalgia can be associated with other conditions, such as irritable bowel syndrome (IBS), chronic fatigue, concentration and memory problems, sleep disorders, and headaches (migraines from trigger point activation) and jaw pain (TMJ). Many of these associated symptoms are also dysfunctional pain types independent of fibromyalgia, which makes the care of a fibromyalgia patient more complex.

Many severely affected fibromyalgia patients are followed by a rheumatologist, and given a full education about their condition, medication treatment, aerobic exercises, and positive thinking strategies, as the mainstay of the pain management strategy. There are many state and federal fibromyalgia pain syndrome associations in America available for patients to help with information, obtain answers to questions, and to meet various groups who suffer with this difficult condition. Fortunately, for many fibromyalgia sufferers the painful symptoms improve through time following a conservative care plan.

Forming a **P-I-T-S** *treatment protocol* plan for this difficult dysfunctional pain problem entails a multidisciplinary approach. In terms of **Pills** or medications, the nonsteroidal anti-inflammatory choices are many, including Motrin, Aleve, Mobic, Celebrex, and others. Muscle relaxant options include Flexeril, Baclofen, Robaxin, Skelaxin, and others. Various nerve pain agents are also available, including Cymbalta, Lyrica, and Savella, are other FDA-approved medications for the treatment of fibromyalgia. Elavil and Neurontin are also effective in the treatment of fibromyalgia symptoms. Opioid narcotics are not encouraged for long-term fibromyalgia treatment, because research has shown that opioids can make fibromyalgia symptoms worse. However, some select patients may benefit from low-dose, longer-term, opioid narcotic therapy to maximize their pain control and improve their quality of life.

In terms of **Injections** for fibromyalgia, many soft tissues tender point (like trigger point) injections have been attempted, but for the most part these have limited success and are not the mainstay of treatment protocols. Tender points do not typically respond like active myofascial trigger points to injection therapy. The typical trigger point injections that are given for discreet muscle spasm pathology do not seem to have

the same success for soft tissue fibromyalgia sensitivity and the associated widespread pain pathology.

If patients have associated myofascial spasm as a secondary issue, then trigger point injections could be warranted. When any bursas or other fascia are irritated along with the fibromyalgia, then a local anesthetic or steroid injection can be performed to ease the pain. It is not common to have long-term injection management for strict fibromyalgia symptoms alone.

Therapies, both physical and cognitive-behavioral techniques, are the most important in terms of longer-term treatment in fibromyalgia patients. Patients need to achieve and maintain a positive attitude, get a sufficient amount of sleep, and stay in the best aerobic shape they can for the best mitigation of fibromyalgia pain symptoms.

If chiropractic and traction is limited, then patients will do periods of physical therapy for flexibility, strengthening, and conditioning. The goal should be to have an effective home exercise program or gym-maintenance program once formal physical therapy sessions have ended. Independent physical fitness is the goal as the best treatment option for fibromyalgia and is the best way for the patient to maintain a reasonable degree of comfort and functionality.

In terms of **Surgery** intervention, there is no surgical indication for fibromyalgia, so this treatment option of the **P-I-T-S** *treatment protocol* does not apply. However, there are cases of spinal cord stimulation (SCS) relieving the pain of intractable fibromyalgia, but the SCS device is not FDA-approved for the treatment of this condition.

Lifestyle changes are an important strategy to complement physical exercise when treating pain from fibromyalgia. Restful sleep is a critical component, even if prescription medications are needed to assist along those lines. Some prescription sleep aids can be habituating, so the patient needs to be aware of the risk of dependency and employ techniques to avoid this. Although used off-label, Elavil is a favorite among pain physicians for use as a restorative sleep agent, especially if patients do not have a lot of side effects while taking this medication. Elavil can also help with pain symptom management and mood improvement, as it is an antidepressant by design.

Complementary care techniques are essential for successful fibromyalgia treatment. These will include acupuncture, massage, yoga, essential oils, biofeedback, herbal therapy, Reiki, and low-level laser therapy. Fibromyalgia can be extremely disabling when full body pain complaints take hold.

PATIENT EXAMPLE: A 40-year-old female was otherwise well until contracting a cellulitis infection of the legs. She had a difficult course with antibiotic treatment and hospitalization and was sick for quite some time. After four weeks of antibiotic treatment, the infection was eliminated and she was cleared for discharge from the hospital. However, once she was home, she began feeling very fatigued. She also experienced several bouts of irritable bowel and started feeling a lot of tenderness around her neck, chest, hips, arms, and legs.

She returned to her doctor who felt that she did not have recurrent cellulitis, but that she may have been run down by the infection. She was advised to rest and take Tylenol and anti-inflammatory medications for a week. Her pain persisted and was very disabling to her. She continued to feel very tired and was having concentration issues. It was difficult for her to get a good night of restful sleep. Upon return to her medical doctor, it was felt perhaps that she was suffering from chronic fatigue syndrome. Because of the unclear diagnosis, the internist referred the patient to a rheumatologist.

After a thorough history and examination, the patient was found to have multiple tender points in her neck and shoulder area, upper and lower torso, and even her arms and legs, all consistent with a diagnosis of fibromyalgia. She also had bouts of irritable bowel syndrome and some other symptoms consistent with fibromyalgia. She was also suffering for longer than three months with severe widespread pain, and thus, the diagnosis of fibromyalgia was made based on the currently accepted national diagnostic criteria.

Her rheumatologist started her on Cymbalta. She was started on a low dose, and slowly titrated up over the next two months, and subsequently felt less depressed and more energetic. She wanted to get in better shape, so she joined a gym for some cardio fitness, which helped her as well. She also realized she needed continued treatment for her anxiety and periods of depression. After meeting with her rheumatologist, she became aware that it was important to have a positive attitude, and she understood that fibromyalgia could be a manageable condition.

Her widespread pain was helped by at least 50% with her frequent cardio exercises and daily dose of Cymbalta. She was able to maintain her work status and take care of her children, and again her overall pain and quality of life improved tremendously. Had this patient had a more protracted course of painful symptoms, she could have been tried on different medication combinations and medical cannabis and explored other complementary care options (acupuncture, massage, and yoga for example) to optimize her **PITS Score** and improve her quality of life. The patient in this example had learned that the key to success, as she tried different approaches to control her painful flares of symptoms, was to never give up on optimizing her overall program choices which could help her achieve a longer-term comfort level and an improved activity level.

I trust this chapter will serve as an educational platform, with a patient example of a pain care scenario, so that patients can see where their own pain *"fits in."* I have created a separate chapter at the end of this one, called **PITS Educational Pearls of Pain Care Wisdom**; and at the end of the book there is an extensive **PITS Glossary of Pain Terms** section for added information on specific topics, like pain conditions, medications, procedures, and so forth. Remember not to skip these important sections of the book, because they are vitally important as reinforcers of the overall pain knowledge that will help ensure your success in the **PITS Program**!

Neuropathy

SUMMARY: There are many different **neuropathy** pain states that patients develop for different reasons, whether they are due to medical, post-surgical, post-traumatic, or other etiologies. Pain disorders that are neuropathic in nature can involve peripheral, sympathetic, or the central nervous system (spinal cord and brain) nerves. The other common cause of pain which is non-neuropathic is called nociceptive pain, involving either somatic (biomechanical or soft tissue) or visceral (organs) causes of pain.

Neuropathic pain involves direct nerve pathology from direct nerve damage, changes in how nerves connect to each other, or from changes in nerve signal transmission. It is usually more difficult to treat than nociceptive pain due to the deceptive nature of the pain mechanism.

Firstly, neuropathic pain, in contrast to nociceptive pain, generally does not respond well to traditional analgesics, such as nonsteroidal anti-inflammatory medications and low-dose opioid narcotics. Neuropathic pain usually responds to treatment with *anti-neuropathic pain agents*, of which there are many different categories and many off-label uses. These can include antidepressants and antiseizure medications, as well as local anesthetic and controlled-release opioids.

Secondly, there are many pain conditions that involve both neuropathic and nociceptive pain mechanisms, creating a *mixed pain state*. This often makes it difficult to fully diagnose the root of the pain and to prescribe the appropriate pain treatment strategy in these situations. Additionally, not all neuropathic pain states respond to all the nerve pain agents the same way, so even though ongoing research is advancing our knowledge about these pain conditions, many of the current approaches are by trial-and-error treatment and gauging the patient's response.

The choice of a neuropathic pain agent is always individualized to the patient and their specific neuropathic pain condition, considering what has worked and what has not worked in the past, and any serious medical conditions in the patient's history. Other factors are the side effects of previous medications and potential drug interactions with other medications that the patient is currently taking. If opioid treatment is the recommended course, then the question is should the dosage be short term or long term? Remember, it is a primary goal of the **PITS Program** to optimize treatment through the balance of evidence-based scientific research, the treating pain management team's

expertise, and the patient's desires and preferences for pain care choices.

Now, there are *four lines* of treatment medication choices when it comes to treating a neuropathic pain state in general, with each choice being dependent on current science and research, and the medical societies and groups that report guideline recommendations:

- *First-line agents* include tricyclic-antidepressants (Elavil) and anti-seizure drugs (Lyrica and Neurontin).

- *Second-line agents* include serotonin-norepinephrine reuptake inhibitor (SNRI) antidepressants (Cymbalta and Effexor) and the Lidoderm (5% lidocaine) patch.

- *Third-line agents* include tramadol (Ultram/Ultracet) and low-dose controlled-release opioid narcotics (OxyContin, morphine ER, Nucynta ER).

- *Fourth-line agents* include Topamax and methadone.

These are by no means the only choices of nerve pain agents, but it is a good start for organizing treatment options during ongoing pain care. Neuropathic agents can work on pain receptor activation, peripheral and spinal nerve conduction, and at the brainstem level to help pain adjustment factors that modulate the final brain experience of pain (see **Appendix B, Pain Diagram–Mind/Body Relationship**).

This area of pain management is certainly still evolving and is by no means a perfect science. Pain specialists go back-and-forth academically on what are the appropriate pain medications and in what order they should be offered, especially since many are used off-label and not FDA approved to treat specific neuropathic pain conditions for which they are prescribed. Clinically, many neuropathic pain patients need combination medications from different line therapies anyway, thus it is a matter of starting at the top and working your way down the list to optimize the patient's comfort, while closely monitoring the patient's reactions to differing treatments. It is important to start these medications at low doses and slowly increase them as needed over many days or weeks to minimize treatment side effects.

Specific Neuropathy Conditions

1. Diabetic Neuropathy

Diabetic neuropathy is a condition which commonly affects the hands and feet and can be extremely debilitating for diabetic patients. This is especially true when they do not have good control of their blood sugars and their Hemoglobin A1c percentage levels. The A1C level is a common blood test marker for how well blood glucose is controlled in the body.

Millions of Americans are affected with this painful condition, which can feel sharp and burning in nature, and patients often complain of skin sensitivity in the hands and feet. Internists, endocrinologists, and other physicians are constantly reminding diabetics of the importance of controlling diabetic symptoms in order to help prevent this disabling condition from advancing and leading to a host of complications. Complications can include, not only painful diabetic neuropathy, but also painful diabetic ulcers of the feet and toes.

Without getting too technical, diabetic neuropathy can be both a small nerve-fiber condition (C-fibers and Delta-fibers) causing burning and shooting pain, and a large nerve-fiber condition (Beta and Alpha-nerve fibers) causing sensory numbness changes and motor imbalance. This is all due to the neuro-vascular nature of the disease, which can affect the whole body from head to toe. As mentioned, neuropathy pain of this nature can be burning and lancinating and can feel like a hot stove in the affected area. The diabetic neuropathic pain state usually develops as the severity of diabetes worsens.

In terms of the **P-I-T-S** *treatment protocol* for diabetic neuropathic pain, there are many different nerve pain agent choices that can be trialed to try and ease the pain symptoms. As far as **Pills** or medications are concerned, there are multiple FDA-approved drugs in the United States for the treatment of diabetic neuropathy, including Lyrica (pregabalin), Cymbalta (duloxetine), and Nucynta ER (tapentadol, extended release). All three of these drugs have a different mechanism of action effect to relieve pain and can be considered first-line treatment agents.

Lyrica is an anticonvulsant-type, Cymbalta is an antidepressant-type, and Nucynta ER is an extended-release synthetic opioid narcotic-type medication. Elavil, a tricyclic-antidepressant type medication, has also been used as a first-line nerve pain agent, although it is used off-label –not the original FDA-approved intended use. Other second-line and third-line choices of medications that have been successfully used off-label for years, and include Neurontin (gabapentin), Effexor (venlafaxine), Ultram (tramadol), 5% Lidoderm (lidocaine patch), OxyContin (oxycodone controlled-release), and oral morphine. Anti-inflammatory medications can always be attempted, and frequently are, but not with the great response as seen with the anti-neuropathic-type drugs mentioned above.

If diabetic neuropathy is associated with spasms, then short courses of muscle relaxants can be used. For severe patient cases, opioid narcotics, both of a short-acting nature and a long-acting nature, can be started. Awareness of protecting the hands and feet from injury are important and it is beneficial for the patient to be in the best physical condition possible. Thus, formal physical therapy is ordered to rehabilitate diabetic patients who need this level of care.

Specific **Injection** treatments have a limited role for diabetic neuropathy. If there were a peripheral nerve that was very irritated and inflamed, then a peripheral nerve block could be considered to break the pain cycle, but again, not commonly performed.

Therapy options focus on keeping diabetic limbs as functional as possible despite the pain. Also, many of the other multidisciplinary therapy care options may help, including the development of coping strategies, restful sleep optimization, and all the complementary care techniques that are available for other nerve related pain conditions.

Although no **Surgery** cure technique for diabetic neuropathy exists, if patients have severe polyneuropathy pain that is intractable, then a spinal cord stimulation (SCS) lead trial is indicated to *"block the pain"* and break the intractable pain cycle with the use of mild electrical stimulation. The spinal cord stimulation treatment modality is more commonly used in other chronic severe neuropathic conditions, like failed-back surgery syndrome and complex regional pain syndrome. But research and patient studies have shown that many different neuropathic conditions can respond well with pain relief from a SCS device.

There are medical indications in the U.S. for spinal cord stimulation, like any other procedure that is approved by insurance panels, based on previous research and patient care outcomes for a specific condition. Government agencies, like the Center for Medicare and Medicaid Services (CMS), also set rules, regulations, and restrictions on SCS uses.

PATIENT EXAMPLE: A 45-year-old female diabetic, who had poor control of her blood glucose levels and with her hemoglobin A1C level at 8% (normal range: 4–6%), was noticing progressive burning pain in her feet over the last three months. Her neurologist had diagnosed the start of diabetic neuropathy a year prior, and strongly encouraged better glucose control at that time, which is considered the primary approach in slowing down the advancement of diabetic-related neuropathic symptoms.

She was also given a small dose of Elavil as an anti-neuropathic first-line agent, and monitored for the potential side effects of grogginess and dry mouth. Over the subsequent two weeks the dosage was incrementally increased. She experienced a slightly decreased burning sensation at this time. and tried her best to control her diet. She tried exercise and was committed to following her endocrinologist's recommendations for diabetic care.

She returned to her neurologist still with painful symptoms, and she was subsequently prescribed Lyrica, another first-line anti-neuropathic agent. Initially she started with a low dose to minimize side effects, and gradually titrated to a more optimal level over the next month. This helped an additional 50% with overall pain relief, and improved the patient's overall quality of life. She was more diligent about her diabetic program and had better control of her symptoms.

Now, had this patient continued with pain, a second-line and even a third-line anti-neuropathic agent such as tramadol could be added. In severe cases even a course of opiate narcotics could be used. Also, if she needed to explore complementary techniques, like acupuncture, essential oils, and other approaches, then these would be good options, as well.

2. Complex Regional Pain Syndrome (CRPS)

Complex regional pain syndrome (CRPS), formerly known as reflex sympathetic dystrophy (RSD), is a complex chronic neuropathic pain condition. RSD was the original name given to this neuropathic pain condition, but many years ago, it was renamed complex regional pain syndrome (CRPS) by pain management medical professionals to better describe this pain disease, and the two names are still often used interchangeably. CRPS is a moderate-to-severe neuropathic vascular condition typically of the upper and lower extremities, but can sometimes spread to the face and trunk and result in full body RSD pain. It is a diagnosis of exclusion, where no other medical condition can explain the signs and symptoms, and it typically starts after an acute injury or repetitive motion irritation, or after casting of fractured limbs.

It is an abnormal peripheral and central type of neuropathic pain, associated with variable amounts of swelling or edema of the extremities, stiffness and weakness, skin sensitivity to touch and pressure, hot and cold sensations and skin color changes, sweating, and skin, nail bed, or hair changes. There are international diagnostic criteria for CRPS to help clinicians rule-in or rule-out this pain condition. It is a condition, like shingles, which needs to be treated early to have its best clinical outcome. If treated within three-to-six months, patients can often have their pain put into *remission* and experience a better long-term outcome of pain control and quality of life. Controlling CRPS pain and symptom flares can certainly be a challenge at times for those that suffer from this affliction, and following a comprehensive integrative approach to pain care will always lead to the best long-term relief and functional activity outcomes.

Complex regional pain syndrome pain is treated with the **P-I-T-S** *treatment protocol* using all aspects of care option categories. In terms of **Pills** or medications, anti-inflammatories, muscle relaxants, nerve pain agents, and opioid narcotics can all be used to suppress different symptoms and allow for better rehabilitation. If caught early, medications would be used on a short-term basis, but it is certainly acceptable to use various medications longer-term, if needed.

Injections are known to be very effective in treating this pain condition, especially if performed early in the treatment course. Most often sympathetic nerve blocks with local anesthetic are recommended. CRPS of the upper extremities respond to a neck injection outside the spine, called a stellate ganglion local anesthetic injection, which is performed under fluoroscopic X-ray, with or without IV sedation, in an outpatient setting. CRPS of the lower extremities responds to a lumbar or low back injection outside the spine, called a lumbar sympathetic local anesthetic injection.

The main idea or goal is to do a diagnostic block first, and if successful therapeutically, do a series of desensitization injections to decrease pain sensitivity and to further help with hands-on therapy to promote healing, all in an attempt to put the painful condition into remission. Many CRPS patients have excessive sensitivity of the skin, and often pills and therapy are limited in their effectiveness until the limbs are desensitized with injection therapy. Besides sympathetic nerve blocks, peripheral nerve blocks for certain sensory nerve pains can also be offered in selected CRPS patients, to further desensitize and control painful limbs, hands, and feet.

Rehabilitative **Therapy** is a mainstay of CRPS treatment, both short-term and long-term, to keep the pain of this difficult-to-treat condition in remission. Physical therapy can help with desensitization of painful areas and can facilitate and maintain a patient's flexibility, strengthening and endurance. A home exercise program (HEP) with this pain condition is a must.

Because of the complexity of this condition in selected patients, some need an expert in neuromuscular medicine to consult with, to help with advanced treatment options. Physical medicine and rehabilitation (physiatry) care is another important consultation specialty for those intractable cases that need longer-term rehabilitative care. All the other multidisciplinary therapy approaches are equally important, including psychological care to manage the up-and-down flares of pain, restorative sleep because exhaustion can exacerbate the pain, and any complementary care techniques, like acupuncture, massage, essential oils, yoga, and even hyperbaric chamber therapy, which might help with symptomatic pain control.

If pills, injections, and therapy are limited, then a **Surgery** technique can be offered to patients involving a spinal cord stimulation (SCS) device with adjustable electrical impulses—particularly when there is no further surgical correction of an ongoing physical organic pathology planned, or if a surgical procedure was felt to possibly exacerbate the existing RSD condition. The SCS device has been found to be a successful treatment for CRPS in selected cases that have severe persistent neurovascular symptoms.

A spinal cord stimulation lead modality involves placing wire leads safely through the skin and into the epidural space, and then using mild electric current to desensitize pain through the principals of therapeutic electrical stimulation, akin to the concept of a TENS unit using electrical impulses on the skin to control painful surface sensations. Science and research have discovered that *electricity*, whether delivered through conventional or high-frequency stimulation at a spinal cord action level and brain level, can dampen pain sensation and thus offer long-standing pain relief.

The SCS modality has been found to be very tolerable for patients, easy to control, and can be utilized outpatient for up to one week at home. If patients have a 50% or better pain relief result, along with other criteria during the *test period*—improved pain scores, improved sleep quality, an increase in activity level, and less pain medication usage—then longer-term implantation and use of a pulse generator can be considered to treat intractable CRPS pain, and allow patients a period of relief so they can maximize their therapy and functional status, and of course, have a better overall quality of life.

There are risks and benefits with any kind of minimally invasive surgical procedure, including, but not limited to, infection, bleeding, and nerve injury. Again, if a successful trial is achieved, approximately two weeks later the patient can return to an outpatient surgical setting for implantation of longer-term leads and a pulse generator under the skin. The pulse generator is a type of battery that can be charged for repeated use over a period of years.

Implantation of the SCS device is typically performed by an interventional pain specialist or with a spine surgeon specialist. Besides the percutaneous wires, there are surgical paddle spinal cord stimulation leads that can be sutured in place in the epidural space for more active patients. For patients with upper extremity RSD, the stimulation lead wires are placed in the neck region during the trial and for final implantation. If patients have lower extremity RSD, the spinal cord stimulation leads are placed typically in the thoracic region or middle of the back in the epidural space, for both the trial and permanent lead placement.

PATIENT EXAMPLE: A 50-year-old female was involved in an unfortunate work-related accident where she sustained a crush injury of her foot. She needed surgical repair of multiple fractures and soft tissue. After being in a cast for eight weeks, she started developing increasing burning pain in her foot. Her cast was removed and on examination, a painful, red, swollen foot was revealed. The foot was sensitive to touch and stiff in movement. But after examination, it was determined that she was not suffering from complications due to surgery. A blood clot in her leg was ruled out after ultrasound and angiogram.

The pain persisted, and she was referred by her orthopedist to a pain management expert with the suspicion that she might have CRPS which developed from her foot trauma and subsequent surgery and immobilization. The pain specialist conducted a thorough history and examination, and confirmed that the patient met the diagnostic criteria for CRPS of her lower extremity.

The patient was started on the anti-neuropathic medication Elavil and the opioid narcotic Percocet for the severity of the pain. These medications were both titrated for affect over the next month. As physical therapy was instituted, the pain persisted and the patient noticed changes to her nails and that her skin had become quite sensitive to touch.

It was recommended at this point, that the patient consult with an interventional pain management specialist and consider a diagnostic/therapeutic lumbar sympathetic local anesthetic injection. After a risk-and-benefit discussion, the patient decided to undergo this procedure. It turned out that 90% of the patient's skin sensitivity was reduced after a single injection. The pain returned a week later, and a series of desensitization block injections were subsequently performed, after the appropriate insurance authorizations for medical necessity were obtained.

The patient did well after a total of three additional injections over a six-week period and had a 50% plateau of her overall symptoms. Physical therapy was continued during this time to maximize strengthening and conditioning to help keep the patient's functional status. The patient did well thereafter, and after weaning off the narcotics, was able to return to work.

Had this patient had persistent symptoms despite medical and interventional management, then the patient would be offered a spinal cord stimulation lead trial for ongoing intractable pain. Continuing with this scenario, if a successful spinal cord lead one-week trial was performed the patient may have experienced up to 80% pain resolution of the skin sensitivity (allodynia), and possibly would be able to walk again. After that, the patient would have been returned to an outpatient setting where the longer-term spinal cord stimulation lead wires and pulse generator would have been placed for continued pain care. Under this scenario, the patient's pain would have been controlled enough, but she might not have been able to return to work. In time she would have been considered for a permanent-type disability under a Workers' Compensation system.

Other options available to this patient were cognitive-behavioral psychological techniques, particularly for the suffering component of the pain and to help her with sleep. Complementary care techniques could also have been considered such as supplements and herbal treatments, biofeedback and relaxation methods, yoga if tolerated, or other effective non-FDA-approved treatments like hyperbaric chamber therapy and intravenous ketamine infusion. Patients, in general, should always keep an open mind to the various options available to help diagnose and treat their pain states, especially if they feel troublesome persistent symptoms.

3. Post-Herpetic Neuralgia (PHN)

Post-herpetic neuralgia, or shingles, is a painful condition that can develop in patients who have had the chicken pox virus exposure earlier in their lives. Due to the recurrence of this virus, shingles causes a painful skin disruption of the trunk, chest, or face. Shingles is the acute pain state and is extremely severe and burning. Elderly people are more at risk of developing PHN after shingles.

The key to treatment of the pain symptoms is early anti-viral medical attention to try to shorten the intensity of the pain and to keep from further sequelae in the body. Shingles typically activates in younger patients due to stress and in older patients who become immunocompromised. When shingles starts, it causes an intense inflammatory and micro-vascular reaction in the involved nerves, which can then lead to permanent abnormal sensitivity changes if not treated in the first weeks of the outbreak. Once PHN sets in after three-to-six months, it is much harder to treat. This is similar to complex regional pain syndrome, which is much more difficult to treat once the nervous system has undergone permanent biochemical and anatomical changes.

The **P-I-T-S** *treatment protocol* for treatment of PHN will include all four major categories of care as needed to arrest the painful symptoms in a timely fashion. In terms of **Pills** or medications, nonsteroidal anti-inflammatories, like Motrin and Aleve, are often started early, as well as nerve pain agents, like Neurontin and Lyrica, and topical agents, like 5% lidocaine patch (Lidoderm) or capsaicin cream, which are the primary FDA-approved medications for the treatment of PHN. For severe shingles pain, short courses of an opioid narcotic may be prescribed, typically a short-acting choice, like tramadol, hydrocodone, or oxycodone to start. But for the best possible result, an antiviral and shingles pain medication needs to be started as early as possible.

If pain is persistent after the shingles vesicles heal, and medications are resulting only in limited relief, then patients can consider **Injection** techniques, such as epidural local anesthetic and steroid injection, an intercostal rib block with local anesthetic and steroid, or even a subcutaneous injection of local anesthetic and steroid under the painful skin rash area, can all be offered as interventional pain management relief options. These are safe, outpatient techniques that serve to *desensitize* the area of pain through both a somatic (sharp, shooting pain) and sympathetic (burning pain) nerve treatment approach.

Epidural injection therapy can be performed in patients experiencing cervical, thoracic, or lumbar shingles pain. If epidural steroid injections are contraindicated for whatever reason, then other injection approaches can be taken. As mentioned, a peripheral nerve block can be performed in the thoracic region to block intercostal nerve-related pain. Injecting a local anesthetic and steroid around rib intercostal nerves that correspond to a patient's chest wall pain area can be effective in desensitizing shingles pain. Up to three injections can be performed, about 1–3 weeks apart, depending on the patient's response. If patients have facial shingles, then local anesthetic in the neck, outside the spine in an area called the stellate ganglion, can help desensitize the facial pain.

This is a sympathetic-type nerve block, as opposed to a peripheral nerve block like intercostal nerves for shingles of the ribs. Desensitization involves slowing down abnormal nerve impulses, decreasing nerve inflammation, and restoring blood flow to nerves in the pathologic nerve distribution area. The shingles pathologic nerve changes are of a micro-neurovascular inflammatory nature, which destroy the nerve structures. It is this nerve destruction from the chicken pox virus, when untreated, that causes the patient to have sharp longer-term skin pain.

There are other interventional pain options that can help deaden painful nerves from PHN. These include radiofrequency (using heat) ablation and cryoablation (using cold) for treatment in select patient cases. Both of these techniques use specialized probes that can temporarily keep nerve pain symptoms quiet for weeks, or maybe even months, as patients continue to heal. PHN can be a very horrific type of pain that in some patients persists for many, many years. In some patients PHN pain can lessen through time and burn its way out, so there is hope for patients who suffer from this debilitating condition.

In terms of **Therapy** choices, staying active is the best approach. Some patients develop a frozen shoulder from not moving it or from splinting it because of the pain, especially when PHN affects the upper chest wall under the arm. These patients will need short courses of physical therapy to optimize their range-of motion and strengthening. All the other multidisciplinary therapy approaches are equally important, including psychological care coping strategies, restful sleep approaches, and any complementary techniques, like acupuncture, herbals and essential oils, and yoga.

If pills, injections, and therapies are limited, then there are **Surgery** techniques to explore, such as a spinal cord stimulation (SCS) modality. This can be used along the treatment lines of neuromodulation pain relief. There are also selective neuro-destructive techniques involving lesioning of the nerve roots next to the spine to decrease painful nerve impulses—a procedure that is reserved for only the most intractable pain patients who have failed all other options. The spinal cord stimulation device is trialed with temporary leads for up to one week in an outpatient setting first, and if deemed successful, long-term implantation of permanent spinal cord stimulation leads and a pulse generator can be performed to control pain for years, if necessary.

PATIENT EXAMPLE: A 70-year-old female had a bout of singles after a stressful event in her life. She had a painful rash over the front of her leg and went to her internist who promptly diagnosed shingles, and was subsequently started on a course of antiviral acyclovir medication.

After about ten days, her pain was somewhat better, but she still had a persistent burning and sensitivity over her leg. She returned to her doctor who prescribed a Lidoderm patch and low dose Neurontin. She experienced a 50% resolution of her symptoms and started to walk around with more comfort and an improved quality of life. She was satisfied with this level of relief, and continued to improve over the next year, until her symptoms had completely disappeared.

If this patient had persistent pain despite anti-neuropathic agents, then a course of a short-acting opioid narcotic, like tramadol or Tylenol with codeine, would have been in order, while weighing the risks and benefits of using opioids for an older patient. If opioid therapy failed, a referral to a pain management specialist to consider interventional pain management therapy would be in order, to further treat intractable pain symptoms. This type of specialist could offer a lumbar epidural steroid and local anesthetic injection to desensitize the shingles pain and to speed up the healing process. A series of three-to-five injections could be considered to fully desensitize the painful area and help the patient achieve a better quality of life. If this is achieved successfully, then through time, the severe pain typically lessens and the patient improves overall, as the pain eventually plateaus to more manageable levels. In the most intractable cases, a spinal cord stimulator lead modality would be the next step, but this is not usually necessary if shingles is treated aggressively early on from the onset of the vesicular rash.

4. Intercostal Neuralgia

Intercostal neuralgia is a painful neuropathic condition involving the chest wall. Ribs have nerves that run under the lower border of them, and if ribs sustain fractures or if patients have had thoracotomy chest surgery, then rib nerves can be irritated and entrapped and cause chronic pain of a sharp, shooting, burning nature. Intercostal neuralgia can be very uncomfortable for patients and involves a lot of sensitivity especially in the surgical incision area. Typically, the pain wraps around from the back to the front on the affected side.

The **P-I-T-S** *treatment protocol* can utilize all the major treatment options for this type of pain. In terms of **Pills** or medications, nonsteroidal anti-inflammatories, like Motrin and Aleve, and nerve pain agents, like Elavil, Neurontin, and topical lidocaine, are typically started first. Sometimes, if there is associated spasm with intercostal muscles from nerve irritation, patients are prescribed a muscle relaxant, such as Flexeril, which is an FDA-approved medication for muscular spasm. Centrally-acting analgesics, like the mild opioid tramadol, can be effective and in severe pain cases stronger opioid narcotics, both short-acting and long-acting, can be initiated.

If persistent pain continues despite medications, then desensitization **Injection** therapy and physical therapy are the next steps to be considered. Injections such as intercostal nerve blocks with a local anesthetic and steroid are employed to desensitize pain and break the pain cycle. These are injections performed under a fluoroscopic X-ray in an outpatient setting that block and desensitize the intercostal nerves. These blocks are administered from a posterior back approach to the ribs. With repeated injections, the pain reaches a lower plateau pain level that is typically much easier to manage with the rest of the **PITS Program**, especially when it comes to medication adjustments and optimal patient rehabilitation to stay comfortable and functional.

Therapy choices are mainly physical therapy options for those patients who will benefit from hands on desensitization and myofascial stretch release techniques, especially for post-surgical scar tissue. The other multidisciplinary pain management therapy choices of psychiatric care, restful sleep options, and complementary care techniques, all apply. All therapy choices are very important and helpful with this condition, much like any neuropathic pain ailment.

Again, **Surgery** techniques are reserved for ongoing intractable pain, and the spinal cord stimulator is the typical option here, especially if the origin of pain is from post-thoracotomy pain syndrome with a large neuropathic pain component. Spinal cord stimulation lead modality is not commonly needed for this condition, but again, remains an option in carefully selected intractable pain patients.

PATIENT EXAMPLE: A 20-year-old male was involved in an unfortunate car accident shattering several ribs in his left chest. After full healing over the ensuing three months, he still had persistent pain along his ribs and through his chest. The pain was sharp and shooting in nature and aggravated by activity. It was suggested by his medical doctor that he could have intercostal neuralgia due to the injury from the accident, and internal scar tissue that may have developed.

He was given a course of anti-inflammatory medication with Motrin and the anti-neuropathic agent Lyrica, but his pain persisted over the next four weeks. At this point, the patient was referred to a pain specialist. The pain specialist offered him an intercostal nerve block to desensitize his pain and break the pain cycle, in hope of allowing him to better rehabilitate with some physical therapy.

After a risk-and-benefit discussion, the patient underwent a series of intercostal nerve injections with local anesthetic and steroid combination, under fluoroscopy and intravenous sedation at an outpatient surgi-center. The patient had several injections, two weeks apart, and the pain improved to a 50% level. The patient was pleased with this result and continued to heal with a month of physical therapy. One year later, his pain level was down to 10%, which did not hamper his quality of life.

Now, had this patient experienced recurrent severe pain, even after nerve blocks, then he would be a candidate for radiofrequency (burning) or cryoablation (freezing) of the intercostal nerves, for longer-term relief. Ultimately, he would be a candidate for a spinal cord stimulator (SCS) trial if he ever developed intractable neuropathic pain that failed both aggressive medical and previous interventional pain management attempts at comfort.

5. Carpal Tunnel Syndrome (CTS)

Carpal tunnel syndrome is a painful neuropathic condition involving entrapment of the median nerve at the wrist in the carpal tunnel. The carpal tunnel can be constricted and inflamed and cause pressure on the median nerve causing a great deal of numbness and pain in the hand. This can happen with repetitive motion activity, like constantly typing on a computer keyboard, or after sustaining a traumatic injury to the wrist area.

In worse case scenarios, patients develop muscle wasting of the affected hand(s) from severe nerve compression and ischemia. It is important to begin treatment before this muscle wasting occurs, or it is typically too late to fully reverse. The pain can be severe and is accompanied by stiffness, numbness, and motion disability. Patients can go for many years with off-and-on symptoms of CTS, but once the pain and numbness advances, patients will seek medical attention.

The **P-I-T-S** *treatment protocol* for carpel tunnel syndrome involves all four major categories of pain care. In terms of **Pills** or medications, the choices are anti-inflammatories, like Motrin and Aleve; nerve pain agents, like Neurontin and Cymbalta; muscle relaxants, like Flexeril and Robaxin; centrally-acting analgesics, like the mild opioid tramadol and Tylenol; and stronger opioid narcotics, like hydrocodone and oxycodone. All choices are applicable depending on the frequency and severity of the symptoms.

Injection techniques are peripheral nerve injections into the carpal tunnel using local anesthetic and steroid. Patients usually will do one injection, which can offer weeks-to-months of relief, then decide either to repeat it at some point or move on with other options.

In terms of **Therapy** options, physical and occupational therapy techniques are important in restoring and maintaining functional use of the hands. Wrist bracing of the carpal tunnel and wrist during the day or at night will immobilize the painful area and promote healing.

Minimally invasive **Surgery** techniques performed by a hand specialist, typically an orthopedist or other hand specialist, involve *releasing* the carpal tunnel pressure through cutting the tendinous tissue that overlies the carpel tunnel. This safe outpatient minimally invasive procedure is very effective at decompressing the excessive pressure pathology and offering patients long term relief. CTS is usually a slow progressive syndrome, but again, patients move along the treatment protocol as needed based on the advancement of the pathologic process.

PATIENT EXAMPLE: A 65-year-old male, active all his life as a landscaper, had periodic episodes of previously diagnosed right-handed carpal tunnel syndrome. He experienced his first symptoms twenty years earlier,

and had an electromyogram (EMG) and nerve conduction study (NCS) confirming the diagnosis. The numbness and tingling in his fingers would worsen when he performed excessive hedge cutting and other physical tasks that required a continuous hand grasp of his gardening equipment.

He had since retired from his landscaping profession, but his pain symptoms became severe again when he slept on his hand the wrong way. This pain persisted despite anti-inflammatory medications. He went to his orthopedist who advised a wrist splint at night. The pain continued, despite wearing the brace for two weeks. He was given the centrally-acting mild opioid Ultram, which also has anti-neuropathic benefits through norepinephrine and serotonin receptor relief activity, and was able to reduce his pain by about 50%.

Over the next couple of months, he still felt that he did not have the quality of life he desired, so he returned to his orthopedist who now suggested an injection procedure using a steroid mixed with a local anesthetic. The patient agreed, and the injection was placed directly into his carpal tunnel during that office visit under ultrasound guidance. This helped with 50% of the overall pain symptoms for about one month.

Several months later his pain returned, and he again went back to his orthopedist who suggested a carpal tunnel release (CTR) at this point for longer-term relief, to be performed in an outpatient ambulatory surgical setting. After a risk-and-benefit discussion, the patient decided to proceed with the surgery, and did well experiencing near complete resolution of his severe symptoms after a short course of physical therapy. He was soon back to his normal activities and was very satisfied with his results.

I trust this chapter will serve as an educational platform, with different patient examples of pain care scenarios, so that patients can see where their own pain *"fits in."* I have created a separate chapter at the end of this one, called **PITS Educational Pearls of Pain Care Wisdom**; and at the end of the book there is an extensive **PITS Glossary of Pain Terms** section for added information on specific topics, like pain conditions, medications, procedures, and so forth. Remember not to skip these important sections of the book, because they are vitally important as reinforcers of the overall pain knowledge that will help ensure your success in the **PITS Program**!

I. The "ITIS" Conditions

SUMMARY: Painful conditions due to inflammation are numerous throughout our bodies. But at the risk of oversimplifying the *"itis"* conditions, we will focus on three common painful diagnoses that can flare acutely or become a chronic pain state. The first is **bursitis** or inflammation of a bursa, the second is **tendonitis** or inflammation of a tendon, and the third is **fasciitis** or inflammation of a fascia. The **P-I-T-S** *treatment protocol* is applicable for each of these pain conditions. This inflammatory pathology pain type is one of the major groups of chronic pain affecting millions of patients by on a regular basis. Patients typically develop these conditions when they partake in excessive activities and sports, or they are unfortunately injured in accidents.

Specific "itis" Conditions

1. Hip Bursitis

Hip bursitis, or medically known as greater trochanteric bursitis, is the inflammation of a bursa on the outside of both hips. This type of bursitis is not in the joint itself, like the inflammation that occurs within the hip joint from osteoarthritis. The bursa is a protective shock absorber sac on the outside of each hip bone that can get inflamed with trauma, repetitive activity of the extremities, or excessive pressure on the hips from lying on your side for extended periods. When hip bursas get inflamed from different irritating causes, they swell and start to hurt.

In the **P-I-T-S** *treatment protocol*, all four major categories of care apply, depending on the severity and chronicity of the painful symptoms. Nonsteroidal anti-inflammatory **Pills** or medications, like Motrin and Aleve, are the mainstay of treatment, but sometimes a short course of an oral steroid is used in severe cases that do not respond to NSAIDs. If there is associated spasm, a muscle relaxant, like Flexeril or Robaxin, can be used. Centrally-acting analgesics, such as Tylenol, are also options if patients cannot take anti-inflammatories because of stomach or kidney issues. In severe flare-ups, short courses of opioid narcotics, like hydrocodone and oxycodone, can be offered.

Injections for persistent hip bursitis pain involve injecting local anesthetic and steroid directly into the bursa using a needle technique through the skin under ultrasound guidance, often performed as a minimally invasive office-based outpatient procedure. Orthopedists and sports medicine specialists, rheumatologists, and pain specialists offer these injections to try to slow down the pain and inflammation directly in the bursa, to allow patients better rehabilitation and more complete healing. Hip bursa injections can be offered every three-to-six months as needed, always remembering that too much injected steroid in one area too quickly can lead to bone demineralization and tissue softening.

Therapy options include the patient gently stretching and exercising on their own, or they are placed in physical therapy for the use of modalities, like heat and ice, stim and ultrasound, and the TENS (transcutaneous electrical nerve stimulator) unit. Additionally, professional instruction in body mechanic awareness and posture, stretching, strengthening, and conditioning are very important to maximize a patient's functional status. Other multidisciplinary pain management options include acupuncture and low-level laser therapy, cognitive-behavioral therapy (CBT)—with approaches of stress management, positive thinking, and coping skill development—and maximizing restorative sleep through lifestyle modification, supplements, and medications to promote healing. These approaches, with medication, injection, and therapy, work in most patients for control of painful symptoms. However, in severe recurrent cases, even if osteopathic manipulation or physiatrist approaches have failed, some patients turn to their orthopedist for a surgical option.

A **Surgery** option, although rarely necessary, involves release of bursa impingement and compression by decompressing the restrictive iliotibial (IT) band fascia that overlies the hip bursa. This is only used for the most intractable pain patients.

PATIENT EXAMPLE: A 26-year-old female professional basketball player started developing right hip pain, without specific injury. She could not lie on her right side for any extended periods of time. She was experiencing a lot of sensitivity over the outer aspect of her hip, but had no history of osteoarthritis of the hip, and was also concerned about the possibility of a medical illness.

She made an appointment with her team medical doctor, who after a history and physical exam, discovered exquisite palpable pain directly over the greater trochanter bony prominence –the outside hip bone— and felt that she was suffering from an acute case of greater trochanteric bursitis from her sports activity. The doctor recommended a course of Advil and ice, and she was advised to rest and limit her activity for three days.

After this week, she improved 75%, but upon resuming her active workouts the pain returned. Her doctor then referred her to the team orthopedist for revaluation and possible intervention. When she saw the orthopedist, it was felt that she might benefit from a hip bursa injection of local anesthetic and steroid to speed up the pain control and recovery process, and get her back on the court. The patient had undergone this injection with ultrasound guidance, and felt 90% better overall over the next week. She had no side effects from the steroids. She was able to resume her athletic activities, with some additional Advil, ice, and use of the team Theragun percussive therapy device from time to time while on the bench.

2. Elbow Tendinitis (tennis and golfer's elbow)

Elbow tendinitis is pain that can appear on the inner side of the elbow known as medial epicondylitis or golfer's elbow, and when the pain is on the outside of the elbow known as lateral epicondylitis or tennis elbow. These common inflammatory conditions typically flare with excessive sports activity, hence their common sports names.

With tennis elbow, the tendinitis develops in the common extensor tendon on the outside of the elbow. Patients develop a tender point just below the elbow on the outer part, especially when they flex their wrist back and forth. It has a lot to do with repetitive motion, such as swinging a tennis racket, or other repetitive action involving wrist extension. With golfer's elbow, the tendonitis develops from tendons in the forearm that attach on the inside of the elbow, and is typically brought on by repetitive swings of a golf club, or by other repetitive action involving wrist flexion. If these lateral and medial elbow tendons become inflamed and irritated in patients, then all four categories of the **P-I-T-S *treatment protocol*** are available for care.

All of the inflammatory conditions in this chapter benefit from anti-inflammatory **Pills** or medications, such as Motrin and Aleve, as well as ice and rest initially. Muscle relaxants, Tylenol, and opioid narcotics are used depending on lingering severity of symptoms, similar to the treatment of hip bursitis discussed previously.

For persistent cases of elbow tendonitis, **Injections** can be given with local anesthetic and steroids directly into the tendon just below the elbow, to try and break the pain cycle and allow for more comfort, function, and rehabilitation. Orthopedists and pain specialists typically perform these safe minimally invasive office-based procedures, and they can be repeated once or twice as needed depending on the extent of relief they offer. Too many steroid-based tendon injections can lead to tendon rupture, so up to three in a lifetime for any one tendon area is generally considered safe in most medical practices.

Strengthening with **Therapy** can be helpful, as well as the use of physical therapy modalities; heat, ice, stim, ultrasound, and TENS. Other care techniques, such as magnets and acupuncture, psychological approaches for anxiety and depression, and restorative sleep strategies can all be used to treat tendinitis.

Surgery procedures for this condition are rarely necessary but are always reserved for the most intractable pain patients. Orthopedic surgeons can do a tendon release, where they rotate the tendon laterally around the elbow to decompress the pain. This is not a common procedure. Usually all these *"itises"* are self-limited and, although they can be chronically recurrent, the majority respond to conservative treatment options.

PATIENT EXAMPLE OF TENNIS ELBOW (LATERAL EPICONDYLITIS): A 30-year-old male recreational tennis player started out with pain in his right elbow after a long, hard-fought, five-set tennis match. He was right-hand dominant, and had a powerful overhand serve that put severe strain on his elbow area. He had a history of tennis elbow, but this current episode was worse than before.

He was experiencing tenderness just below the lateral part of his elbow especially with flexing his hand backward. He iced it and took some Advil and put a medical magnet over his elbow, but it was no better in two weeks. He went to a sports medicine specialist he knew from his college days, and was diagnosed with an acute flare of lateral epicondylitis—tennis elbow.

The sports medicine physician gave him a choice of continued rest, ice, anti-inflammatories, and therapy, or for him to consider injection therapy. With little or no improvement with the first course of action with Motrin, the patient decided to have injection therapy with a minimally invasive procedure.

In the office, the doctor injected the local anesthetic Marcaine, along with the steroid Depo-Medrol, into his common extensor tendon atraumatically, which gave the patient about 25% relief initially in the first week after the shot. Over the next several weeks, he improved to 50% resolution of his symptoms, and was able to get back to playing tennis. Occasionally, he would feel some pain and continued taking Advil as needed, and did well with magnets as a complementary therapy technique. Over the ensuing months his pain completely resolved.

PATIENT EXAMPLE OF GOLFER'S ELBOW (MEDIAL EPICONDYLITIS): A 32-year-old female pro golfer on the LPGA tour had recurrent medial epicondylitis. After a difficult second round at Augusta National, she iced her elbow and took Advil, which helped reduce her pain to about 50%. She played the next day still experiencing some residual pain and continued treatment with Advil and ice.

That night she was treated for the first time with a course of low-level laser therapy (LLLT) by her sports physician's staff. This achieved nearly 90% relief of the acute pain symptoms, and allowed her to play in the final round with some degree of comfort. Not only did she finish up with a respectable final score, but she also gained a newfound appreciation for the potential power of laser light therapy relief, and its place in her pain control options for the future.

3. Plantar Fasciitis

Plantar fasciitis is a common inflammatory condition of the heel and arch of the foot. This condition affects millions of patients in the United States. Patients often irritate the connective tissue—the plantar fascia—and muscles in the bottom of the foot, which causes the mechanical and inflammatory pain. Patients at more of a risk of developing plantar fasciitis, include those who do not have proper arch support, are obese, and who partake in repetitive sports that involve a lot of running. Podiatrists and orthopedic foot surgeons typically treat this condition.

All four categories of the **P-I-T-S** *treatment protocol* apply to the treatment of plantar fasciitis based on the severity and chronicity of the painful symptoms. Initially, **Pills** or medications, such as the nonsteroidal anti-inflammatories Motrin and Aleve, and muscle relaxants, like Flexeril and Zanaflex, are used to decrease the flare of inflammation and spasm that is associated with the fascia and muscle irritation. Tylenol can be effective, and in severe cases, short courses of short-acting opioid narcotic can be added, until patients are up and walking around more comfortably.

For persistent cases, despite medications, ice, orthotics, and rest, patients are offered **Injection** therapy with steroid and a local anesthetic with a foot specialist, utilizing the anti-inflammatory power of steroids to suppress the inflammation process and to break the pain cycle to allow patients to better rehabilitate.

In the **Therapy** option for pain care, many patients will choose physical therapy with modalities—heat, ice, stim, ultrasound, TENS—and stretching and conditioning exercises. Also, some patients will undergo shockwave therapy to break up fasciitis adhesions. Other multidisciplinary choices for therapy are also available, and they include low-level laser therapy (LLLT), acupuncture, massage, and so forth.

Surgery techniques are reserved for the most intractable cases, and are performed by a trained podiatrist or orthopedic foot specialist, where surgical release or cutting of the constricted plantar fascia is performed. This is not a common procedure, as it may lead to other support issues in the foot, so it reserved for patients who literally cannot walk.

PATIENT EXAMPLE: A 60-year-old man had bought a new pair of hard leather shoes, and after two weeks at work where he is on his feet all day, he started having an ache in both feet. He tried to stay off of his feet at night, but the pain and stiffness persisted, especially upon awakening in the morning and when first starting to walk.

He did not have any history of previous foot problems, and he attributed this uncomfortable pain to his new shoes. Over the next couple of weeks, he still had increasing pain and tightness in his feet despite heel inserts. He went to his family doctor who diagnosed possible plantar fasciitis, and suggested a podiatrist for further evaluation and treatment. Upon visiting the podiatry specialist, plantar fasciitis was confirmed, and he was subsequently prescribed Naprosyn, which is an anti-inflammatory medication. He was also given a prescription for orthotics.

His pain subsequently got better over the next month, and resolved completely within two months. Now, if the patient had continued with persistent pain, even at this point in his treatment course, then he would be a candidate for interventional management considering a local anesthetic and steroid injection by his podiatrist. In the worst-case scenario, after a risk-and-benefit discussion, surgical release procedures could be offered to the patient to treat intractable pain symptoms.

I trust this chapter will serve as an educational platform, with different patient examples of pain care scenarios, so that patients can see where their own pain *"fits in."* I have created a separate chapter at the end of this one, called **PITS Educational Pearls of Pain Care Wisdom**; and at the end of the book there is an extensive **PITS Glossary of Pain Terms** section for added information on specific topics, like pain conditions, medications, procedures, and so forth. Remember not to skip these important sections of the book, because they are vitally important as reinforcers of the overall pain knowledge that will help ensure your success in the **PITS Program**!

Coccyx Pain (Coccydynia)

SUMMARY: Coccyx pain, known medically as coccydynia, is typically caused by some kind of traumatic event to the tailbone area of the spine. This could be from a slip or fall on the buttock during daily life, during a sports activity, or by some type of work or motor vehicle-related accident. In females, the pain could result from a painful vaginal birth where the coccyx is strained or sprained resulting in a persistent pain condition.

Coccyx pain is usually of an acute mechanical and inflammatory nature, and is typically self-limited. If it extends beyond the acute and sub-acute phases and into the chronic recurrent phase of pain recovery of more than six months, then longer-term pain management strategies should be considered. Damage to the coccyx causes irritation and scarring of the sacro-coccygeal ligament and coccygeal nerves around the coccyx bones—five small, fused bones making up the lowest part of the spine. Conservative treatment with medications, injections, and therapeutic strategies offers adequate relief in nearly all patients.

Considering the **P-I-T-S** *treatment protocol* for coccyx pain, all four categories of care apply depending on the severity of the initial event and intensity of lingering chronic symptoms. In terms of **Pills** or medications, the usual anti-inflammatory medications, such as Motrin, Aleve, diclofenac, Mobic, and others, are usually quite effective. Muscle relaxants, like Flexeril, Zanaflex, Robaxin, Baclofen, and others, are typically started immediately to decrease painful inflammation and spasm in the injured area. For moderate-level pain, the mild opioid tramadol can be dosed, and for severe cases, a stronger opioid narcotic can be prescribed, like hydrocodone and oxycodone, among others.

For persistent pain, despite applications of ice and heat, and a donut pillow to take pressure off the coccyx area when seated, **Injections** of a local anesthetic and steroid combination can be offered. Coccyx injection of the ligamentous and nerve area is performed under fluoroscopic X-ray guidance in an outpatient setting and is considered safe and minimally invasive, to desensitize and break the pain cycle. Typical of any steroidal injections, they cannot be performed too frequently, or bone and tissue can become demineralized and softened. Typically, chronic care can consist of injection therapy every three-to-six months as needed for recurrent flares of severe pain.

If the pain cycle can be broken and allow for more healing with medications and injection management, then physical **Therapy** for coccydynia can consist of pelvic floor exercises to strengthen and stabilize the area.

In very few cases, and only if the coccyx is fractured and impinging important structures in the rectal-pelvic area, will a **Surgery** corrective procedure be necessary. Surgery on the coccyx is rarely performed and can distort surrounding tissue structures.

PATIENT EXAMPLE: A 40-year-old female was skating with her children at a local park when she slipped and fell hard on her buttock. She experienced a severe sensation of pain in her lower spine, but without sciatica symptoms. After leaving the ice rink, she went home and soaked in a warm tub and applied an ice pack to her tailbone area afterwards. She took a dose of Aleve that night, but woke up the next morning with more severe pain.

The next day the area was sore to touch, but there were no neurologic symptoms in her legs. She had a hard time sitting and had to lean toward one buttock cheek or the other to avoid direct contact on her tailbone region, so she went to see her internist.

Her internist immediately diagnosed acute coccyx pain from her fall at the skating rink. She was told to sit on a doughnut pillow to take pressure off her coccyx, to do Epsom salt baths twice a day, and to take Motrin 800 mg three times a day for the next five days. After this, she felt a 40% improvement in her pain while up and moving around, but still had persistent pain while specifically sitting and lying flat.

She was then given a course of Vicodin (hydrocodone/Tylenol combination) for more severe pain especially if she was having difficulty sleeping at night due to the pain. Her pain persisted for two more weeks, and again after returning to her medical doctor, she was given a pain management referral to consider injection management to try to break her pain cycle. After meeting with her pain specialist, who was board-certified in interventional pain management, she was offered a coccyx injection of local anesthetic and steroid to speed the healing process.

After insurance approval was obtained, she underwent a coccyx injection under fluoroscopy X-ray guidance as an office outpatient, with 75% of her pain relieved a few days later. She was very satisfied with this relief result at this point in her treatment protocol. As a principle of pain management, an injectable local anesthetic works fast but of shorter duration and an injectable depo-steroid works slowly but for a longer duration. The patient subsequently fully healed over the next month, again using her doughnut pillow and taking anti-inflammatory medication on an as-needed basis.

I trust this chapter will serve as an educational platform, with a patient example of a pain care scenario, so that patients can see where their own pain *"fits in."* I have created a separate chapter at the end of this one, called **PITS Educational Pearls of Pain Care Wisdom**; and at the end of the book there is an extensive **PITS Glossary of Pain Terms** section for added information on specific topics, like pain conditions, medications, procedures, and so forth. Remember not to skip these important sections of the book, because they are vitally important as reinforcers of the overall pain knowledge that will help ensure your success in the **PITS Program**!

Central Pain Syndrome

SUMMARY: Central pain syndrome (CPS) is an uncommon state of severe nervous system disruption, such as stroke or other medical disease that affects the central nervous system—brain and spinal cord—and leads to abnormal pain pathways and sensations. CPS is a type of neuropathic pain that can have both central and peripheral nerve involvement. Besides post-stroke pain, other types of central pain syndrome can arise from multiple sclerosis, Parkinson's disease, spinal cord injury (SCI), traumatic brain injury (TBI), and from injury resulting in phantom limb pain.

CPS pain is typically constant and burning in nature, and usually moderate-to-severe in pain intensity. It is typically worse with high emotional states and cold temperatures. A central pain state can develop right away after an accident or medical event, or it can develop months or years later. If patients have thalamic ischemia and stroke in brain areas where pain relay fibers travel, then these are the patients at greater risk of developing a central pain state. CPS is one of the more difficult neuropathic pain states to treat.

There are several **P-I-T-S** *treatment protocol* options for treating CPS and to try and minimize the pain and suffering from central pain conditions. **Pills** or medications are the mainstay of treatment to reduce pain and anxiety levels for most patients. Surgical implants with motor cortex brain stimulation and intrathecal spinal pump pain medication infusion, are options for advanced intractable cases. Other medication choices are anti-neuropathic agents, like certain antidepressants, anticonvulsants, and opioid narcotics. Successfully used antidepressants include Elavil (amitriptyline) and Pamelor (nortriptyline), as well as Cymbalta (duloxetine) and Effexor (venlafaxine).

Anticonvulsants, like Neurontin (gabapentin) and Lyrica (pregabalin), have been used with successful relief. Opioid narcotic therapy is often needed to manage severe pain, and it turns out that methadone and Nucynta (tapentadol) have been shown by science and research to have anti-neuropathic pain control properties. In terms of stress and anxiety reduction, the benzodiazepine Klonopin (clonazepam) has been used with selected patients. Even with an optimal combination of pain medications for central pain patients, relief is typically only partial, so patients need to explore additional relief options.

There are no specific **Injection** therapies for most of the central pain states, except for phantom limb pain. This could be treated with sympathetic nerve blocks to control burning pain and desensitize skin pain, and somatic (peripheral) nerve blocks to help with sharp shooting pain sensations. Also, if there is associated secondary spasm pain, then trigger point injections can be considered.

Physical **Therapy** is important to maximize functionality in the affected body part(s), with the aid of modalities of heat, TENS unit, and so forth, to lessen symptoms. Other multidisciplinary pain management therapy choices include cognitive-behavioral therapy (CBT) and stress management, and these options can play a vital role for patients who struggle with the day-to-day pain and emotional distress from this difficult pain state.

Optimizing restorative sleep is typically a struggle with this condition, but a very important focus, so patients are not always waking up exhausted. Complementary care techniques, such as acupuncture, massage, and relaxation strategies, are popular approaches that patients often pursue, when conventional medical approaches offer only partial or limited relief.

Surgery techniques are reserved for the most intractable central pain patients. In the past, thalamic neurosurgical destructive lesioning was performed to interrupt the pain pathway transmission to the brain. Today, this ablative destructive procedure is rarely performed, especially with the development of neuromodulation technology involving brain cortex stimulation—akin to spinal cord stimulation, but for the brain.

Highly trained *functional specialty* neurosurgeons are finding a lot of success with placing a specialized plate on the outside of certain brain areas, which when stimulated, can block pain signal transmissions without causing damage to the brain. Also, implanting an intrathecal spinal pain pump is another option, where opioid and anti-neuropathic spinal fluid medication can be given by continuous infusion to block central nervous system pain. As challenging as a central pain condition can be for the healthcare team, the good news is it is not very common, compared to other kinds of chronic pain states that afflict patients.

PATIENT EXAMPLE: A 69-year-old female who suffered an unfortunate stroke and experienced weakness on the left side of her body. She was in a rehabilitation center, with an outpatient neurologist who was overseeing her care, and was slowly starting to recover over the ensuing months. About three months after her stroke, she started experiencing a burning sensation in her left arm, which became very sensitive to touch and movement. This pain and sensitivity were making her quite nervous.

When she returned to her neurologist after discharge, it was felt that she was starting to experience neuropathic pain that was consistent with a diagnosis of central pain syndrome due to her earlier stroke. She was started on the anti-neuropathic medication Lyrica for her pain, and the antianxiety medication Klonopin. Within two weeks, she felt at least a 50% improvement in her symptoms.

She was satisfied with this level of improvement because now the pain was not consuming her every day. With less pain and sensitivity, she was able to devote more time to her outpatient physical therapy to improve her muscle strength. She had tried some complementary techniques, such as acupuncture and massage, which also helped an additional 20%, and was taught some cognitive-behavioral therapy techniques to help deal with her residual pain. She continued to do well with her quality-of-life gains, thereafter.

I trust this chapter will serve as an educational platform, with a patient example of a pain care scenario, so that patients can see where their own pain *"fits in."* I have created a separate chapter at the end of this one, called PITS Educational Pearls of Pain Care Wisdom; and at the end of the book there is an extensive PITS Glossary of Pain Terms section for added information on specific topics, like pain conditions, medications, procedures, and so forth. Remember not to skip these important sections of the book, because they are vitally important as reinforcers of the overall pain knowledge that will help ensure your success in the PITS Program!

Peripheral Vascular Disease (PVD) Pain

SUMMARY: The pain of **peripheral vascular disease** (PVD) arises from nociceptors—specialized pain receptors that exist in many structures in the body including in the arms and legs—when vascular ischemia and lack of adequate blood flow affects these receptors, especially in the lower limbs. This condition involves the vasculature and soft tissue, muscles, and even peripheral nerves, and can result in ulceration of the feet and toes.

Most PVD is secondary to atherosclerotic plaques in leg arteries which causes a lot of intermittent leg pain or claudication, usually when patients walk extended distances. If blood flow is drastically reduced to the point of gangrene with tissue death and breakdown, then this situation typically mandates a surgical option to amputate. If this process is repeated time after time resulting in repeat amputations, then it becomes a difficult nociceptive and neuropathic pain state to control.

Considering the **P-I-T-S** *treatment protocol*, all four categories of pain care are available. In terms of **Pills** or medications, the anti-inflammatory choices, such as Motrin, Celebrex, Tylenol, and the mild opioid tramadol, are available. Stronger opioid narcotics, like hydrocodone, oxycodone, morphine, and hydromorphone, can be introduced if pain is severe in nature. Also, anti-neuropathic medications, like Neurontin and Lyrica, and muscle relaxants, like Flexeril, Baclofen, and Zanaflex, can be quite helpful when trying to control skin sensitivity and leg spasm pain.

In terms of **Injection** options, a sympathetic local anesthetic injection outside the spine on the affected leg side, may provide some symptomatic relief. The idea is to open blood vessels and restore some blood flow to try and help with ischemia and small ulcer healing. If this is limited, sometimes chemical neurolysis injection of a phenol chemical for nerve destruction, or a radiofrequency heat probe ablation procedure of sympathetic nerves, is performed to destroy the nerves outside the spine, for longer-term improved blood flow. These are not permanent blocks, because the sympathetic nerves can grow back to certain degrees within months after these procedures.

As far as **Therapy** is concerned, if patients maintain some strengthening and conditioning in their leg muscles, then this will aid in the muscular-pump squeeze effect on the vasculature to promote blood flow. This may be limited because most severe PVD patients cannot walk very far.

Surgery is a viable option for PVD. If vascular surgeons can restore blood flow through a bypass procedure, this is optimal treatment because it allows longer-term blood flow correction. In patients who have non-operable PVD and a small ulcer, and where other pain management remedies have been less effective, then the spinal cord stimulation (SCS) modality can be offered as a minimally invasive surgical option for pain control and ulcer healing. Research has shown that the spinal cord stimulation device has the capacity to heal small ulcers because of its positive effect on blood flow and the improved oxygen content of tissue.

PATIENT EXAMPLE: A 70-year-old male who had severe peripheral vascular disease (PVD) for years, and had an amputation in his right leg below the knee and a femoral bypass graft in his left leg, started developing left leg ulcer pain in his ankle. He had a 1-cm wide, round ulcer that his vascular surgeon felt was not re-operable, because of the relatively high risk-to-benefit of re-operation in this particular patient. He was on Duragesic patch opioid narcotic medication as a long-acting baseline agent, and Percocet as a short-acting breakthrough pain medication to attempt to control his high pain scores. Despite the aggressive use of pain medication, he still was experiencing periods of 9/10 pain, on a 0–10 pain scale, especially at night.

It was suggested by his vascular doctor to consider longer-term advanced interventional pain management options. After his evaluation with the pain specialist, he was felt to be a spinal cord stimulation lead trial candidate for vascular ischemia, with the hope of not only controlling pain symptoms better, but also, having a chance at healing the small ulcer on his ankle. After a risk-and-benefit analysis, the patient decided on a SCS trial, which was successful in controlling 50% of his pain over the ensuing week. It was also helping him to sleep better. Shortly thereafter, he elected to undergo permanent implantation of the SCS device, and six months later much to his amazement, the ulcer was completely healed. The patient was very satisfied with this result, and continued to use his spinal cord stimulator to control vascular pain symptoms successfully, for many years thereafter.

I trust this chapter will serve as an educational platform, with a patient example of a pain care scenario, so that patients can see where their own pain *"fits in."* I have created a separate chapter at the end of this one, called **PITS Educational Pearls of Pain Care Wisdom**; and at the end of the book there is an extensive **PITS Glossary of Pain Terms** section for added information on specific topics, like pain conditions, medications, procedures, and so forth. Remember not to skip these important sections of the book, because they are vitally important as reinforcers of the overall pain knowledge that will help ensure your success in the **PITS Program**!

Psychogenic Pain

SUMMARY: Psychogenic pain is an uncommon pain category type, and is diagnosed when patients complain of chronic headache, back ache, stomachache, and pelvic pain, in the absence of a physical cause. When the healthcare team conducts a thorough physical exam and obtains tests with blood work, X-rays, CT-scans, MRIs, or other pertinent tests, and there is no apparent organic reason to explain the persistent pain complaints, this is basically the nature of psychogenic pain. To put it simply, the pain derives from psychological and behavioral reasons, like depression and anxiety, and reveals itself as real bodily symptoms, sensory and motor dysfunction, numbness, aching, and spasm.

This condition is commonly diagnosed as a *Somatoform Pain Disorder (SPD)*, which is a real type of pain characterized by symptoms that suggest a physical illness, but cannot be explained by a likely medical condition, any planned malingering, the patient deliberately harming themselves, or any substance abuse problem.

Good appropriate psychiatric care is the primary treatment of psychogenic pain, with a focus on psychotherapy, use of medications that are in the antidepressant group, avoiding medications in the opioid narcotic group, and pursuing other nonpharmacologic approaches to help patients, such as lifestyle changes, stress management strategies, and cognitive-behavioral therapy (CBT).

A diagnosis of psychogenic pain is hard for patients to accept and harder to treat, compared to other types of pain with physical pathology. Patients often hear that their pain is *"in their head,"* and that is the key. The pain is a real issue to the patient and can greatly affect their quality of life, but patients will learn to use their brain to control the physical body symptoms they experience, to ultimately improve their situation.

Science and research are revealing more and more about the mind-body connection of pain and how the *emotional state* can affect the *physical state* of patients. We now have functional brain MRIs that show how the emotional suffering component and sensory physical pain component pathways cross, and share common nerve pathways in different parts of the brain, where the final *pain experience* is perceived. It turns out, that a lot of psychogenic pain patients unfortunately have a history of physical and sexual abuse, and are full of repressed anxiety and anger which manifests as physical symptoms.

In terms of the **P-I-T-S** *treatment protocol* for the treatment of psychogenic pain, **Pills** or medications and psychological **Therapy**, as opposed to physical therapy, are the key choices. **Injection** or **Surgery** category options are generally not considered because the diagnosis of pain has no physical *organic* source.

Although there are many categories of psychiatric medications to adjust the psychiatric outlook of afflicted patients, three main types of antidepressant medications or **Pills** stand out:

- The *first group* is the tricyclics, like Elavil (amitriptyline) and Pamelor (nortriptyline).

- The *second group* is the selective serotonin reuptake inhibitors (SSRIs), like Zoloft (sertraline) and Paxil (paroxetine).

- The *third group* is the serotonin-norepinephrine reuptake inhibitors (SNRIs), like Cymbalta (duloxetine) and Effexor (venlafaxine).

Patients typically are treated by a psychiatrist or neurologist, who select choices for antidepressants based on their medical assessment and judgment. Nonsteroidal anti-inflammatory, muscle relaxant, and anti-neuropathic medications are also used in selected patients, but not opioid narcotics, due to their high risk versus lack of benefit and the fact that there is no primary organic pathology indication for this class of medication.

In terms of **Therapy**, it is the psychological therapy approach utilizing cognitive-behavioral strategies for care. These may include talk therapy to treat symptoms of the psychogenic pain, lifestyle changes to reduce stress, or well-being therapy to change ill thoughts and attitudes. Other complementary strategies can be effective, such as acupuncture, massage, and hypnosis. These can be helpful in ensuring that patients achieve restorative sleep, because fatigue and exhaustion affects a patient's mood, and the way they think about their pain.

Fortunately, psychogenic pain with somatoform pain disorder is not commonly seen in everyday outpatient pain management practices. It is a diagnosis of exclusion when all the tests do not suggest a clear etiology for the pain symptoms. Although the pain is a real functional-type of pain, and not organic in nature like a broken bone, it is treated conservatively with a lot of supportive psychological and psychiatric therapeutic approaches which could take months or even years to achieve a satisfactory outcome.

PATIENT EXAMPLE: A 32-year-old female, who had suffered from being raped as a child by her uncle, started to miss a lot of days at work, because of vague pelvic pain symptoms and associated back pain. This continued for six months, and was getting her depressed. She eventually made an appointment with her internist, who after a thorough review of the patient's history, physical exam, blood tests, a pelvic ultrasound, and abdominal-pelvic CT scan, could not discover any physical ailment.

Her doctor noticed she was depressed, so he prescribed a low dose of Elavil antidepressant for a month. After a month, she returned for a re-evaluation with ongoing pain complaints of spasms in her back and pelvic area. She was started on Flexeril muscle relaxant, and a home exercise program, but this did not help much. When she started complaining of severe pelvic pain, she was given a prescription for Vicodin narcotic, and told to see her OBGYN physician.

After her OBGYN exam, it was recommended that she wean off the Vicodin and undergo a laparoscopy, which is a surgical procedure involving a lighted scope placed in the abdominal-pelvic cavity for diagnostic and therapeutic purposes, to see if a condition was not picked up on by the previous ultrasound and CT scan. It turned out that the laparoscopy was negative, and this left both the patient and physicians involved puzzled as to what was the source of all the painful symptoms.

She was then referred to a pain psychologist, despite the patient's reluctance, who took a much more detailed patient history about the patient's family dynamics. The unfortunate rape incident was discovered during one of the follow up sessions, and the patient broke down crying. At this point, she was referred to a psychiatrist for possible medication treatment and psychotherapy concerning this childhood incident.

She was placed in an outpatient support group with other rape victims at this point, and started on the antidepressant Effexor, to help with anxiety and depression. Within a month, much to the surprise of the patient herself, her pain symptoms started to lessen, and she was able to stop the Flexeril and wean off the Vicodin narcotic.

After two months her spirits were greatly improved and her work was more enjoyable. She was able to make peace with her uncle, and all her original pelvic and back pain symptoms soon disappeared. Helped by her psychiatrist and her psychiatric therapy sessions, she came to realize that she had repressed her anger about the rape incident which eventually caused the Somatoform Pain Disorder that previously consumed her—but not anymore!

I trust this chapter will serve as an educational platform, with a patient example of a pain care scenario, so that patients can see where their own pain *"fits in."* I have created a separate chapter at the end of this one, called **PITS Educational Pearls of Pain Care Wisdom**; and at the end of the book there is an extensive **PITS Glossary of Pain Terms** section for added information on specific topics, like pain conditions, medications, procedures, and so forth. Remember not to skip these important sections of the book, because they are vitally important as reinforcers of the overall pain knowledge that will help ensure your success in the **PITS Program!**

Cancer Pain

SUMMARY: Cancer pain can be very debilitating to patients, not only from the disease itself, but also from going through all the treatments in hope of long-term remission or even a cure. Cancer itself hurts, especially when tumors invade bones, organs, and nerves. But some of the cancer treatments themselves can give transient pain states, especially certain chemotherapy agents which can cause some nerve pain while administered, like cisplatin to treat bladder and ovarian cancer, vincristine to treat leukemia and lymphoma, and paclitaxel to treat breast cancer. This treatment-related cause of neuropathic pain typically resolves slowly once the chemo-agent is discontinued. Additionally, if the chemo-agent causes muscle pain symptoms, then this also lessens once the course of chemotherapy is finished. Thus, in general, cancer pain can result in a mixed nociceptive and neuropathic type of pain state.

As mentioned, cancer itself can hurt bones and muscles and organs and nerves through local spread and by spreading or metastasizing to other parts of the body. Radiation therapy, when targeted to certain abdominal cancers, can cause radiation enteritis or painful injury to bowels. It can cause scarring in tissues which can also lead to pain states that can persist with moderate-to-severe pain levels. The number one fear that patients typically have with any kind of cancer news is, *"Am I going to die?"* The second question is, *"Is this cancer going to hurt me?"*

Everyone is afraid of dying from cancer, but it is the fear of uncontrolled pain from the cancer that preoccupies a lot of patients, just as much as the prospect of death, when they first get cancer news. The diagnosis needs to be addressed in a compassionate and informative multi-disciplinary manner.

Cancer pains can be non-nerve nociceptive in nature, including soft tissue, muscle, bone, and organs, as well as, neuropathic in nature, including peripheral nerves, spinal cord, and brain nerve pathways—or mixed with both types of pain. Many patients experience acute pain at the onset of painful cancer, but if the pain continues for more than six months, and most do, then pain specialists are prepared for chronic pain management as a major treatment focus during the patient's cancer battle.

The **P-I-T-S** *treatment protocol* applies to cancer pain like any other benign pain condition. In terms of **Pills** or medications, anti-inflammatory nonsteroidal and steroidal type medications can help most cancer pains, especially if bone and organs are involved. If cancer is causing muscle spasm, then muscle relaxants can be added. If cancer invades nerves and creates neuropathic-like pain, then nerve pain agents in the antidepressant and anticonvulsant groups can be prescribed.

Tylenol and the mild opioid tramadol may play a role in early treatment of mild-to-moderate pain symptoms. For severe pain levels, stronger opioid narcotic medications for cancer are instituted earlier rather than later. Short-acting narcotics can be used as needed initially and titrated to affect. If cancer pain persists, and long-acting narcotics are needed as a baseline of pain relief, then two narcotics can be used—one serving as a baseline and one for breakthrough pain as needed. Sometimes, a cancer patient will experience incident movement pain, at which time a course of narcotic analgesia can be prescribed. A lot of the medication choices come in oral, intravenous, and pain patch forms, all depending on whether the patient is capable of eating and drinking.

In terms of **Injection** choices, there are many specific types of interventional pain management options, depending on the type of cancer pain and its severity. If patients start to develop discrete areas of muscle spasms, then local anesthetic trigger point injections (TPIs) can help to break the spasm cycle and allow patients to better rehabilitate. TPIs are safe and minimally invasive, and typically performed in an office setting or right at the patient's bedside if they are hospitalized. The skin is cleaned with an alcohol swab, a small injection needle is placed through the skin and into the taut spasm. The local anesthetic, usually either lidocaine or bupivacaine, is then injected with a short-lived stinging or burning sensation, and then the needle is removed. TPIs can be repeated as needed if severe spasms return.

If patients start to experience radiating pain in the spine and legs from metastatic cancer lesions which are irritating spinal nerves, then epidural steroid and local anesthetic injections can be considered to decrease pain and inflammation to break the pain cycle. Hopefully, this can offer enough relief until other measures can be taken to treat the spinal cancer involvement. If cancer invades organs, such as the pancreas or stomach, and this leads to a lot of abdominal and flank pain, then these patients might benefit from a *celiac plexus block* using local anesthetic or neurolytic nerve killing injection that can offer both diagnostic and therapeutic relief from severe pain symptoms.

When it comes to injectable neurolytic agents for longer-term relief of typically months in duration, 100% medical grade alcohol can be used to destroy the celiac nerve plexus safely to get patients extended relief from their intractable abdominal pain. This plexus injection is performed in a sterile outpatient or hospital inpatient setting, under fluoroscopic (X-ray) or CT scan guidance, and typically with an IV sedative for patient comfort. These blocks work better earlier in the cancer pain treatment course, when patients cannot get enough relief with opioid narcotics, or who are too symptomatic with opioid side effects. Abdominal and pancreatic cancer can be very disabling to patients, and if there are limited treatments, then palliative care needs to be more aggressively sought, especially in advanced cases.

As far as **Therapy** choices are concerned, a lot of cancer pain patients explore physical therapy and rehabilitative choices to maintain their independent functional status for as long as they can. All the major principles of physical therapy need to be considered, depending on the level of an individual patient's debilitation, to optimize functional care, including biomechanics, posture, flexibility, strengthening, and conditioning. Modalities are also helpful to patient care, including heat, ice, electric stimulation, ultrasound, and TENS unit. These can help with swelling, inflammation, spasms, and any other general neuromuscular issues. In addition, many cancer patients explore psychological and sleep therapies to improve their pain, along with complementary care therapies, like acupuncture, massage, and essential oils, for full integrative care.

As far as **Surgery** options are concerned, this option makes sense for any individual patient considering the likelihood of success, the risk-and-benefit discussion, and possible recovery time. There are oncology cancer surgeons who are very skilled at dissecting tumors before or after chemotherapy and radiation, to give the patient a much better chance of survival with certain cancers.

Another surgical implant option for pain control is the *intrathecal infusion device (IID)*, also referred to as *spinal narcotic pain pump*. If patients require high dose oral narcotics and are either still uncomfortable or symptomatic from side effects, such as nausea and sedation and other side effects, then they may be candidates for morphine spinal testing. This option is usually done in a hospital setting, where the patient receives a dose of opioid narcotic in the spinal fluid space under X-ray guidance, and then monitored for effectiveness and any side effects.

With an inpatient opioid testing protocol, patients can stay for one, two or even up to three days or longer. During the testing phase, if narcotic testing in the spine is deemed beneficial, then the patient may have a longer-term intrathecal pump and catheter system implanted with a continuous infusion of narcotic, typically starting with morphine, delivered directly to the spinal fluid. This involves placing a plastic tube in the spinal fluid through a spinal needle, which is then connected to a subcutaneous catheter under the skin, which is then connected to a narcotic pump reservoir under the skin in front of the abdomen.

These morphine devices can be very effective in controlling symptoms and minimizing side effects of systemic opioids, especially high dose oral narcotics. A patient only needs a fraction of the morphine narcotic in the spinal fluid to equal hundreds of milligrams of oral morphine equivalent! The morphine in the spinal pump is delivered right to the spinal nerves that need to be treated for comfort, rather than taking a large oral dose and having it be metabolized by the liver and then traveling in the blood stream and going eventually to the spinal cord and brain.

Spinal morphine pumps are safe to test and place in patients who suffer from intractable cancer pain, and even used in chronic benign pain intractable states that would have otherwise failed other modalities of treatment, such as the spinal cord stimulation device. The spinal morphine pump can be run by the physician team and with an infusion agency, and certain patients are allowed a hand-held programmer device that allows them to bolus small doses of additional narcotic through the pump and into the spinal fluid, for times of breakthrough pain. With cancers that may be causing recurrent severe pain in patients who are projected to live for years, like stabilized metastatic breast cancer cases, the intrathecal infusion device narcotic pump may be the best option for prolonged pain management care.

Multiple myeloma is a specific type of cancer that can come and go during a patient's lifetime, and is a type of blood cancer that can cause a lot of bone pain and kidney problems. There are several oncology treatments approaches to put this disease into remission and offer patients a more comfortable life. During treatment, and because of the moderate-to-severe bone pain that can arise with progression, the **P-I-T-S treatment protocol** involves mainly the **Pill** or medication category. The treating medical team will utilize anti-inflammatory medications and opioid narcotics, like methadone for example, for strong bone pain cases. The use of long-acting and short-acting opioids are important to cover both baseline pain and breakthrough pain when it occurs. Bone pain is exacerbated through *prostaglandins*—fatty acid substances in the body—and treatment with nonsteroidals, like ibuprofen and Toradol, and steroidal medications, like prednisone and Decadron, are some of the anti-inflammatory medications that are used to inhibit these prostaglandins. By combining anti-inflammatory with narcotic medication, this results in a synergistic or booster effect, to give a patient better relief compared to just using one or the other medication alone. Treating pain with more than one drug-mechanism of relief is a helpful treatment principle to remember.

Also, the side effect profile of drug treatment can be lowered if you can reduce the overall levels of individual medications. Again, opioid narcotics alone may be limited, and anti-inflammatories may be limited if used alone, but when combined patients can have additive relief effects and do better with certain bone pain control. Excessive use of anti-inflammatory medications poses the risks of gastrointestinal bleeding, kidney issues, and central nervous system issues. So, anti-inflammatory usage is always balanced with a risk-and-benefit analysis reviewing the patient's condition and other co-existing problems that may be non-cancer related.

With certain bone cancer pain, oncologists have other agents that can be directed to strengthen bones and to fight bone cancers to give patients palliative care relief. For example, Strontium, a common radioactive metallic isotope, is used to strengthen bones in multiple myeloma patients. Bone pain also responds well to radiation therapy, but there are limits on how much radiation each bony segment can get during a patient's treatment.

With the treatment of cancer pain, the healthcare team tries to provide hope and be supportive when patient situations are less likely to end up with a cure. Thus, psychiatric and psychological care options are often needed to help patients cope with the diagnosis of cancer. Most complementary care techniques are available if patients are willing to explore this area of care choices. It turns out that many cancer patients are eager and willing to consider all available integrative options to improve their treatment situation, and why a lot of oncology programs have developed complementary and alternative medicine (CAM) programs, to assist the traditional conventional medical approaches. For example, a lot of cancer patients seek treatment with vitamins and minerals and holistic approaches to boost their immune system and give them every hope of survival and achieving a longer life.

Many cancer patients have other comorbid disease states that can cause pain from a non-cancer standpoint, and this needs to be addressed along with the ongoing cancer treatment. If patients start developing other pain problems not related to cancer, such as mechanical and radicular low back pain from a herniated disc or spinal stenosis, then these treatment needs can be addressed within the usual **P-I-T-S *treatment protocol*.** Keeping any pain under control throughout the cancer treatment process is vital to give the patient comfort, maximum function, and hope in fighting the cancer itself.

As cancer advances, and there are no medical cure options remaining, then patients move from a *primary oncology care* treatment focus to a *palliative care* focus and optimizing a patient's remaining quality of life. When patients reach an end-of-life care stage, then *hospice care* is available until a patient's ultimate demise. Thus, the typical continuum of cancer care is first being treated primarily by the oncologist, and then if the situation does not resolve despite the various cancer care approaches, a palliative care specialist team can get involved. This team will ensure that the patient's ongoing medical, spiritual, and nutritional care needs are being met when a cure is not possible. Hospice care is then typically provided when a patient has two weeks or less to live.

Hospice care can mean an enormous difference as to whether a patient suffers from intractable pain at the end of their life. The use of palliative care and hospice care options, especially with end-of-life issues, has been an important improvement in medical practice in America over the last twenty years. This type of care is available whether a patient suffers from cancer or a non-cancer illness. If you have end stage cardiopulmonary disease, a patient can still be a candidate for palliative care and eventually hospice care if they choose.

PATIENT EXAMPLE #1: A 40-year-old female was diagnosed with pancreatic cancer. After this devastating news, a team of multidisciplinary specialists was assembled to give the patient her care options. She had moderate pain and was comfortable with oral morphine doses, until a more definitive plan of treatment was formulated.

She began chemotherapy to shrink the tumor prior to a planned surgical resection. In the meantime, she was maximizing her nutritional status and taking some stress management classes with a local psychologist. Within a month, she was felt to be a surgical candidate to remove as much cancer as possible for best survival moving forward. She underwent a Whipple procedure with her oncology surgeon, and made a good recovery in during the next four weeks.

She was on oral morphine at discharge for residual pain, and her spirits were good. She was told that she had negative nodes and that an expectation for survival was reasonable. Her cancer was smaller than usual and the patient had a lot of hope and optimism.

The patient subsequently did well and was disease free for five years. She had her life back, and thanked God every day, and was grateful for her cancer team that gave her a second chance at life. This is an excellent patient outcome scenario.

Another possible scenario with this patient might have involved being told after her initial evaluation, that her cancer was non-operative and had spread all over her body, and that palliation would be given to improve her quality and length of life. She might have had palliative chemotherapy and given narcotics and herbal supplements.

If the patient had persistent pain with her palliative care moving forward, then she might have become a candidate for interventional pain management considering a celiac plexus neurolytic injection. The patient would then have been referred to a pain specialist for a risk-and-benefit discussion and told how the procedure worked, the likely pain relief result, and potential side effects. Had the patient decided for this, then in an outpatient setting, under fluoroscopic or CT scan guidance, a needle procedure with a neurolytic agent could be performed percutaneously through the skin to block the nerves to the abdomen that were responsible for the pain. This could result in weeks or months of relief as the patient continued to control symptoms, especially if the patient had less than six months to live.

For patients who are expected to live for only three months or less, an intrathecal spinal morphine pump is typically not considered. The intrathecal pump in a cancer care scenario is offered for patients on high dose narcotics who are very symptomatic or not well controlled, and who have typically greater than a three-month life expectancy.

PATIENT EXAMPLE #2: A 50-year-old female was diagnosed with metastatic breast cancer to her bones. She had a pathologic fracture of her femur leg bone that was fixed by her orthopedist with a plate and screws. After rehabilitation, she still had persistent pain, but from other bone metastases from her cancer.

She was on a high dose Duragesic fentanyl patch while taking oxycodone for breakthrough pain. She started to get sleepy and nauseous with slow increased titration of the medication. It was felt that she could be an intrathecal morphine pump candidate and subsequently was referred to a pain specialist for evaluation.

After a thorough discussion, the patient decided on an in-hospital intrathecal morphine test trial. She was in the hospital for three days and felt tremendous relief with no excessive side effects after two trial doses of medication. She decided on the permanent implantation of the spinal fluid catheter and morphine pump, to

take place one week from her hospital discharge date.

After successful implantation, and over the next two months, the patient was titrated to a 2 mg daily dose of continuous infusion intrathecal morphine, which was successful in controlling 90% of her pain without side effects. She was able to eliminate her Duragesic patch and took only an occasional Percocet for breakthrough pain. She used this pump for the next two years as her cancer advanced, and she expired comfortably in a hospice care setting with her family around her. Her family considered this to be a satisfactory resolution to the potential for end-of-life intractable pain, which was the primary concern once she had the diagnosis of cancer.

PATIENT EXAMPLE #3: An 80-year-old man who had developed metastatic lung cancer which had spread to his ribcage had been suffering with persistent intractable pain for two weeks. After bone scan imaging studies, the patient was found to have bony lesions in his right 7th and 8th ribs.

After evaluation, it was determined that the rib involvement represented the main area that was causing the most pain to the patient, even though he had been undergoing active cancer treatment for the lung cancer. Oral and intravenous narcotics were not effective in controlling this pain. In addition, the patient was on a muscle relaxant, anti-inflammatory medication, and anti-neuropathic medication. He was also symptomatic on these medications, with drug interactions which started to become intolerable.

It was suggested by his pain specialist that he might benefit from local anesthetic and steroid injections to desensitize his pain, and to help isolate diagnostically the exact pain source(s). After successful injections to the rib area which provided more than 50% relief for a week, the patient was thought to be a candidate for longer-term relief of his rib pain with a cryoanalgesia nerve freeze procedure.

The patient was told about the procedure, which involved placing a probe under each of the two involved ribs and freezing the intercostal nerves, and that it could offer weeks to months of relief. The patient had undergone the procedure and was satisfied with the result. With control of his symptoms, he was able to stop taking some of the medications that were giving him side effects.

He subsequently moved into a hospice care unit where he died comfortably two months later. The family was most grateful to the oncology and pain management team for providing their loved one with excellent end-of-life comfort care.

I trust this chapter will serve as an educational platform, with different patient examples of pain care scenarios, so that patients can see where their own pain *"fits in."* I have created a separate chapter at the end of this one, called **PITS Educational Pearls of Pain Care Wisdom**; and at the end of the book there is an extensive **PITS Glossary of Pain Terms** section for added information on specific topics, like pain conditions, medications, procedures, and so forth. Remember not to skip these important sections of the book, because they are vitally important as reinforcers of the overall pain knowledge that will help ensure your success in the **PITS Program**!

Pediatric and Obstetric Pain

SUMMARY: The management of **pediatric and obstetric pain** are part of the many medical care requirements for both pediatricians and obstetricians. These physicians, as well as their staff, have to deal with many different challenging painful conditions in their patients on a daily basis. Pediatric pain management is especially difficult in the very youngest infants and small children, and obstetric pain control needs to be timed just right so as not to slow down labor and delivery.

Specific Pediatric and Obstetric Pain Conditions

1. Pediatric Pain

Pediatric (newborn and children) pain should never be underestimated. When babies are born, they are born with a complete nervous system and can sense, transmit, and experience pain like any other adolescent or adult. Their pain receptors and pathways are fully developed and are susceptible to nociceptive and neuropathic pain states. Pediatric patients can experience the onset of pain from receptor activation in their skin. From the skin, pain is transmitted into the nervous system from peripheral nerves to the spinal cord. Upon reaching the spinal cord, the pain transmission moves up to the thalamus—a relay station on top of the brainstem—and then up to the brain cortex for interpretation and the final experience of the painful signals. There are modulating pathways and connections up and down the brain and spinal cord, which can adjust the pain transmission signals to a less intense level.

Neonates and children are given the same **P-I-T-S** *treatment protocol* options as adults and are typically treated by pediatric pain-trained physicians. Most children's hospitals in America have a pain expert on staff, typically a pediatric anesthesiologist who consults on difficult cases beyond the scope of the pediatrician.

For the sake of definition, it is assumed that adulthood begins at 18 years of age. Fortunately, chronic pain states are not as common in children as adults. They suffer from a lot of acute post-surgical and post-traumatic pain that is mostly of a nociceptive soft tissue pain type. Chronic pain can be due to a host of reasons, including sports injuries, post-surgical pain states, painful medical conditions, musculoskeletal problems like scoliosis and juvenile rheumatoid arthritis, childhood migraines, Crohn's disease and bowel obstruction, endometriosis, juvenile diabetes and neuropathy, complex regional pain syndrome (CRPS), cancers, and so forth. Back and neck are common pain areas. Abdominal pain in children from a psychogenic somatoform cause is a common scenario, particularly when children connect abdominal pain with the likelihood of missing school. Children who are raped can develop a lot of chronic pelvic pain. Certain painful cancers in kids are more common than in adults. Post-surgical pain from scarring can be a problem, especially after severe multi-surgery trauma victims or burn victims. Certain neuropathic pain states can also be a problem, especially if they develop a lot of CRPS-type of pain in their extremities after injury or surgery.

As far as the **P-I-T-S** *treatment protocol* is concerned, all four areas of pain care apply, depending on the pain condition. **Pills** or medications, even though many are not FDA-approved in neonates and children, are the mainstay of an initial pain management strategy. Many of the choices have been used safely in clinical pediatric pain management for years. Nonsteroidal anti-inflammatory medications, like ibuprofen, naproxen, and ketorolac, and opioid narcotics, like codeine, oxycodone, morphine, and hydromorphone, are the usual combination for most types of pain states that affect children. Antidepressants, anti-neuroleptics, and anti-spasm medication choices for neuropathic and nociceptive pains are used with wide frequency, again with off-label indication but with a clinical history of success and safety. The key is watching the patient closely, and when it comes to increasing doses, titrate slowly with time and monitor for potential side effects.

Injection options are peripheral and spinal nerve blocks with local anesthetic for surgery and trauma, trigger point injections for muscle spasms, epidural steroid injections for radiculopathy usually from herniated discs in the spine, and sympathetic local anesthetic injections for treatment of CRPS of the arms and legs. For the most part, the types of injections that help diagnose and treat adults can also help children.

Therapy is an important option that helps children maintain their functional status, and this is where physical and occupational therapy care can be vital. Also, the modalities of ice, heat, electrical stimulation, ultrasound, and TENS unit are helpful in treating painful recurrent conditions. Regarding multidisciplinary therapy options, there is psychological care for anxiety and depression, restorative sleep approaches, and complementary care techniques, like acupuncture, massage, music therapy, and the use of natural products—Echinacea, fish oil/omega-3 fatty acids, and flaxseed oil.

In terms of **Surgery**, there are many procedures that offer millions of acute and chronic pediatric pain patients a chance at a better life, especially when they have a chronic illness at an early age. Orthopedic, neurosurgeons, plastic, urology, cardiothoracic and general pediatric surgeons are all very active with new cases to offer operations for intractable pain in those pediatric patients who fail both medical and interventional pain management options.

A general surgeon may correct a newborn's pyloric stenosis, which is narrowing of a part of the small intestine resulting in abdominal pain and projectile vomiting. A urologist may repair a child's painful inguinal hernia. An orthopedist may repair a teenage torn ACL knee ligament from a soccer injury. A neurosurgeon may correct a teenager's advanced painful scoliosis curvature of the spine. Finally, a plastic surgeon may perform multiple skin grafts for a child's severe third-degree arm and leg burns or facial deformity.

PATIENT EXAMPLE: A 7-year-old child with sickle cell disease had a recurrent sickle cell crisis with severe leg and back pain. After admission to the hospital, the patient was given a low dose of Elavil for pain and sleep at night, and intravenous morphine every three hours titrated to relief effect. The patient's pain was slowly resolving after hydration and antibiotics and sickle cell care with his pediatrician.

After three days, the patient converted to a short course of Percocet, and did well in the subsequent days that followed. One week later, the boy was discharged from the hospital with complete resolution of the pain condition.

Now, if the patient in this example were older, had severe pain, and could understand the operation of an intravenous patient-controlled analgesia (IV-PCA) pump, then he could have been a candidate for starting an IV-PCA morphine pump on a low dose per button push. The older patient could then titrate his dose of comfortable morphine on his own, with the usual safe monitoring by nurses, staff, and physicians. The IV-PCA pain pump could be used for a short course of two-to-three days or longer if needed, and then after control of the painful symptoms, the patient could be converted to oral analgesics and then subsequently discharged.

In still another scenario, this patient could have received intravenous Toradol (ketorolac) every six hours for a few days to serve as a powerful anti-inflammatory pain medication, to work synergistically with the morphine narcotic. This is an example of one medication increasing the effectiveness of another medication when taken together.

2. Obstetrical Pain

Obstetrical (OBGYN) pain should never be accepted as a part of life that is a *"necessary evil."* The pain of childbirth can be quite severe when measured in women who experience other pain states, such as muscular pain or sciatica pain or arthritis pain. A lot of attention has been given to making childbearing more comfortable for women and to improve the inpatient birthing experience which is usually a joyous time.

There are many painful conditions that pregnant woman can suffer from, but the main focus of this chapter will be on labor and delivery (L&D) obstetrical pain. One of the tricky aspects of women who are pregnant is that as their uterus expands, and their abdomen increases, it may cause strain and sprain to the spinal structures. If a patient had a bad back to begin with prior to becoming pregnant, then this can be exacerbated during pregnancy. Sciatica symptoms may flare at any time in the pregnancy period, and can be quite debilitating at times. These symptoms need to be treated conservatively, because chronic pain injections of steroid and local anesthetic that may have been offered before the pregnancy, are rarely performed during a pregnancy due to the risk of precipitating a miscarriage.

During labor, early pain is due to the uterine contractions and later pain comes as the cervix dilates and the infant moves through the birth canal for delivery. Strategies for pain control are formulated by the obstetrician and anesthesiologist around these two kinds of L&D pain.

In terms of the **P-I-T-S** *treatment protocol* options, all four categories of care apply. However, this is based on the specific patient's medical condition at the time of delivery and the patient's personal pain control desires. **Pills** or medications are used initially to control early labor. Common medication choices are in the opioid narcotic category, and include Demerol (meperidine), morphine, Dilaudid (hydromorphone), fentanyl, and Stadol (Butorphanol-IV and inhaled form). Doses of intravenous (IV) or intramuscular (IM) opioid narcotic are often given by the obstetrical nurses in the OBGYN suite—as written by the OBGYN physician or nurse practitioner. Intravenous patient-controlled analgesia (IV-PCA) narcotic pain pumps are also available, where the patient gives themselves a dose of pain medication as needed, per a specified interval of time.

In terms of **Injections** or interventional pain techniques, the lumbar epidural catheter technique with a local anesthetic, with or without the addition of an opioid narcotic, infusion is the most common analgesic technique for women in labor right up until delivery. If the woman had a previous lumbar spinal surgery, or a coagulation issue with low platelets from preeclampsia, then she might not be a candidate for this type of injection which could risk spinal bleeding with subsequent spinal cord compression and paralysis weakness in the legs. If patients are not candidates for spinal or epidural analgesia, then intermittent doses of intravenous narcotic are used until delivery.

Pain management **Therapy** choices include psychological care for anxiety and depression around the childbirth period, restorative sleep approaches to avoid exhaustion, and any complementary techniques, like massage and meditation.

Regarding **Surgery** techniques, if women require cesarean sections, then spinal and epidural techniques can be used to block pain from the abdomen down to the feet. If a woman cannot have an epidural for medical reasons, then they have their cesarean section under general anesthesia.

Some women prefer not to have an epidural at all, because of the risks associated with a spinal procedure. They want to deliver their baby naturally, perhaps with a holistic approach that involves deep breathing and relaxation meditation. The degree of pain that a birthing mother can endure varies greatly, and it is up to the individual patient to decide how much interventional pain management they are willing to accept.

However, most women prefer epidural analgesia because of its effectiveness in decreasing labor and delivery pains. Epidural analgesia is not without its potential side effects, like any procedure and treatment process, but on the whole, the labor and delivery process with epidural pain relief typically runs smoothly. Sometimes obstetricians feel that an epidural local anesthetic may delay labor, which may not be in the best interests of the fetus. If the epidural local anesthetic is too late, a patient may miss its window of relief opportunity during the labor-to-delivery transition period. Often, an anesthesiologist will combine a spinal fluid dose of narcotic first to minimize delaying the progression of labor, and then start an epidural local anesthetic continuous infusion later for the rest of the labor and delivery process. This is known as a *combined spinal-epidural technique.*

Once the baby is delivered and the epidural catheter is removed, women may have oral or intravenous narcotics as they move into the postpartum or after delivery care period. If they have some muscle spasms, especially after cesarean section, or low back pain after labor, they may be more comfortable with muscle relaxants to reduce spasm. They may prefer a gentler analgesic, such as Tylenol (acetaminophen) or Ultram (tramadol), for their postpartum pain care. Cesarean sections usually heal up quite well, with a low single incision approach, and it is uncommon for a woman to develop a post-cesarean surgery chronic pain state.

When it comes to the use of pain medications during the pregnancy itself, a very conservative care approach with maternal pain medications is encouraged. This is to avoid the developing fetus from becoming exposed to possible and known teratogenic or birth defect causing agents. Opioid narcotic medications are given a warning in pregnancy that is known as a Category-C risk, meaning that human studies are not adequate to rule out potential problems. There is no way to test the use of opioid narcotics with pregnant humans due to ethical reasons, but animal studies have found birth defect problems in newborns.

Tylenol is probably the safest of all the pain agents, and is given a Category-B (no adverse effects in animal studies) rating in the United States. The safest muscle relaxant is Flexeril (cyclobenzaprine) which is Category-B, but the rest are Category-C, except for Valium, which is Category-D and harmful to the developing fetus. Anti-neuropathic medications (Cymbalta, Effexor, Neurontin, and Lyrica) are all Category-C pregnancy drugs.

As mentioned earlier, chronic pain injections—having an epidural steroid injection for a painful low back lumbar herniated disc—are not performed on pregnant women because of the risk of birth defects and miscarriage. The injectable steroids, Kenalog (triamcinolone) and Depo-Medrol (methylprednisolone), are Category-C pregnancy medications. Lidocaine local anesthetic is Category-B, while bupivacaine (Marcaine) local anesthetic is Category-C. Gentle therapy is most certainly to be used for symptomatic control of back and neck pain. If patients are actively exercising prior to pregnancy, then continuation is okay.

When it comes to a surgery option to relieve a chronic pain condition while undergoing obstetric care, this is almost never done unless there is a true emergency. All elective surgical pain procedures are put off until after the baby is born.

It is controversial for opioid narcotics to be prescribed during pregnancy. There are research studies that show several weeks before pregnancy right up until six-to-eight weeks after a woman becomes pregnant, narcotics can cause birth defects to the developing fetus's organs. This possibility requires a serious risk-and-benefit discussion among the prescribing physician, the obstetrician or other physician, and the patient. If certain women have been on narcotics prior to pregnancy, then the obstetrician may continue a certain amount of it during pregnancy, balancing potential risk to the baby versus the mother's well-being.

If women carry to term and they have been on narcotics, then there are issues of care with the newborn baby, especially narcotic tolerance and possible respiratory depression. Neonatologists and obstetricians are acutely aware of this, and take the proper precautions of post-delivery care in this scenario. The good news is that most pregnant women are minimalists and tend to prefer only the mildest of medications as a last resort.

PATIENT EXAMPLE: A 28-year-old woman and her husband were excited about the upcoming birth of their first baby. She had a history of chronic low back pain from a herniated lumbar disc for two years, and was able to come off her Vicodin narcotic and Cymbalta antidepressant prior to the pregnancy. It was not easy, but she was motivated by the strong desire to have a baby and to minimize the potential risk of a birth defect to the baby.

When it came time to deliver the baby, she was experiencing severe uterine contraction pains, and desired to have a labor epidural placed for pain control. She had been given a dose of IV Demerol earlier in the day, but the relief lasted only a few hours and it made her head feel funny. After discussion with the patient, obstetrician, and anesthesiologist on staff, the anesthesiologist placed an epidural catheter and started a continuous infusion of local anesthetic, with subsequent complete relief of the labor pain. Five hours later, she was ready to deliver the baby, and all went well with a vaginal delivery.

After the epidural catheter was removed and the local anesthetic wore off, the patient ended up taking a few doses of Percocet for pain relief. She and her husband were satisfied with the whole obstetrical and pain management experience and left the hospital two days later.

Now, if this patient had not been a candidate for a labor epidural catheter because of a previous low back operation, then an IV-PCA Dilaudid pump could have been offered for IV narcotic comfort until delivery.

Had the fetal heart rate become dangerously low for whatever reason, and the patient needed an emergency C-section with a crash general anesthetic and breathing tube, then this represents another birthing option in order to deliver the baby as soon as possible.

I trust this chapter will serve as an educational platform, with different patient examples of pain care scenarios, so that patients can see where their own pain *"fits in."* I have created a separate chapter at the end of this one, called **PITS Educational Pearls of Pain Care Wisdom**; and at the end of the book there is an extensive **PITS Glossary of Pain Terms** section for added information on specific topics, like pain conditions, medications, procedures, and so forth. Remember not to skip these important sections of the book, because they are vitally important as reinforcers of the overall pain knowledge that will help ensure your success in the **PITS Program**!

Emergency Room Pain

SUMMARY: Many patients will present to an emergency room (ER) have **emergency room pain**, both acute and chronic in nature. It is the primary job of the emergency room physician and staff to quickly determine the cause and severity of a patient's pain complaint in order to rule out life threatening conditions. True emergency conditions, especially with acute pain around the head and neck, chest, and abdominal areas, need rapid diagnosis and treatment for best patient outcome.

A cerebral aneurysm presenting with severe headache pain or an actual intracranial bleed is an emergency and needs neurosurgical attention. Any discovery of a space occupying lesion in the brain causing pain, whether it is tumor or infection, is an emergency and needs prompt neurosurgical care. Likewise, acute chest pain due to a myocardial heart attack needs cardiology care. A pulmonary embolism blood clot in the lungs causing chest pain and shortness of breath, is an emergency. A ruptured organ in the abdomen, like the appendix for example, resulting in acute peritonitis inflammation of the abdomen and pain, is another type of emergency.

These scenarios of acute pain in a life-threatening etiology are recognized and treated urgently in emergency room medicine, and again the appropriate specialty of medicine is consulted to deal with the presenting medical situation on an emergency basis. In most scenarios, true emergency pain management situations are ruled out, and these patients experience non-life-threatening conditions that are typically treated conservatively. Emergency room doctors are not meant to be chronic pain management doctors.

After most non-life-threatening pain diagnoses are evaluated and treated, ER physicians will then advise patients to follow up with their primary care physician (PCP) or other specialist as appropriate, their chronic pain management team—if they have one, or given a list of pain management doctors in the area. While patients are in the ER, their pain is typically treated with non-opioid narcotic medication first, like IV Tylenol or IV Toradol (ketorolac), but sometimes IV lidocaine or IV ketamine are administered, through a bolus or *IV push*, followed by a local anesthetic continuous infusion.

After this, if patients still have significant moderate-to-severe pain, they are typically given short courses of oral or intravenous opioid pain medication. If outpatient prescriptions are needed, a very short course, perhaps three days or up to a one week, are written until patients can follow up outpatient for continued pain management care. Unfortunately, many patients will be recurrent visitors to emergency rooms looking for additional opioid medications. Hopefully with better education and monitoring of opioid usage, this burden on the emergency rooms in America will lessen, and patients will follow up with outpatient pain providers for legitimate long-term care pain care. Hopefully, patients will continue to understand the healthcare crisis surrounding opioid prescriptions, and not be lured into *"doctor shopping"* anymore to obtain their medications.

Thankfully, true addiction is not common with chronic pain patients who are revaluated on a monthly basis by a pain management team, where potential problems can be picked up earlier rather than later. Most patients are generally concerned about their well-being, and are well connected with society, where they trying to work and raise kids and stay functional—and only go to an emergency room for a good reason. For these patients, basic history, physical examinations, and tests can be run in the emergency room situation to rule out emergencies, and then patients are given treatment and reassurance, and given basic instructions to return to their outpatient medical team. Sub-specialty referrals are commonly needed for certain rheumatologic conditions, neurological conditions, and surgical orthopedic conditions. With complicated pain management patient scenarios, these patients can be directly referred to a pain specialist in the community.

In terms of the **P-I-T-S** *treatment protocol* in an emergency room setting, acute pain management care choices dominate rather than chronic stable ailments, because of the nature of patient pain complaints. **Pill** or medication choices are typically of an IV variety, and mostly include IV Tylenol or Toradol, and IV morphine, Dilaudid, or fentanyl.

Injection management is mostly local anesthetic infiltration of skin lacerations that need to be sutured. Occasionally, the anesthesia pain specialist will be called to perform a peripheral nerve local anesthetic block, or place an epidural catheter for intermittent bolus or continuous infusion of a local anesthetic for anticipated extended periods of inpatient pain control.

Therapy choices are typically developed on an outpatient basis for patients who need it unless the patient is admitted to the hospital. However, more and more emergency rooms are offering short courses of acupuncture or massage for patients, as non-opioid complementary care approach. Otherwise, the therapist evaluates and treats the patient once they are admitted and on the hospital ward. Other pain management therapy choices in an ER setting include psychological care strategies to reduce anxiety and depression, restorative sleep techniques, and other options such as deep breathing, meditation, and guided imagery. More and more hospitals are setting up complementary and alternative medicine (CAM) departments to assist with hospital-based care issues.

In terms of **Surgery** choices, as mentioned earlier, the ER staff will contact the appropriate surgical specialty if a patient needs immediate or urgent surgical correction of an acute pain condition, like appendectomy for acute ruptured appendicitis.

PATIENT EXAMPLE #1: A 25-year-old female with known history of migraines with aura –visual and auditory changes preceding the migraine—started experiencing the worst headache of her life with persistent pain and numbness in her left arm and jaw, while she was at work. She was under a lot of stress at work, and trying to make a deadline with an important project. Her regular abortive triptan headache medication and backup Dilaudid opioid narcotic were ineffective in bringing the symptoms under control, so a colleague drove her the nearest emergency room for evaluation.

The patient had never been to the ER for a migraine before, but she was worried that she may be having a stroke or heart attack because of the severity of the pain and symptoms. Right after the ER triage process, the patient was told she needed a brain MRI to rule out the possibility of an intracranial bleed or cerebral neurologic event—since this was the worst headache of her life and it was associated with neurologic symptoms of numbness.

She was also told she would need an EKG electrocardiogram and blood work to rule out a possible cardiac event, since she was experiencing left arm and jaw pain, as well. When all the tests came back negative, the migraine pain was eventually stopped with a combination of 100% oxygen, a dose of 1 mg IV dihydroergotamine (DHE), and a dose of 60mg IV Toradol (ketorolac nonsteroidal anti-inflammatory medication). The patient was reassured and told to follow up with her headache neurologist in a week for outpatient reevaluation and possible medication adjustments.

Now, had this same patient unfortunately experienced a rare bleeding aneurysm, then she would have been seen urgently by a neurosurgeon for emergency care options. Ruling out secondary-headache emergency conditions is always the key in the ER, especially if a patient ever complains of the very *first* severe headache of their life, the very *worst* headache of their life, or any headache that is associated with *neurological* changes they may be experiencing.

PATIENT EXAMPLE #2: A 45-year-old male with chronic low back pain was otherwise stable on his monthly outpatient Percocet opioid narcotic medication. He suffered a slip-and-fall accident on ice outside his back door and had to be brought to the emergency room for evaluation. While in the ER, he was complaining of new numbness and weakness in his right leg, associated with 8/10 level of pain—on a scale from 0–10, where 0 is *no pain* and 10 is the *worst pain imaginable.*

He was smart to have remembered to bring a note from home outlining his chronic pain management care from his outpatient pain specialist, and when he asked for pain medication for his symptom exacerbation, the ER staff was reassured that the patient was legitimate, and not drug seeking.

When an emergency lumbar MRI came back as showing a large right-sided L4-5 level disc herniation, the orthopedic spine surgeon on call was notified to see the patient before discharge. When the surgical evaluation was completed, the patient was given the option of outpatient interventional pain management to consider a lumbar epidural steroid injection (LESI), or a surgical discectomy to be performed as an inpatient.

He decided on continued outpatient care, and thus was discharged from the ER with a three-day supply of stronger Percocet for his increased pain symptoms, until his pain specialist could reevaluate his situation. Had this patient developed true *cauda equina* herniated disc spinal nerve injury with bowel and bladder changes, then he would have needed urgent spinal surgery decompression to prevent permanent nerve damage.

PATIENT EXAMPLE #3: An 8-year-old male sickle cell patient, with a history of four ER visits per year, returned to the hospital emergency room complaining of severe leg pain. He had become terribly dehydrated while playing basketball with his friends, and this is what he felt sent him into acute physical distress. An intravenous was inserted and aggressive hydration was started. He rated his leg pain at a range of 7–10/10 and was given IV Toradol and oral oxycodone.

An hour later, he still complained of significant pain and was given a total of three IV doses of morphine 15 minutes apart. It was decided at this time that the patient should be admitted for a few days, to monitor the acute sickle cell crisis event. The acute pain anesthesia team was consulted to consider starting an IV-PCA morphine pain pump for the patient to use for a few days, until the pain settled down to the point of oral narcotic control levels. The patient did indeed do well with excellent use of the IV-PCA pain pump without side effects for three days, before converting to low dose Percocet and Motrin for pain control at discharge. Three days after being home, he was able to stop the Percocet and got back to his active life.

I trust this chapter will serve as an educational platform, with different patient examples of pain care scenarios, so that patients can see where their own pain *"fits in."* I have created a separate chapter at the end of this one, called **PITS Educational Pearls of Pain Care Wisdom**; and at the end of the book there is an extensive **PITS Glossary of Pain Terms** section for added information on specific topics, like pain conditions, medications, procedures, and so forth. Remember not to skip these important sections of the book, because they are vitally important as reinforcers of the overall pain knowledge that will help ensure your success in the **PITS Program**!

Acute Pain

SUMMARY: Four of the most common types of **acute pain** that we experience are post-operative pain, post-traumatic pain, acute burn injury pain, and acute medical illness pain. These pain conditions involve inflammatory, nociceptive pain types, but neuropathic pain can also play a part in *mixed* acute pain state conditions—both soft tissue and nerve involvement, for example. Acute pain sensations with their normal physiological responses serve a protective bodily function, and immediately remind patients that they need to stop and treat the acute cause of the discomfort, or they put themselves at risk of worsening illness or death.

Acute pain is different than chronic pain, which does not serve a protective and survival purpose. Acute pain is usually self-limited to hours, days, weeks, or months, depending on the cause, from a thorn prick to the thumb versus sustaining multiple long-bone fractures in a car accident, and finally resolves after full healing. Chronic pain conditions—although all chronic conditions first start out as acute pain episodes—are long-lasting, can last for months to years, and may never go away or fully heal for many patients.

In general, the **P-I-T-S** *treatment protocol* involves all four categories of **Pills**, **Injections**, **Therapy**, and **Surgery**, depending on the timing and need for individual patient situations.

Specific Acute Pain Conditions

1. Post-Operative Pain

Post-operative pain is an acute inflammatory nociceptive pain, with or without a neuropathic pain component. Nociceptive pain can be of both a somatic and visceral nature after surgery, depending on the type of surgery. Somatic pain involves skin, soft tissue, fascia, bone, tendons and ligaments, and muscles. Visceral pain typically involves the internal organs. If patients undergo an orthopedic bony surgery, this is an example of somatic pain. If patients undergo an appendectomy or gallbladder removal, then this is a type of visceral pain. Also, when surgeons open the abdomen, this causes a somatic pain component involving the abdominal wall tissues. Most surgery is done on an outpatient basis, but if patients are inpatient there are more options available to control post-operative pain.

For outpatient surgery, when pain is expected to be mild-to-moderate, patients typically are discharged on oral analgesics, whether anti-inflammatory, like

Motrin, Mobic, Celebrex, or an opioid narcotic, like the mild opioid-like drug tramadol, and Tylenol #3, Vicodin, or Percocet. Also, muscle relaxants, like Flexeril, Baclofen, Robaxin, or Zanaflex, are used, and in some cases anti-neuropathic agents, like Neurontin, Lyrica, Cymbalta, or Elavil, are prescribed. Some patients have indwelling disposable local anesthetic continuous infusion pumps that are removed at home a day or two later.

In terms of inpatient care, depending on the severity of pain, patients have options of intermittent intravenous opioid narcotic medications given by nurses, an intravenous patient-controlled analgesia (IV-PCA) pump, or indwelling epidural catheters with continuous infusion local anesthetic and opioid. Patients can also be offered local anesthetic nerve blocks to aid in post-operative pain control. These common and safe nerve blocks, often performed by the anesthesiology team, typically last for many hours and can control the vast amount of initial severe pain, while narcotic levels are being adjusted. As the block wears off slowly, the patient can stay ahead of the pain that returns by taking oral pain medication as directed.

After surgery that has severe pain associated with it, patients will start with titrated intravenous narcotic for several days then switch to oral narcotic in anticipation of outpatient use. If patients start with an epidural catheter pain control managed by the hospital anesthesiology team, then they will be converted to oral narcotic after the epidural catheter is removed.

There are a few choices for intravenous narcotic, like morphine, Dilaudid, or fentanyl, and a lot of choices for oral narcotic, both long-acting and short-acting, depending on an individual patient's severity of pain. Long-acting choices include, OxyContin, a Duragesic patch, MS Contin, and others. Short-acting choices include, Tylenol #3, Percocet, Vicodin, and Dilaudid by mouth, and many others. After certain surgeries patients will undergo a period of post-operative physical therapy, such as after total knee or hip replacement. The key will be to try to wean down on your opioid as soon as you can, as surgical recovery progresses.

In anticipation of severe post-operative pain, prior to the surgery patients can receive what is called *pre-emptive medication*. Choices include anti-inflammatory medications in the form of Celebrex (a nonsteroidal drug) or Decadron (a steroid drug), anti-neuropathic medications in the form of Neurontin (gabapentin) and Lyrica (pregabalin), or intravenous Tylenol or IV ketamine, all of which can aid in a smoother post-operative pain control experience. There is research showing that this preemptive analgesia approach may translate into the need for less narcotic use post-operatively, which may lead to less side effects of treatment.

The concept is that by blocking the pain mechanism pathways before incision and surgery, patients will feel less post-operative pain sensitivity at the surgical and surrounding tissue site. This multimodal approach, with using different medication types that work on different types of pain mechanisms for pain management, is being better understood for treating both acute and chronic pain scenarios. Where local anesthetic nerve blocks can be employed during an operation as preemptive analgesia, this will also aid in a smoother surgical recovery period.

Many patients will choose to undergo general anesthesia combined with a nerve block or epidural catheter, especially for major abdominal-thoracic, vascular, and joint replacement surgeries. Research has shown that aggressive control of pain after major surgery, such as vascular and thoracic in an intensive care setting, can translate into decreased post-operative cardio-pulmonary complications, such as heart attack and pneumonia. Research has also shown that aggressive control of acute post-operative pain can decrease the likelihood of developing a chronic pain state, even after healing from the initial surgery.

PATIENT EXAMPLE #1: A 34-year-old female had undergone an abdominal hernia operation with mesh repair. She had 7/10 pain in the hospital recovery room, where on a 0–10 verbal pain scale, 0 is *no pain* and 10 is the *worst pain imaginable*. An anesthesiologist started an IV-PCA pain pump with morphine and titrated this to the patient's comfort. She was satisfied with this pain control modality, as her pain settled down to a 3/10 level.

She continued the IV-PCA for the next two days on the surgical floor, without excessive side effects. Her oral intake status returned, and she was switched off the

IV-PCA and on to Percocet successfully. She was discharged from the hospital on day five with a prescription of Percocet to use as needed at home, until her first outpatient follow-up 7 days later with the surgeon.

PATIENT EXAMPLE #2: A 69-year-old male had entered the hospital for an elective total knee replacement. Prior to the surgery, after a risk-and-benefit discussion between the anesthesiologist and patient, a femoral nerve block with long-acting local anesthetic was performed to offer improved post-operative pain control, along with a combined general anesthetic.

The patient was given an IV-PCA Dilaudid pump after surgery and did well for the next two days in his continuous passive motion (CPM) machine. Thereafter, he was started on the long-acting narcotic OxyContin in anticipation of rehabilitation pain control. He experienced some breakthrough pain of 6/10 after the IV-PCA was discontinued, so small doses of Percocet were used for immediate-release pain control, which knocked the pain down to 2/10, a much more manageable pain score for this patient. He was discharged from the hospital at day five and did well thereafter in outpatient therapy, weaning off all his opioid narcotic within a month.

PATIENT EXAMPLE #3: A 70-year-old female had an elective abdominal aortic aneurysm repair with a combined epidural catheter infusion of local anesthetic and general anesthetic. The epidural anesthetic helped control a lot of immediate pain during her ICU care. She was able to deep breath and cough, and was comfortable enough to make a smooth transition out of the ICU and on to the post-operative surgical floor. The epidural was discontinued prior to leaving the ICU, and she was placed on an IV-PCA Dilaudid pump. After a few days she was again transitioned to oral narcotic, and did well thereafter with 2/10 pain at the time of discharge.

2. Post-Traumatic Pain

A **post-traumatic pain** cause, whether it is due to a motor vehicle accident, slip-and-fall, work-related accident, or recreational sports, can present with acute pain of a moderate-to-severe nature that mandates immediate attention. In a motor vehicle where patients may have sustained multiple bone fractures, this can present as a very painful acute inflammatory nociceptive somatic type of pain. Once patients are stabilized in the emergency room or trauma room, small amounts of intravenous narcotic can be titrated to reasonable comfort, again if their vital signs are stable and there is not a great concern for possible head injury—intracranial bleeding or abnormal cranial neurologic signs.

If a patient's mental status is okay, the patient may be slowly given small amounts of narcotic to reasonable comfort effect. This is preferred to patients spiking with 8–10/10 pain. Small amounts of narcotic, such as morphine, will calm down the stress response that trauma puts on the body and brain of these unfortunate patients. A whole host of pain control devices and techniques become available to trauma victims as they stabilize in the ICU and later in the hospital ward. These include opioid narcotic pumps, intermittent intramuscular and intravenous injections, long-acting oral opioids and transcutaneous opioids, and peripheral nerve blocks with local anesthetic.

Patients should realize that nearly all hospitals have a pain management service for consultation and treatment, and as such, if they feel their pain is not adequately managed by the surgical team alone, then the pain specialist on staff should be consulted to help with the case—especially if current therapies are failing to get pain scores below 5/10 levels.

In addition to a lot of somatic pain that trauma patients may experience, they can also experience visceral or organ-related pain, especially if they injure the liver or spleen and develop hematomas. Depending on the type of trauma pain, patients can experience nociceptive, neuropathic, or mixed nociceptive-neuropathic pains. It becomes important for the pain management team to follow a multi-modal treatment approach, using appropriate analgesics based on the mechanism of action specific for the type of pain(s) involved. We have anti-inflammatory medications, opioid narcotics, muscle relaxants and anti-neuropathic agents. Patients are often anxious and/or depressed and cannot sleep well in the hospital, so there are many choices of medications to utilize for addressing these issues.

PATIENT EXAMPLE: An 18-year-old male was involved in an automobile accident and sustained multiple injuries to his bones and internal organs. He was stabilized in the emergency room and X-rays and CT scans revealed fractures of his right humerus in the upper arm and left femur in the leg. An abdominal CT scan revealed a liver hematoma, but no major hemorrhage.

The patient was complaining of 8/10 pain in his abdomen and arm and leg. After stabilization, he was given small doses of intravenous morphine, 2 mg every 5–10 min, until the pain level was a 4/10. His vital signs remained stable. His blood cell count was low, and he needed a blood transfusion. The surgical trauma team felt that he might need exploratory abdominal surgery for the liver if the blood cell count continued to drop. He was brought to the ICU and monitored. He was not allowed to eat or drink at this point. The nurses in the ICU brought the patient IV narcotic every 2–3 hours as needed for his comfort.

He was subsequently placed on a Duragesic fentanyl narcotic patch as a baseline analgesic for continuous comfort, as he began his healing process. He was fortunate to have avoided surgery. At this point, the orthopedic team had casted the two fractured bones. By the first week, his pain was better controlled and he was deemed stable, so he was transferred to the floor on oral Vicodin for pain, along with the Duragesic patch. He was given ibuprofen for inflammatory pain which helped in addition to his narcotic.

He experienced spasms at times in his arm and leg and was prescribed Flexeril three times a day, as an antispasmodic drug. He had some difficulty sleeping at times and was given a sleep medication for a more restorative rest. With further healing, he was discharged from the hospital at day fourteen, to follow up the following week for the start of outpatient rehabilitation.

3. Burn Injury Pain

Burn injury pain is a type of acute inflammatory nociceptive somatic pain that is typically severe to patients, in terms of all the repetitive dressing changes that need to be done, as the burns slowly heal. This is a type of severe acute pain that need immediate control, typically with intravenous opioid narcotic, either by IV-PCA machine or given in intermittent bolus by the burn unit team. Also, IV ketamine is used as an anesthetic-type drug for pain control, which works differently to control pain compared to opioids. Many patients go on to surgical skin grafting of their wounds. This is very difficult, especially in children, who need frequent dressing changes, as the pain can get intolerable and become quite frightening. Doses of intravenous propofol, ketamine, and Versed (midazolam, a valium-type drug) can be given for burn dressing changes. Eventually skin grafting speeds up the healing process and allows for full recovery.

PATIENT EXAMPLE: An 11-year-old boy had inadvertently knocked over a pot of boiling water on the kitchen stove, while playing tag with his sister, and sustained severe burns to his left arm. He was brought to the local hospital burn unit where it was felt that the boy had suffered third-degree burns on most of his forearm. He had undergone multiple dressing changes for one week, followed by skin grafting.

He had horrible pain initially, and was given IV narcotic analgesics and valium-type drugs for the pain and anxiety while in the burn unit. This was successful in controlling pain down to 3/10 as a baseline comfort, but he did need additional medication after each dressing change. He was given IV Toradol (ketorolac), a potent nonsteroidal anti-inflammatory medication, to aid in his pain control, as he started to wean off the narcotic. One of his parents was always in attendance and this also aided in controlling the emotional pain component and the mental trauma associated with such burns. The parents were concerned about possible addiction developing to all the Fentanyl narcotic pain killer and Versed sedation medication their child had received, but were reassured that that likelihood was small compared to the medication treatments needed to control all the severe pain and anxiety that their child would have had to endure—which was not acceptable.

The child made a speedy recovery and was discharged from the burn unit on day 12, to follow up with the plastic surgeon for continued outpatient care and therapy. He required a short course of Tylenol with codeine at home, and then was able to switch to Motrin as needed.

4. Acute Medical Illness Pain

There are many types of **acute medical illness pain** conditions that are associated with moderate-to-severe pain. Nociceptive and neuropathic pain types can arise, including acute gout, shingles, gallbladder and kidney stone attacks, acute pancreatitis, and so forth. Anti-inflammatory and oral narcotics are the mainstay of pain treatment, but intravenous narcotic is often needed when trying to get the visceral-type pain of pancreatitis and kidney stones under control, especially in a hospital setting. Acute pancreatitis is an example of severe visceral nociceptive pain, typically due to gallstones or alcohol, or other etiology.

Patients are frequently put on intravenous narcotic when admitted to the hospital, hopefully for a short course, but can drag on for many weeks with severe pain cases. Only when patients are able to tolerate liquids and soft foods again, can they be successfully converted to oral narcotics or narcotic patches, like the Duragesic and Butrans patches.

Patients who have alcohol as the cause of their illness are always advised that this behavioral habit has to cease, in order for their pancreatitis to heal fully and to decrease future attacks. Otherwise, these patients are at serious risk of morbidity—illness symptoms and signs—and mortality or death with the pancreatitis disease pathological process. Unfortunately, many patients with acute pancreatitis go on to develop chronic pancreatitis, necessitating frequent hospitalizations throughout the year.

PATIENT EXAMPLE: A 57-year-old alcoholic male was admitted to the hospital for acute abdominal and flank pain and was diagnosed with acute pancreatitis. His liver function tests (LFTs) were markedly elevated. He was given intravenous morphine in intermittent IV boluses by the nursing staff for two days until his pain settled down. He was not allowed to anything by mouth at this point, and with continued need for analgesia, he was given a Duragesic patch. He was given aggressive medical care and he slowly gained his appetite back at day five, and was taken off the IV narcotic component in favor of oral narcotic. By day six, he was eating again, his liver enzymes improved, and was discharged home to come off narcotic altogether in the next week as an outpatient.

I trust this chapter will serve as an educational platform, with different patient examples of pain care scenarios, so that patients can see where their own pain *"fits in."* I have created a separate chapter at the end of this one, called **PITS Educational Pearls of Pain Care Wisdom**; and at the end of the book there is an extensive **PITS Glossary of Pain Terms** section for added information on specific topics, like pain conditions, medications, procedures, and so forth. Remember not to skip these important sections of the book, because they are vitally important as reinforcers of the overall pain knowledge that will help ensure your success in the **PITS Program!**

Post-Surgical Pain Syndromes

SUMMARY: Post-surgical pain syndromes are a multifaceted type of chronic pain that develops beyond six months after an original operation. Unfortunately, patients develop persistent pain soon after certain types of surgery even though they were fully expected to improve with the surgical correction. This can happen for a host of different reasons involving different types of surgery. It can happen after surgery involving herniorrhaphy hernia repair, after surgery when the chest wall is opened from a thoracotomy, and even after a total joint replacement. The pain that develops can be nociceptive, neuropathic, or mixed in nature, and can persist for months-to-years, or may never go away.

All four categories of the **P-I-T-S** *treatment protocol* apply to the treatment of various post-surgical pain syndromes. In terms of **Pills** or medications, all drug groups can help with medical pain management, including:

- Nonsteroidal and steroidal anti-inflammatories: Motrin, Aleve, Mobic, Celebrex, diclofenac, prednisone, Medrol Dosepak, and many others. Keep in mind Tylenol –although not an anti-inflammatory—has good centrally-acting pain relief.

- Anti-neuropathic medications: Elavil, Pamelor, Neurontin, Lyrica, Cymbalta, 5% Lidoderm patch, and others.

- Muscle relaxants: Flexeril, Zanaflex, Skelaxin, Robaxin, Baclofen, and others.

- Opioid narcotics: *Short-acting*, like Tylenol#3, Vicodin, Percocet, Dilaudid, and others like the mild centrally-acting opioid-like medication tramadol; and *Long-acting*, like OxyContin, MS Contin, Nucynta ER, Duragesic and Butrans patches, and others.

By combining different drug types, patients will benefit from synergistic boosting medication effects to improve overall pain relief potential.

In terms of **Injections**, if pain can be desensitized like the neuropathic pain component of a nerve entrapment injury, then local anesthetics like lidocaine and Marcaine can be combined with the steroids Depo-Medrol or Kenalog, and injected as treatment with the expertise of an interventional pain specialist. Patients who receive these injections often have a lowering of their pain intensity, which then makes it easier to manage the pain with medications and therapy. Other interventional techniques include, radiofrequency burning lesioning or ablation of certain sensory nerves, usually around the knee after painful total knee replacement, and cryoablation freezing of painful nerves, typically performed for a neuroma scar after a hernia operation.

In terms of **Therapy**, there are many choices that can aid patients in achieving maximum comfort and function. These include physical therapy options with or without myofascial release techniques, chiropractic manipulation with or without *manipulation under anesthesia (MUA)*, occupational therapy as needed, a home exercise program with or without going to the gym, and seeing a rehabilitation physician or neuromuscular physician in consultation. Medications and injections will help break the pain cycle, allowing patients to better rehabilitate and maximize their pain control and overall quality of life. Other multidisciplinary therapy choices for post-surgical pain are, psychological care for anxiety and depression, restorative sleep techniques, and other complementary care techniques, such as acupuncture, massage, herbal therapies, and low-level laser therapy (LLLT).

Regarding **Surgery**, keep in mind that it was the original surgery that started the post-surgery pain syndrome, and to re-operate is a difficult decision to be pursued, so a detailed risk-and-benefit discussion about the re-operative healing process and post-operative pain management plan would need to be set before proceeding. Only in intractable pain cases, or patient cases where there is some element of ongoing neurologic compromise or entrapment, will an exploratory re-operation be considered, with the hope of finding and decompressing the ongoing structural problem that is underlying the painful symptoms.

Specific Post-Surgical Pain Syndromes

1. Post-Herniorrhaphy Pain Syndrome

Post-herniorrhaphy pain syndrome is a condition that occurs after an inguinal hernia operation. With this condition, patients can frequently have ilioinguinal neuralgia and myofascial scarring, with persistent numbness along the scar, and through the groin area. This type of pain happens frequently in patients who undergo multiple hernia repairs.

Conservative treatment starts with ice packs and anti-inflammatory medication or **Pills**, like Motrin and Aleve, and an anti-neuropathic agent like 5% Lidoderm patch, Neurontin, and Elavil. If there is a spasm pain component, then a muscle relaxant like Flexeril, Baclofen, Robaxin, Zanaflex, and others, can be added. Patients left with moderate-to-severe pain will frequently be placed on a short course of an oral opioid narcotic medication, like Vicodin or Percocet, or another type of opioid, like Nucynta. Also, analgesic creams like 4% lidocaine cream, CBD oil, and menthol/camphor sprays can also be attempted to desensitize the painful area.

Sometimes for persistent pain, **Injections** of steroid and local anesthetic can be placed into painful neuroma sites—sensitive areas of nerves and tissue. These injections can be done 1–2 weeks apart with up to three injections in total. If these injections are helpful but the pain reduction is only temporary, then neuromas can be frozen in an outpatient procedure using a cryo-analgesia probe. Freezing of a neuroma may offer many weeks or even months of relief.

In terms of **Therapy** choices, physical therapy myofascial release techniques can be attempted to break up scarring and soft tissue pain, and complementary care acupuncture, vitamins, and supplements may help control painful symptoms.

As mentioned earlier, only in extreme cases of intractable pain will patients undergo **Surgery** wound exploration, and only after risk-and-benefit discussion with an experienced reoperation hernia surgeon. Sometimes nerves get scarred during the healing process or nerves get caught up in sutures or in the implanted mesh repair. Fortunately, this is not a frequent problem encountered by skilled surgeons.

PATIENT EXAMPLE: A 30-year-old female had an elective left inguinal hernia repair with mesh reinforcement as an outpatient, and did well until one month into her recovery. Although the procedure had gone smoothly, and her scar was healed, she began to notice an increased sensitivity in the middle of the scar, and severe pain was reproduced when she pressed the scar in toward her stomach. When she returned to her hernia surgeon for evaluation, it was discovered on physical examination that she had developed a scar neuroma.

She was given treatment options of medications or injection desensitization, and she opted for medications at first. She was started on 5% Lidoderm patch and tramadol for two weeks, and she experienced a 50% overall improvement. However, she still had discomfort while wearing jeans, so she returned to the surgeon to consider injection therapy for additional comfort in the neuroma area. After a risk-and-benefit discussion, it was decided that she would undergo up to three injections of steroid and local anesthesia as needed into the neuroma to reduce the residual pain. After just one injection however, there was a dramatic reduction in the pain level and she was quite pleased. Over the next two months, the pain gradually subsided and she was back to her full activity and lifestyle.

Now, had injection therapy resulted in only temporary pain relief, then she would have been a candidate for cryoablation freezing of the neuroma for longer-term pain relief. And if even cryoablation proved to be ineffective, or even worse pain developed through time, then she could have considered exploratory reoperation to find the neuroma, excise it, and bury the exposed nerve area in deeper tissue to protect it more from external pressure.

2. Post-Thoracotomy Pain Syndrome

As for **post-thoracotomy pain syndrome**, thoracic chest wall surgery can involve damage to ribs, muscle, and intercostal nerves—the small nerves that run under each rib from the back to the front—due to the nature of the surgical procedure involving opening and stretching the ribs and tissues. When patients undergo long complicated chest surgery procedures, or if a surgery requires multiple rib areas to be removed, these scenarios represent some of the main risk factors that can give rise to residual longer-standing pain symptoms, long after the surgical wound site has healed. This type of persistent pain after a thoracotomy procedure is what is termed post-thoracotomy pain syndrome. This post-operative pain syndrome can involve both a nociceptive type of bone and muscle and fascia pain and a neuropathic type of intercostal nerve pain, and therefore, different strategies need to be directed to treat both these types of pain mechanisms.

As for **Pills** or medications, anti-neuropathic and muscle relaxant medications are commonly used to decrease intensity and frequency of pain symptoms. Opioid narcotics can also be prescribed for more intense pain occurrences.

Intercostal nerve **Injection** blocks can be offered to desensitize sharp shooting nerve pain sensations that can wrap around the chest wall. This is accomplished with steroid and local anesthetic injections, placed under each of the affected rib levels under fluoroscopic guidance, on an outpatient basis. Patients can typically undergo up to three injections, a week apart, to reach optimum relief effect. Cryoablation freezing of intercostal nerves is also an option for longer-term relief, if needed.

Therapy should be focused at keeping the patient's respiratory status optimized and to prevent frozen shoulder syndrome, which happens when patients do not want to move their arms due to *guarding* or protecting themselves from the thoracotomy pain.

Physical therapy is the mainstay of treatment here, but complementary therapy care is often utilized, as well, such as acupuncture and massage to desensitize pain.

Surgery reoperation for pain control is rarely done. Rather, the spinal cord stimulation (SCS) modality is offered for the most intractable patient pain cases.

PATIENT EXAMPLE: A 63-year-old male had a left sided thoracotomy incision to remove a small lung mass that was found to be benign. He did well with the two-hour operation without complication, and healed fully in a month following the surgery.

During this first postoperative month, the patient noticed a tingling sensation along the thoracotomy scar and did not think too much about it. By the start of the second postoperative month however, the patient started to experience sharp shooting rib pain that sent him immediately back to his thoracic surgeon for evaluation. Since the tumor was benign, and there was no cause for alarm that he might have cancer. His wound appeared well healed, but he had decreased skin sensitivity along the scar line. His surgeon felt that he may be experiencing neuropathic pain from irritated rib nerves, so he prescribed Neurontin (gabapentin) 100mg three times a day. After a week he was 40% improved with less sharp pain, but still had a lot of sensitivity pain from his back, through the scar area, and right up to the front of his chest wall area.

At this point, his surgeon referred him to an interventional pain specialist to consider desensitization injection therapy. After consultation with the pain specialist, and after undergoing three intercostal nerve injections a week apart, the pain intensity was dramatically reduced, and he was back to his normal activity level. Over the next six months, the residual discomfort diminished to 2/10, which was an acceptable level compared to his original discomfort.

3. Post-Total Joint Replacement Pain Syndrome

Post-total joint replacement pain syndrome involves the development of persistent pain after total joint replacements of the shoulder, hips, knees, or ankles. Pain from these syndromes can be from a nociceptive cause from bone, muscle, fascia, ligaments, and tendon involvement, or due to a neuropathic peripheral nerve cause, or both. Orthopedic joint replacement surgeons are very skilled, and do an excellent job at implanting prosthetics. But despite their level of skill, joint replacement patients sometimes experience persistent pain outside the joints that may be due to soft tissue scarring, contracture of muscles, and/or peripheral nerve injury.

This can be unnerving to patients who had expected near complete pain relief after the joint replacement, only to feel persistent pain, albeit less pain than prior to the surgery, when they were previously feeling bone-on-bone grinding pain. Conservative courses of oral medication or **Pills**, and limited **Injections** to outside the joint capsule or a radiofrequency ablation procedure of certain nerves called genicular nerves, can usually get patients back to manageable pain levels.

Physical **Therapy** is also important to stretch and improve mobility while reducing adhesions. If there are issues of contractures and adhesive capsulitis, then manipulation under anesthesia (MUA) can be an option, to *release* these pathologies and regain full mobilization. MUA is done by orthopedists, osteopaths, and certified chiropractors in a safe outpatient setting, usually in a hospital or surgi-center. MUA is performed under intravenous anesthetic to achieve an optimal stretching through a normal range-of-motion (ROM) manipulation, and of course, without a patient hurting as much during the manipulation.

Patients who elect to have MUA, will typically undergo three consecutive outpatient daily sessions under monitored IV sedation, followed by a series of office-based manipulations to maintain the added range-of-motion gained after the MUA sessions. After joint replacement, expert rehabilitation will help ensure maximum flexibility, strengthening and conditioning in the rehabilitative period to decrease the incidence of contracture and scarring.

It is not uncommon with postoperative healing in patients, that scarring which develops can result in limited range of motion, as mentioned. This is where early rehabilitation and patient motivation have the biggest impact in decreasing *static* scar formation, or

scar tissue that does not stretch or move functionally as it naturally forms. The goal is to optimize *dynamic* healing of scar tissue so that patients keep their full range-of-motion and maintain their functional status.

Surgery reoperation on previously replaced joints is typically reserved for the return of intractable pain and when the implanted device is too old or worn to continue to be effective and comfortable. Other uncommon reasons for repeat surgery include traumatic injury to the joint and implant, infection in the joint, and loosening of hardware or other internal derangement.

PATIENT EXAMPLE: A 70-year-old mail carrier was recently retired and was scheduled for a long-awaited right hip replacement. His orthopedist performed a total hip replacement—also known as total hip arthroplasty (THA)—that was technically challenging, but everything went well during the two-hour surgery. The patient had a smooth postoperative course, and was discharged to a nearby rehabilitation center for the next week.

During outpatient physical therapy over the next two months after leaving the rehabilitation center, he noticed a persistent muscle spasm in back of his right hip near the buttock region. When he returned to the hip surgeon, it was discovered on examination that he had an active trigger point in his piriformis muscle, which is a deep muscle underneath the gluteus muscles that overlies the sciatic nerve. All this pain was causing him to limp and not walk properly as instructed by his physical therapist. He was also starting to develop pain in the front of his hip, and this started to worry him, as well.

After more therapy and anti-inflammatory and narcotic medication failed to relieve the pain symptoms, he was referred to a pain specialist for evaluation. The pain specialist offered him a piriformis muscle spasm trigger point injection of a steroid and local anesthetic, which the patient promptly accepted. The outpatient X-ray guided injection was able to reduce the buttock pain by 50%, but the pain in the front of the hip persisted.

The hip surgeon repeated X-rays and the implant

appeared to be in good anatomical position and alignment. The ongoing pain was eventually attributed to post-operative soft tissue scarring outside the hip joint, and that the future treatment plan would be very conservative. Although the pain persisted for years, its periodic 5–8/10 pain episode intensity was managed with tramadol and Advil as needed, and with the use of a TENS unit.

Post-surgical pain syndromes are an ongoing major problem in the United States, as many susceptible patients develop persistent pain or experience worsening of their original pain problem after a surgical operation. Research has shown that aggressive post-operative pain management may aid in decreasing the incidence of developing post-surgery pain.

The nervous system seems to get overly sensitized by chemical changes due to uncontrolled pain signals from the surgical wound, where the peripheral nerves exist, that constantly bombard the spinal cord and brain. This leads to permanent structural and neuro-physiological changes in the nervous system that set up circuits (nerves and synapses) of persistent pain in a vicious cycle, even after full healing of the original inciting issue.

Frequent surgical causes of persistent pain are soft tissue scarring and localized peripheral neuropathic injury, and it is less likely that the pain is from the original surgical procedure. Many patients undergo repeat surgeries for the same condition, and this is a prime setup for a post-surgical pain syndrome, especially with multiple repeat abdominal, joint, and back surgery procedures.

I trust this chapter will serve as an educational platform, with different patient examples of pain care scenarios, so that patients can see where their own pain *"fits in."* I have created a separate chapter at the end of this one, called **PITS Educational Pearls of Pain Care Wisdom**; and at the end of the book there is an extensive **PITS Glossary of Pain Terms** section for added information on specific topics, like pain conditions, medications, procedures, and so forth. Remember not to skip these important sections of the book, because they are vitally important as reinforcers of the overall

pain knowledge that will help ensure your success in the **PITS Program**!

Chronic Abdominal and Pelvic Pain

SUMMARY: Chronic abdominal and pelvic pain affects millions of Americans and significantly impairs their quality of life. These are chronic pain patients who have persistent pain from a variety of different etiologies, and these types of pain are usually difficult to treat on a chronic basis. Much of the pain is visceral in nature, which means it originates in organs from within the abdominal and pelvic cavities. Different medical conditions can cause these pains, as well as post-surgical disorders.

A majority of abdominal-pelvic pain can arise from chronic bladder cystitis problems, endometriosis, or pelvic inflammatory disease (PID). The pain could also be from recurrent cholecystitis gallbladder attacks, pancreatitis, or inflammatory bowel disease, like ulcerative colitis or Crohns disease. Many patients will undergo surgical procedures in attempt to control these types of pains, but these procedures can sometimes fail to alleviate the symptoms, or in some cases make the symptoms worse, especially if abdominal-pelvic adhesions form.

Medications and lifestyle changes are the mainstay of chronic treatment, along with cognitive-behavioral care strategies to better cope with the stress of a chronic pain condition. Many patients do not want to accept that that have a chronic problem—they continue searching and hoping for a cure.

While there will always be miracle stories to tell, the majority of patients will experience years of chronic pain with little hope of it ever being completely eliminated. The best strategy for them is to *prepare* for expected exacerbations pain, so that their quality of life is impacted as little as possible. The **PITS Program** can help these patients manage their painful conditions proactively, and hopefully keep the spikes of severe pain to a minimum. Pelvic floor exercises and other exercise therapies for chronic pelvic pain are an important part of the multidisciplinary approach to overall wellness. Surgical options exist, but to be pursued only in specific clinical scenarios to optimize the best possible outcome, where benefit outweighs the risk of surgical intervention.

The **P-I-T-S** *treatment protocol* applies fully for the treatment of abdominal and pelvic pain conditions. As for **Pills** or medications, patients often in time will develop a multimodal oral analgesic mix of medications that often include nonsteroidal anti-inflammatories, such as Motrin and Aleve. To help manage spasms a muscle relaxant, like Flexeril and Zanaflex can be effective, as well as anti-neuropathic agents, like Elavil and Cymbalta or Ultram (tramadol) and Ultracet (tramadol and Tylenol combination). For severe recurrent pain cases, a non-oral opioid narcotic such as the Butrans patch or Duragesic patch can be considered.

When it comes to narcotics, there is always a need for a risk-and-benefit evaluation, because as much as opioids can help with the pain, they can also have serious negative side effects on the bowels and other parts of the GI tract. There is a risk of constipation and nausea. There is also the risk of limited organ sphincter function because of increased sphincter spasm—with the bladder it could be more difficult to urinate. High dose opioids are really a *double-edge-sword*—they can help but they can hurt. Balancing these opioid effects is the key to long-term beneficial narcotic management.

Abdominal-pelvic pain patients will often undergo diagnostic and therapeutic **Injections**, where interventional pain specialists place a local anesthetic and steroid around nerve plexuses in the abdominal-pelvic cavity, performed under fluoroscopic-needle guidance and intravenous sedation in an outpatient setting. This is attempted when medications have not controlled the pain adequately, and aims to target and block the origin of the painful sensations. These types of nerve blocks often reset a patient's pain threshold, and give them a physical and psychological break from the previously high pain levels.

Patients are encouraged to stay as functional as possible with various forms of **Therapy**, which include a lot of pelvic floor exercises and aerobic exercises to help keep up energy levels. The other multidisciplinary therapy choices are also important to consider, and include psychological care for pain-related anxiety and depression, restorative sleep approaches to ensure effective REM sleep quality, and other care options, such as acupuncture, massage, stress management and biofeedback, and herbal supplements.

In terms of **Surgery** options, exploratory surgery with laparoscopy, either by using a lighted wand-scope placed in the abdominal-pelvic cavity or by an open laparotomy (surgically opening the abdominal cavity), are performed for intractable pain cases to surgically correct the problem—for example, lasering pelvic endometriosis tissue or painful adhesions. If patients fail high dose oral narcotic medications, or they are too symptomatic on the narcotics, then they may be candidates for a trial of intrathecal spinal narcotic test dosing, and if successful, eventual implantation of an intrathecal morphine continuous infusion device. These spinal pain control devices are surgically implanted in the abdomen and spine by an interventional pain management team, and are only for the most intractable pain scenarios.

PATIENT EXAMPLE #1: A 26-year-old female had been suffering with what her obstetrician felt was a case of severe recurrent endometriosis. She had tried hormonal therapy and different oral analgesics, without success. She eventually underwent a laparoscopy with laser burning of endometriosis pelvic tissue, which resulted in significant relief. There was better control of the severity of the pain symptoms—from 8/10 pain down to 4/10 average pain—and was grateful to have her life back again. She was able to wean off all her pain medication in the following month, and did well thereafter.

PATIENT EXAMPLE #2: A 59-year-old male with Crohns disease had been on medication with his gastroenterologist and pain specialist physician for many years. He was watching his diet, but he had increasing episodes of more frequent and intense pain. He sought surgical evaluation with a colorectal surgeon who felt he was a surgical candidate at this point, to get control of his severe recurrent symptoms. He subsequently underwent resection of a portion of inflamed bowel, and recovered well. His pain had subsided 90%, and he was satisfied when he was able to completely wean off his narcotic medication two months later, with a much better quality of life.

PATIENT EXAMPLE #3: A 30-year-old female businessperson had unfortunately needed multiple abdominal surgeries surrounding a complicated gallbladder removal, and two repeat lysis of adhesion surgeries. This resulted in her having 8/10 abdominal pain flares every month. She started seeing a chronic pain specialist who recommended monthly methadone narcotic prescriptions to control this level of pain. She had failed Motrin, Flexeril, Lyrica, and Effexor medications through the years, as well as, failing multiple other narcotics, including Percocet, Vicodin, and the Duragesic patch, either due to lack of results or excessive side effects.

She slowly worked her way up to 5 mg of methadone, four times a day, over the next three months and this helped keep her usual chronic pain level at 4/10, which was acceptable to her. Once in a while she took Tylenol if she felt additional pain in between methadone doses. She was able to keep her job and take care of her family. Her husband was not thrilled that she was on methadone, but realized that she had a real pain problem, was certainly not an addict, and was not abusing the medication in any way. Thankfully, the patient did well on this regimen of pain control for many years and never needed any repeat surgery.

I trust this chapter will serve as an educational platform, with different patient examples of pain care scenarios, so that patients can see where their own pain *"fits in."* I have created a separate chapter at the end of this one, called **PITS Educational Pearls of Pain Care Wisdom**; and at the end of the book there is an extensive **PITS Glossary of Pain Terms** section for added information on specific topics, like pain conditions, medications, procedures, and so forth. Remember not to skip these important sections of the book, because they are vitally important as reinforcers of the overall pain knowledge that will help ensure your success in the **PITS Program**!

CHAPTER 7

PITS Educational Pearls of Pain Care Wisdom

This chapter will offer many insightful pieces of **P-I-T-S** *educational information* that can serve as pain care wisdom, to help a pain patient with their diagnosis and treatment progress, and with their overall pain management knowledge. In many ways, this chapter will serve as a *highlight review* of what has been examined in this book. It has been demonstrated over-and-over that the **PITS Program** can lead to better patient education and motivation, which in turn, can lead to better pain control treatment outcomes and an improved quality of life. At the very least, these pearls of wisdom will serve as ongoing reminders that there are many different integrative approaches to managing your pain and improving your quality of life. At best, these helpful bits of information will help you become, what I call, a *critical patient thinker*. This will allow you to participate in a more meaningful way with your healthcare pain provider team—your doctors, nurses, therapists, and so forth—so you can adjust your **P-I-T-S** *treatment protocol* as needed to best maximize your personal **PITS Score**—your **PITS Pain and Quality-of-Life Score** (see **APPENDIX A**). *Get motivated!*

The **Pain is the PITS Program** is an educational pain management program utilizing a disease-model clinical pathway and protocol for both the assessment and treatment of chronic pain, and for acute pain as well. This disease model is much like following a disease program for other medical conditions, like diabetes and hypertension. The **PITS Program** uses a structured

multi-disciplinary integrative chronic pain guideline, so that patients get the best coordinated comprehensive care possible based on their specific pain problem.

Any *PAIN* that a patient experiences can start the **PITS Clinical Pathway & Protocol for the Assessment & Treatment of Chronic Pain** (see **APPENDIX G**). Knowing that *all CHRONIC pain first starts out as ACUTE pain*, the treatment options will be based on an initial assessment and plan for that pain, as typically outlined by their physician-lead healthcare team. Any patient who remains in a state of persistent, continuous, chronic pain *needs a comprehensive medical care pain evaluation*—a history, physical examination, examination of radiology studies and other tests, followed by an assessment and plan—so they can begin to start their much-needed longer-term pain management care. This long-term pain care is typically accomplished under the care of a pain specialist, especially for difficult and complicated cases.

In terms of conducting an **Assessment** for pain management, it is very helpful to have a pain management specialist structure a multidimensional evaluation, focusing on pain and quality- of-life issues. This assessment leads to the **PITS Pain and Quality-of-Life Score**, also called the **PITS Score**, for short. Remember, the **P-I-T-S Assessment** sections include **P for Physical Function, I for Intensity of Pain, T for Thoughts and Behaviors,** and **S for Social**

Interactions. Each section focuses on key elements of the pain and quality-of-life assessment:

- The *Physical function section* of the **PITS Score** assessment focuses on your ability to work and take care of your home and children, your ability to do some exercise, and your ability to carry out activities of daily function like cooking, shopping, bathing, and so forth.

- The *Intensity of pain section* of the **PITS Score** assessment focuses on acceptable pain levels, the duration of pain relief, and any side effects of treatment from medications, injections, and so forth.

- The *Thoughts and behaviors section* of the **PITS Score** assessment focuses on control of anxiety and depression, getting restful sleep, and keeping your energy levels OK.

- The *Social interactions section* of the **PITS Score** assessment focuses on getting out with friends and family, traveling and doing hobbies, and having enough money and insurance coverage for your pain care.

Realize that a **CHRONIC** *pain assessment* requires, not only the evaluation of the pain itself, but also everything else in a patient's life that it affects—hence a 12-question assessment of the bio-psycho-social issues—not just the original 0–10 scale pain intensity score alone. The 0–10 pain scale that we are all accustomed to is best utilized for an **ACUTE** *pain assessment*, like for postoperative and traumatic pain clinical situations, when a quick one-dimensional assessment is needed before dosing an opioid narcotic for quick relief, for example.

In terms of developing a **Treatment** plan for pain management, it is very helpful to have a structured protocol plan for a multidisciplinary integrative approach to chronic pain care, and the **Pain is the PITS Program** provides that framework. Remember, the **P-I-T-S** *treatment protocol* sections include **P for Pills** or medications, **I for Injections, T for Therapy,** and **S for Surgery.** This integrative approach will balance all of these treatment options using the **PITS Program** *philosophy of care.*

When planning an acute or chronic back and neck pain program, as an example, it is important to involve the *necessary specialties of medicine*, including anesthesiology interventional pain management, physical medicine and rehabilitation, neurology and psychiatry, and spinal surgery. Depending on other types of pain, a patient may need rheumatology, palliative care and oncology, or OBGYN and pediatrics. Emergency room physicians provide their own assessment of pain, to rule out possible critical disease events that cause pain. Internal medicine and family practice physicians see most of the pain management patients in this country at initial evaluation, so they are critically involved with the initial plan for pain management. Their practices have thousands of patients with all kinds of chronic diseases that lead to chronic pain, so they often work in concert with a pain management specialist for the more complicated advanced pain patients.

The patient **Education** *component* to pain management is critical to the success of the **PITS Program**, so that patients can best understand what is wrong with them and how to get better, both on their own and with the help of their healthcare team. Patients themselves eventually will realize their true comfort path, through the combination of self-management and professional management as their pain is put into *remission.* Remember, acute pain is often curable but chronic pain is rarely curable, it is manageable—so you can get on living your life with more relief and overall quality.

The implementation of the treatment part of the program involves the **P-I-T-S** *treatment protocol* options of *P* for *Pills* or medications, *I* for *Injections, T* for *Therapy,* and *S* for *Surgery*—but realize that the **Therapy** *component* of the program is actually composed of four different areas of care:

- physical care options

- psychological care approaches

- restorative sleep strategies

- complementary pain management techniques

All four of these therapy treatment components taken together is what forms the **Pain is the PITS** comprehensive multidisciplinary *integrative therapy approach* to the management of all pain in general.

Pills or medications are frequently needed to treat pain, and, pharmacologic choices in the **PITS Program** include four basic categories: **anti-inflammatory medication**, **muscle relaxants**, **nerve pain agents**, and **opioid narcotics**:

- The two major *anti-inflammatory categories* are nonsteroidal anti-inflammatory drugs (NSAIDs) and steroids, both oral and injectable. NSAIDs are used to maintain anti-inflammatory comfort during time periods between powerful steroid dose injections—patients need to space steroid injections for pain control, to not only avoid localized bone and soft tissue damage where the injections are administered, but also to minimize the potential negative systemic or whole-body side effects of excessive steroids.

- *Muscle relaxants* and spasticity agents can be used to treat muscle spasms, depending on the specific pain condition.

- *Nerve pain agents* can be used directly for an approved pain condition, as approved by the FDA, or as *off-label medication usage*—off-label meaning not specifically studied for the approved use but used with clinical safety by physicians extensively for years with positive pain relief results.

- *Opioid narcotics* are of both short-acting and long-acting varieties. A typical approach to pain of a moderate-to-severe intensity would be to try short-acting opioid first to find the narcotic level needed to control the pain symptoms and, if necessary, add or switch to a long-acting opioid to maintain patient comfort for an extended period of time—all depending on the specific patient and their clinical situation.

Considering *America's opioid crisis*—or opioid epidemic—from years of heavy physician prescribing, patient misuse and abuse, unscrupulous pharmacy activity, and not enough government oversight, the **Pain is the PITS Program** always tries to minimize the tendency to keep escalating opioid therapy through time—by implementation of both a multidisciplinary

assessment approach and the many integrative treatment protocol options. This is a foundational tenet of the **PITS Program**. *THIS PITS OPIOID TREATMENT PHILOSOPHY IS A CRITICAL ELEMENT OF THE PITS PROGRAM'S COMPANY MISSION STATEMENT:*

"…a privately held pain management company dedicated to creating a universal educational pain program for America to bring patient and healthcare provider together for better understanding and compliance of care. In light of the opioid crisis and pain epidemic in America, the **PITS Program** approach utilizes simplified **P-I-T-S** *acronym* guidelines for the assessment and treatment of pain to avoid the need for continually escalating opioid narcotic therapy. The overall goal is to achieve a lifetime of improved comfort and quality of life, while focusing on the use of multidisciplinary opioid-sparing integrative strategies for individualized patient long-term care."

When opioid narcotics are being considered in a patient's longer-term care plan, it is important to conduct an *opioid risk assessment evaluation*—the **PITS Opioid Risk Screening (PORS) Assessment** (see **APPENDIX E**). Questions about a patient's history of opioid, alcohol, and drug abuse; history of psychiatric problems, like anxiety and depression, PTSD, and ADD; current use of sedative-hypnotic medication, like Valium or Ambien; patients less than 50 years old, history of sleep apnea, social alcohol drinking and tobacco smoking, and history of multiple car accidents, all put patients at different risk levels of respiratory depression and accidental death when taking opioid narcotics.

Depression screening is also very important in the **PITS Program**. The program has a **PITS Depression Screening (PDS) Assessment** (see **APPENDIX F**) that includes six 0–10 Agree-to-Disagree questions where *0 is totally disagree* and *10 is totally agree*, which follows the simple *M-E-E-S-I-C acronym*:

M = **MOOD** down all the time?

E = **ENERGY** levels low all the time?

E = **EATING** too much or too little?

S = **SLEEPING** too much or too little?

I = INTEREST in life is lacking?

C = CONCENTRATING difficultly?

The higher your depression score, the higher your risk of an adverse event when taking long-term opioids for control of chronic pain. Remember, taking opioids as a class of medications can worsen depression through drug interactions, and through direct depressive effects on the body and mind.

Ever since physicians, the government with the CDC opioid guidelines for the United States, and insurance companies started paying closer attention to opioid levels as measured in what is referred to as **MME (Morphine Milligram Equivalent)** or **MED (Morphine Equivalent Dose)**, there has been a firestorm of adjustments in how the whole medical system is handling opioid therapy for patients. What MME essentially does, is that it compares all the strengths of other opioids to that of morphine, where 1 milligram (mg) of morphine = 1 MME. The MME is calculated by *adding up ANY opioid a patient may be taking on a Daily basis*, and many patients are on more than one daily opioid. As examples: Oxycodone—the opioid in Percocet—is 50% stronger than morphine, and therefore 1 mg of oxycodone is 1.5 MME comparison. Likewise, hydrocodone –the opioid in Vicodin and Norco—is equal to morphine in potency, and therefore 1 mg of hydrocodone is 1 MME comparison—get it? What the CDC really wants is for physicians in general to be more aware of MME levels, and the intendent risk of patients having an adverse event. So, they want MME levels not to exceed 90 MME, based on overall risk and benefit analysis, or else refer to a pain specialist for future prescribing, or try a different approach to treating the pain.

In terms of the **PITS Program** MME levels, my suggested guideline intended for pain specialists—based on years of academic study and expert clinical patient treatment experience—is an upper dosing MME of 180, with sometimes up to 25% more if needed individualized to a patient—for factors like an opioid-tolerant severe pain state, their **PITS Opioid Risk Screening (PORS) Assessment**, their **PITS Score Assessment** status, and previous response to non-opioid therapies in the **P-I-T-S** *treatment protocol*. It

turns out statistically in the **PITS Program**, that only historically high opioid patients—those on large opioid doses over 10–20 years—remain above the 90 MME levels, and many have weaned down on their levels considerably in recent years.

Typically, all the new opioid-naïve patients that enter and adopt the **PITS Program** *philosophy of care* who need long-term opioid prescribing, *usually stay below a daily 90 MME (Morphine Milligram Equivalent)*. These new patients are strongly encouraged to embrace a more multidisciplinary integrative philosophy of chronic pain care from the start, considering different non-opioid medications, therapy options, injection options, and possible surgical options, rather than resorting to the *"old"* way of continually escalating opioid therapy based solely on a patient report of subjective pain feeling. This is the new reality in America when it comes to assessing and treating persistent long-term pain. The bottom line, we can still use opioid narcotic to treat pain, just not *"the sky's-the-limit"* philosophy anymore!

Injections are often needed to treat pain, and there are a lot of interventional pain management techniques, both minimally invasive and more invasive, that can be offered to patients who fail to get enough relief with medications and therapy alone. After medical and interventional pain management, there is surgical intervention as it applies, reserved for ongoing intractable pain and/or progressive neurologic symptoms, like bowel and bladder incontinence and worsening numbness and weakness. Here are some basic interventional care options:

- *Epidural steroid injections (ESIs)* are one of the more common safe, minimally invasive outpatient pain management injections to treat spinal inflammatory pain, from a typical bulging or herniated spinal disc. Epidural injections of steroid have both an anti-inflammatory and a nerve membrane stabilizing effect as its mechanism of action to treat pain. ESIs are performed under fluoroscopic X-ray guidance by interventional pain management specialists—anesthesiology, physiatry, and neurology physicians—and some interventional radiologists, as well.

- *Nerve blocks*, including peripheral, sympathetic, and spinal, are effective both diagnostically and therapeutically for pain diagnosis and treatment. These local anesthetic injections—with or without the addition of a steroid—are often performed in conjunction with ongoing medication and physical therapy methods, with the goal of desensitizing a pain state, to allow more healing and better rehabilitation care moving forward.

- *Joint injections*, with local anesthetic and steroid or viscosupplementation, can provide a minimally invasive method to control pain, which persists despite medications and therapy techniques. Ultimately, joints can be replaced if they become completely degenerated and patients are in intractable pain.

- *Trigger point injections (TPIs)* are muscle spasm injections of mostly local anesthetic, like lidocaine and bupivacaine, for breaking the pain cycle of persistent myofascial pain syndromes, and are very common and safe. The addition of other medical substances to these injections, such as steroids, vitamins, tissue enzyme to promote spread, can also be considered depending on the preference of the treating healthcare provider. TPIs are most effective if followed up with exercises to strengthen muscles, to keep active trigger points from returning as frequently and as intensely.

- *Minimally invasive injections of tendons and bursas and fascia* can be very effective in breaking the pain cycle, if conservative management fails with rest, medications, ice and heat, and exercise.

- *Radiofrequency lesioning (RFL)* or *burning of nerves*, also known as *Radiofrequency ablation (RA)*, can be effective for longer-term control of certain pain conditions, when previous local anesthetic and steroid injections were helpful, but limited in duration of relief. RF is commonly performed for persistent back pain, due to spinal facet and sacroiliac joint causes, and more recently for even persistent knee pain in certain clinical situations. Likewise, *Cryoablation* or *freezing of nerves* can also offer longer-term relief of certain neuropathic pain conditions, such as intercostal neuralgia or for traumatic neuromas, again, if previous local anesthetic and steroid injections are effective but short-lived.

- *Diagnostic cervical and lumbar discography* can be helpful in discovering discogenic pain, or which spinal disc levels hurt, in certain patients. This is often considered prior to procedures, such as percutaneous discectomy, nucleoplasty, intradiscal electrothermal therapy (IDET), and prior to certain spinal fusion procedures. Also, a CT scan myelogram imaging study can be an effective way to diagnose spinal nerve root compression, again prior to surgical planning to better identify which level(s) to decompress in the spine.

Both medications and injections will be very helpful in "breaking the pain cycle" so that patients can better rehabilitate and maintain their functional status. One of the primary focuses of pain treatment in general is to **suppress inflammation,** which is the primary cause of most chronic pain states. Medications, injections, therapy, and supplements can all reduce the toxic inflammatory process that slowly wears our bodies down, and perpetuates a chronic pain state.

Therapy approaches are almost universally used to treat pain and involve *Mind/Body techniques* including, **physical therapy**, **chiropractic care**, a **home exercise program (HEP)**, and **psychology and complementary care therapy** approaches—all considered the most important parts and the *top priority* of the **P-I-T-S treatment protocol**. Once medications and injections break the pain cycle, **then mind/body therapy and self-directed exercise will strengthen the area and help decrease recurrent pain**, all with the goal of helping patients function better. These therapy-based strategies are really long-term solutions to controlling pain flares and maintaining optimum activity levels. Here are the overall basic therapy care group options:

- *Physical therapy and Chiropractic/traction care* will help to strengthen and straighten our body's painful issues when they arise, like decompressing and stabilizing a patient's spine from a disc problem, to help decrease the frequency and severity of symptoms. The combination of chiropractic or osteopathic manipulation therapy (OMT) and physical therapy will often be better than the individual use of just chiropractic or therapy alone. Rehabilitation's focus is to straighten and strengthen, and optimize biomechanics and posture, so physical therapy and chiropractic care can be thought of as helpful together. Physiatrists—rehabilitation doctors—all know this secret of success.

- *Occupational therapy* can be used as well, so consider this therapy especially for hand injuries that need basic and more advanced rehabilitation.

- A *Home exercise program (HEP)* is the most self-sufficient therapeutic way to stay in shape, whether you are a chronic pain patient or not—everyone must diet and exercise appropriately for the general maintenance of our bodies. Our bodies were meant to move, by design. Once the pain cycle is broken, many patients if they have access to a gym or home equipment, can maintain their physical strengthening, flexibility, and conditioning for life. Always try to live a healthy lifestyle.

- *Physician care*, including *neuromuscular medicine or osteopathic physicians* and *physical medicine and rehabilitation doctors (physiatrists)*, can be consulted, especially if patients have persistent pain despite chiropractic and physical therapy care, and need a longer-term therapy-based physician care program. The key to this physician level of therapy is to continue to adjust a program, focusing on strengthening and conditioning of neuro-muscular structures, to further decrease the chance of recurrent pain that keeps patient's from achieving their maximum functional gains.

- *Psychological care* of the chronic pain patient should never be ignored or minimized, because of its importance on the final perception of the physical pain itself. Patients with a positive outlook and free of a lot of anxiety and depression, will often feel less pain, and generally will stay motivated and focused on the wellness aspects of their **PITS Program**. Remember, pain is both physical and emotional, so good psychological care will help the emotional component of *perceived* pain in the brain, which in turn will help the physical component.

- *Restorative or restful sleep* is a major area of therapy concern in any pain care plan, as patients who wake up fatigued in the morning tend to have more chronic pain—their bodies have not had sufficient time to rest and repair. The importance of restorative sleep should not be overlooked.

- *Complementary care techniques* can be very effective, alongside conventional medicine, to create an *integrative* care balance, especially when trying to avoid escalating opioid narcotic therapy. Many patients want to seek out these complementary therapy options in their communities, such as acupuncture, massage, yoga and Pilates, hypnosis, Reiki, magnets, low level laser therapy, biofeedback, essential oils, herbal therapies and supplements, and the like.

Surgery indications to help correct painful conditions are always individualized to a patient's specific clinical situation. Here are some basic surgical care option concepts and examples:

- For patients with a bad back and sciatica, for example, surgical intervention is typically reserved for patients who remain in intractable pain, despite aggressive medical and interventional pain management (medications-therapy-injections), or who have persistent neurologic compromise like bowel and bladder incontinence or progressive numbness and weakness in their legs. For patients who do undergo back and neck spine surgery, realistic expectations should focus on better overall management of the pain symptoms, rather than expect a cure of all the pain. Some patients do feel that their pain is completely gone, but many patients, especially after *multilevel spinal fusions*, can feel some intermittent flares of mild-to-moderate discomfort from time-to-time, even after full healing. This is typically a pain that is much easier to manage at this point, as modified care options move forward, as needed.

- When patients consult spine surgeons, they should look toward *minimally invasive* options at first if they apply, like discectomy or laminectomy—removing pieces of disc and bone—and then to more aggressive strategies, such as spinal fusion with instrumentation hardware placement for persistent spine pain.

- When patients consult orthopedic surgeons for persistent joint pain, they should look toward minimally invasive treatment options at first if they apply. Or, they can consider a *joint replacement* surgical option, for example, if they fail more conservative approaches with medication, therapy, joint injections, and joint arthroscopy.

- Patients with chronic abdominal pain or pelvic pain can consider undergoing *diagnostic laparoscopy or laparotomy* as a surgical option, if a surgeon offers this level of care at any point, especially when other conservative measures have failed.

- *Implantable spinal devices*, such as *spinal cord stimulation (SCS)* or *spinal narcotic pump*, are reserved for patients who remain in intractable pain, despite aggressive medical, interventional and/or surgical techniques, or for patients who need an advanced pain management technique to break their intractable pain, because they either have non-operable disease, or where a reoperation is not likely to benefit them. Varying degrees of electrical current through a spinal cord stimulator has been shown to treat somatic and neuropathic pain states, from an implantable modality standpoint. Likewise in selected patients, spinal delivery of opioid narcotic can be very effective in controlling pain and minimizing systemic whole body side effects, by using very small dosing amounts of drug delivered directly into the spinal fluid space where the pain receptors exist.

In terms of Evaluation of patients, after patients have been through their assessment and plan and implementation clinical pathway process, it is very important at this point to make sure a patient's individual goals are being met as much as possible, and to a degree that is acceptable to that patient. Afterall, the whole focus of the **Pain is the PITS Program** is to maximize your **PITS Pain and Quality-of-Life Score—PITS Score**, where the higher your score—maximum 120 points —the better pain control and improved quality of life you will experience!

The overall **Goals** of staying functional and resuming productivity, improving comfort, having better control of the pain itself and minimizing side effects, controlling anxiety and depression and keeping energy levels up, and improving social events with friends and family, are some of the key elements of the pain and quality-of-life treatment focus in the **PITS Program**.

The **motto of the Pain is the PITS Program** is: "**Feel better and live your life, because pain is the PITS!**" Improving your **PITS Pain and Quality-of-Life Score** is the "Holy Grail," or ultimate objective of the **PITS Program**. Just like a weight loss program philosophy of diet and exercise to reach your desired weight goal, the closer a patient follows the **PITS Program** *philosophy of care*, the better opportunity there will be to reach a desired level of improved pain control and quality of life as the outcome. Patient adherence and compliance and keeping to the program course is the key, and lack of patient adherence is the number one reason why any medical care plan fails, not just with pain management.

The **Pain is the PITS Program** provides **PITS Sample Worksheets** (see **APPENDIX C**) to help keep patients on track with their assessment and treatment progress, as well as keeping track of their pain treatment timeline. Also, within the worksheets there is a patient information and medical history page, as well as a questions-and-concerns page for patients to take notes. The key is following the program progress on a weekly or monthly basis and taking your **PITS Score** regularly, to keep you motivated and on target to reach your desired level of comfort and quality of life. *You must own your pain management program and be proactive to get your best results*, much like following a weight loss program. If you do not follow your weight loss program you get heavy again, and if you do not follow your **PITS Program** you start hurting again.

The **Pain is the PITS Program** is a multi-disciplinary integrative approach to all types of pain and for all patients. In fact, it applies to acute, chronic and cancer pain. It is for biomechanical and soft tissue nociceptive pain, inflammatory, neuropathic, dysfunctional, and psychogenic pain. It is for the young and old, men and women, educated and non-educated, and the poor and rich. The **PITS Program** is a universal educational pain program for America, to bring patient and pain care health professionals together on the same page for better education and clinical best-practice pain management care, with a focus on minimizing the need to keep escalating opioid therapy in a patient's long-term care. It can certainly help the one hundred million people who suffer from chronic pain in America and need this type of program guidance.

There are only so many board-certified pain specialists in the United States from accredited programs available to treat the one hundred million people who suffer from chronic pain. Therefore, the **PITS Program** can be used as a guide for patients to bring to any physician or healthcare provider that can help them with their chronic pain management needs. There are many more primary care physicians in America, but they are not fully trained to handle the complexities of many chronic pain sufferers. So, the **PITS Program** will help bridge that gap for improved knowledge, as well as providing a level of motivation that is badly needed for effective pain care.

To reemphasize, the **Pain is the PITS Program** will follow an integrative clinical pathway and personalized assessment and protocol treatment plan of care:

1. Conducting an initial assessment using the **P-I-T-S** *acronym*:

   P for *Physical Function*

   I for *Intensity of Pain*

   T for *Thoughts and Behaviors*

   S for *Social Interactions*

2. Developing the treatment plan with patient education.

3. Implementing the treatment plan with the protocol options using the **P-I-T-S** *acronym*:

   P for *Pills* or medications

   I for *Injections*

   T for *Therapy*

   S for *Surgery*

4. Conducting evaluations to ensure the treatment goals are being met.

As a matter of course, pain care progresses from conservative to more aggressive management until the patient reaches his or her goals. In other words, *patients move from medical pain management → interventional pain management → surgical pain management as needed*, following a **PITS Treatment Timeline** (see **APPENDIX H**), until the pain is controlled. After any pain care sequence of treatments, a reassessment is performed to keep patients maximizing their **PITS Pain and Quality-of-Life Score**.

The *clinical triangle* involving the interactive relationship of **pain, mood, and sleep** cannot be overstated. If pain is not controlled, mood and sleep are more disturbed. If mood is not right, then sleep is disturbed and pain is exacerbated. If sleep is not restful, then a patient's mood is anxious and pain is out of control. So, if symptoms in any one area worsen, then the other two areas will experience worsening symptoms—all due to the interconnected experience of pain, mood, and sleep in the brain.

Another important *triangle of care* is putting together the **best pain specialist expert, with the best available evidence-based scientific pain management research, with the individual patient's experience and preferences for care**—what a patient's pain and suffering means to them. Pain care cannot follow a 100% scientific direction or a 100% patient preference direction or a 100% pain specialist preference of care. Instead, the development of a pain care program needs to be more of a 50-50 split between the pain physician and patient working closely together—as half the equation—and what science and research evidence says is the best course of action—as the other half of the equation. The pain specialist who can best coordinate this will be the most successful! The **key will be to do the right pain management treatment option for the right pain patient at the right time in the protocol**. This is the focus of what is known as *evidenced-based medicine*—using science and research to help guide treatment decisions. The **PITS Program** provides this framework for best treatment and constantly focuses on an integrative-care approach, rather than *higher dose opioids* like in the past, to maximize a patient's **PITS Score**.

The **PITS Program Treatment Priority Table** (see **APPENDIX J**) helps to keep patients focused on the relative importance of different treatment categories:

- The *first priority is T-Therapy*, to maximize mind and body health to keep your functional status, which needs to be long-lasting.

- The *second priority is P-Pills* or medications, to have your daily medication for relief which can be short-term or longer-term, depending on the circumstances and nature of your painful condition.

- *The third priority is I-Injections*, to help break the pain cycle and allow improved rehabilitation moving forward, lasting for weeks to months at a time, when previous therapy and pills or medications are not enough relief.

- *The last priority is S-Surgery*—barring an emergency—which is irreversible and considered at the end of the pain care protocol when and if needed, because the pills, injections, and therapy are not enough relief or not lasting long enough, and intractable pain and ongoing neurologic symptoms are dominating your clinical course.

It is important to understand that all the pain management treatment options are put into the perspective of a patient's *pre-existing* medical problems, especially if they are on anti-coagulants or if they are a brittle diabetic, or at high cardiovascular or pulmonary risk, and so forth. Knowing a patient's major medical conditions, if any, will help to safely fashion the **P-I-T-S** *treatment protocol* options, with an appropriate risk-and-benefit analysis for ongoing care. Remember, first do no harm!

Always remember, when it comes to interventional pain management, ***no procedure is 100% safe***, and unfortunately, *"things"* can always happen no matter how well a patient is selected, or how well a procedure was performed, or how good the doctor is, and so forth. Minimally invasive outpatient fluoroscopic-guided pain management injection procedures are extremely safe in the hands of highly trained, board-certified, experienced interventional pain management medical professionals—abscess infection, excessive bleeding, and nerve injury paralysis are rare events. Nonetheless, it not an exact science with a guaranteed positive outcome. Again, patient selection and a doctor's pain management expertise and up-to-date knowledge are the keys!

PITS Pain and Quality-of-Life Score = PITS Score
(A Multi-dimensional Integrative PITS Assessment Tool)

Directions: For each category question, indicate how much you **Agree** or **Disagree** (on average, *in the last week*), by circling a number from 0 to 10, where **0 is totally Disagree** and **10 is totally Agree**.

Sections	Category Questions			Sub-Totals
P Physical Function	Able to work or take care of home and/or children? 0 1 2 3 4 5 6 7 8 9 10	Able to do some exercise? 0 1 2 3 4 5 6 7 8 9 10	Able to do activities of daily living? 0 1 2 3 4 5 6 7 8 9 10	
I Intensity of Pain	Pain score levels are acceptable? 0 1 2 3 4 5 6 7 8 9 10	Duration of pain relief is adequate? 0 1 2 3 4 5 6 7 8 9 10	Treatment side effects are tolerable? 0 1 2 3 4 5 6 7 8 9 10	
T Thoughts & Behaviors	Suffering from anxiety or depression? 0 1 2 3 4 5 6 7 8 9 10	Getting restful sleep? 0 1 2 3 4 5 6 7 8 9 10	Overall energy level is OK? 0 1 2 3 4 5 6 7 8 9 10	
S Social Interactions	Getting out with family and friends? 0 1 2 3 4 5 6 7 8 9 10	Able to travel or do a hobby? 0 1 2 3 4 5 6 7 8 9 10	Have enough insurance coverage for pain care? 0 1 2 3 4 5 6 7 8 9 10	

SCORING: Add up the totals from each category question and place the answer in the Sub-Total box. Then add the Sub-Total column and place that number in the Total Score box.

Total Score

PITS

Score Ranking

The overall goal is for the PITS score to be above 100

Excellent	100–120
Very Good	81–100
Good	61–80
Fair	41–60
Poor	21–40
Very Poor	0–20

PITS Pain Diagram—Mind/Body Relationship
The Four Phases of Pain

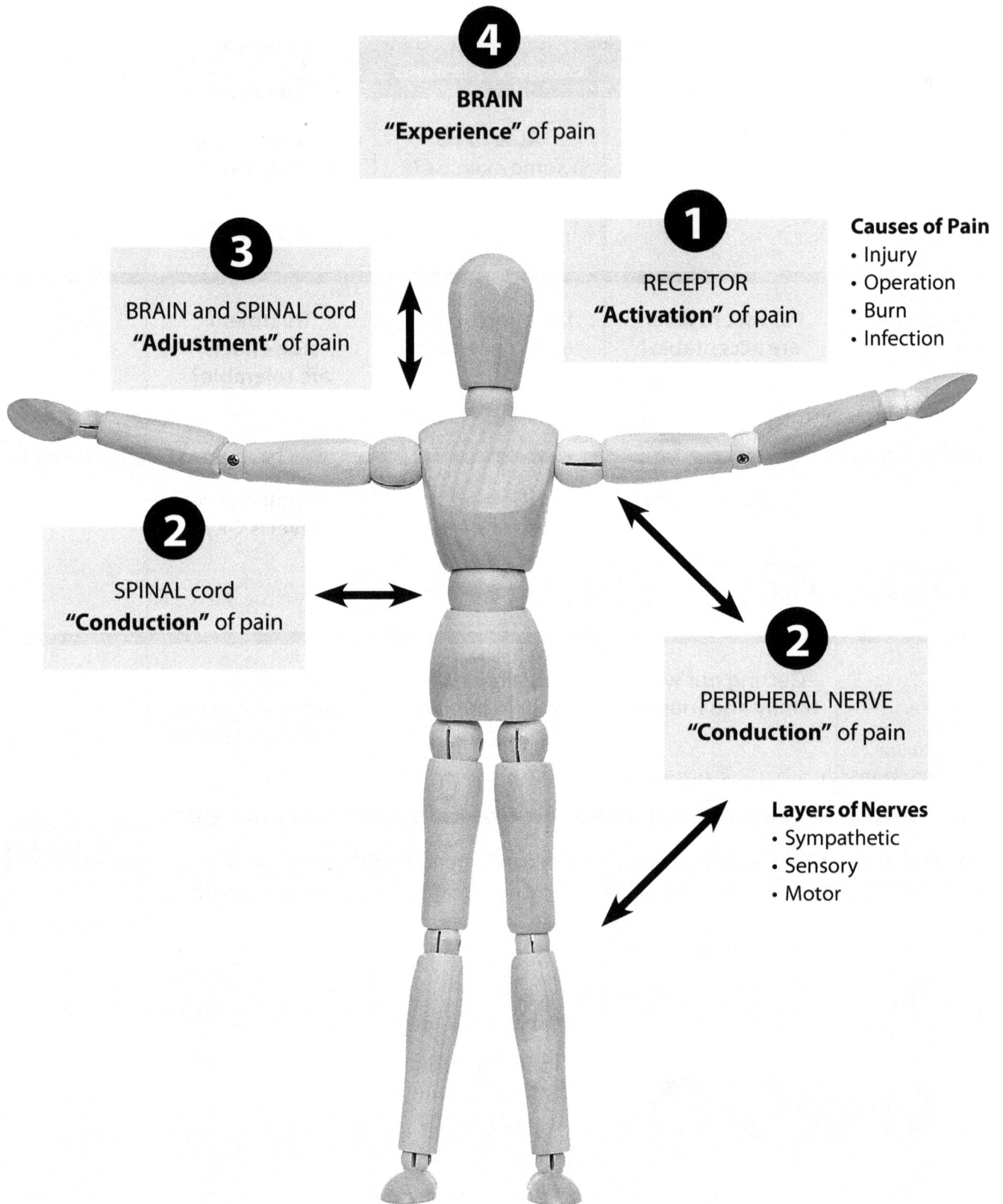

4

BRAIN
"Experience" of pain

1

RECEPTOR
"Activation" of pain

Causes of Pain
- Injury
- Operation
- Burn
- Infection

3

BRAIN and SPINAL cord
"Adjustment" of pain

2

SPINAL cord
"Conduction" of pain

2

PERIPHERAL NERVE
"Conduction" of pain

Layers of Nerves
- Sympathetic
- Sensory
- Motor

PITS Sample Worksheets (page 1) — Patient Information

Name	Phone #	E-Mail Address

All Medications / Dosages

_____

_____

Herbal Drugs / Supplements _____

_____

Pain Problem List

1 _____

2 _____

3 _____

4 _____

Allergies

Contrast _____

Antibiotics_____

Latex _____

Other_____

Pain Management Team

Primary _____

Surgeon _____

Anesthesiologist_____

Specialists _____

✔ Check all that apply:

Medical Issues		Past Surgeries	Lifestyle Issues
☐ Diabetes	☐ Stroke—TIA	☐ Head	☐ Smoking
☐ Blood Thinners (please specify)	☐ Seizures	☐ Neck	☐ Alcohol
_____	☐ Autoimmune disease (please specify)	☐ Shoulder	☐ Recreational Drugs
_____	_____	☐ Chest	☐ Opioid Abuse
☐ Bleeding disorder	_____	☐ Back	☐ Car accidents
☐ Heart attack—stents	☐ Osteoarthritis	☐ Abdomen—Groin	☐ Diet
☐ Hypertension	☐ Headaches (Migraines, etc.)	☐ Hips	☐ Exercise
☐ Emphysema—asthma	☐ TMJ (jaw) pain	☐ Knees	☐ Weight Issues
☐ Sleep apnea	☐ Trigeminal neuralgia (face nerve pain)	☐ Arms	☐ Sleep Issues
☐ Kidney	☐ Depression/Anxiety/ PTSD/Bipolar	☐ Legs	☐ Stress Issues
☐ Thyroid	☐ Infections	☐ Hands	☐ Pregnant?
☐ Liver—Hepatitis	☐ Rashes	☐ Feet	
☐ Stomach ulcer— gastritis	☐ Other medical issue(s)		
☐ Abdominal: gallbladder, pancreatitis	_____		
☐ Cancer	_____		

PITS Sample Worksheets (page 2) — PITS Score Sheet

Directions: For each category question, indicate how much you **Agree** or **Disagree** (on average, *in the last week*), by circling a number from 0 to 10, where **0 is totally Disagree** and **10 is totally Agree**.

Sections	Category Questions			Sub-Totals
P Physical Function	Able to work or take care of home and/or children? 0 1 2 3 4 5 6 7 8 9 10	Able to do some exercise? 0 1 2 3 4 5 6 7 8 9 10	Able to do activities of daily living? 0 1 2 3 4 5 6 7 8 9 10	
I Intensity of Pain	Pain score levels are acceptable? 0 1 2 3 4 5 6 7 8 9 10	Duration of pain relief is adequate? 0 1 2 3 4 5 6 7 8 9 10	Treatment side effects are tolerable? 0 1 2 3 4 5 6 7 8 9 10	
T Thoughts & Behaviors	Suffering from anxiety or depression? 0 1 2 3 4 5 6 7 8 9 10	Getting restful sleep? 0 1 2 3 4 5 6 7 8 9 10	Overall energy level is OK? 0 1 2 3 4 5 6 7 8 9 10	
S Social Interactions	Getting out with family and friends? 0 1 2 3 4 5 6 7 8 9 10	Able to travel or do a hobby? 0 1 2 3 4 5 6 7 8 9 10	Have enough insurance coverage for pain care? 0 1 2 3 4 5 6 7 8 9 10	

SCORING: Add up the totals from each category question and place the answer in the Sub-Total box. Then add the Sub-Total column and place that number in the Total Score box.

Total Score

Score Ranking		
	Excellent	100–120
	Very Good	81–100
Score Ranking The overall goal is for the PITS score to be above 100	Good	61–80
	Fair	41–60
	Poor	21–40
	Very Poor	0–20

PITS Sample Worksheets (page 3) — PITS Treatment Protocol

Category	Integrative PITS Treatment Protocol
P Pills	**Anti-inflammatory:** NSAIDs (nonsteroidal anti-inflammatory drugs): Motrin–Advil (ibuprofen), Aleve, etc.; Steroids = Prednisone or Medrol Dosepak; Tylenol (acetaminophen); Immunosuppressants
	Muscle Relaxants: Flexeril (cyclobenzaprine), Robaxin (methocarbamol), Zanaflex, Baclofen, etc.
	Nerve Pain Agents: Neurontin (gabapentin), Lyrica (pregabalin), Cymbalta (duloxetine), etc.
	Opioid Narcotics—Short-Acting: Hydrocodone (Vicodin, Norco), Oxycodone (Percocet), Tramadol
	Opioid Narcotics—Long-Acting: MS Contin (morphine), Duragesic Patch (fentanyl), Oxycontin (oxycodone), Nucynta ER (tapentadol), Zohydro ER (hydrocodone)
I Injections	**Epidural Steroids** (ESIs)—Cervical + Lumbar (midline), Caudal (sacral), Transforaminal (side)
	Joints: Spinal (facet and sacroiliac), Major Joints (shoulder, hip, knee, ankle)
	Muscle: Trigger point muscle (TPIs), **Other:** nerve blocks, tendon + bursa injections, etc.
	Neuroablative: Radiofrequency (RF) burning nerves (spine, sacroiliac), Cryoablation freezing nerves
	Diagnostic: Lumbar + cervical discography for the spine; **Prophylactic:** Botox for migraines
T Therapy	A. **Physical Care:** Chiropractic/Traction, inversion tables + cervical inflatable cuff Physical Therapy (PT): flexibility, strength, endurance, posture/biomechanics Home Exercise (HEP) or Gym: Independent self-management focus Physical Medicine and Rehab (PM&R—physiatry), Neuromuscular medicine—Osteopathic (DO)
	B. **Psychological Care:** Anxiety: Xanax (alprazolam), Klonopin (clonazepam), Talk therapy Depression: Effexor (venlafaxine), Cymbalta (duloxetine), Elavil (amitriptyline), Talk therapy Cognitive Behavioral Therapy (CBT): Changing thoughts and behaviors (distraction, relaxation, etc.)
	C. **Sleep Care Strategies:** Lifestyle changes (quiet, dark, cool bedroom), no caffeine at night Supplements: Chamomile tea, Melatonin, Valerian root, Kava, etc. Prescription Medications: Ambien, Lunesta, Klonopin, Trazodone, Elavil, Pamelor, Sinequan, Flexeril, Baclofen, etc.
	D. **Complementary Care Techniques:** Acupuncture, massage, yoga/pilates, hypnosis, guided imagery, herbals/supplements, vitamins/minerals, probiotics, essential oils
S Surgery	**Minimally Invasive:** Spine (disc), Joints (arthroscopy), Abdomen (laparoscopy), Face (trigeminal ablation)
	Decompressions: Spine Laminectomy (remove bone), and Discectomy (remove disc material), etc.
	More Invasive: Lumbar and Cervical fusions (hardware placement), Joint Replacement (knee, hip, shoulder, ankle), Hysterectomy, etc.
	Implantable Devices: Spinal Cord Stimulation (SCS), Intrathecal Infusion Device (IID)—spinal narcotic pump

GOALS	
Staying Functional — Work, homemaker/childcare, exercise, and daily activities of living
Improve Comfort — Better day-to-day pain control levels, duration of comfort, and minimizing side effects
Mood/Sleep — Control anxiety and depression, improve sleep patterns, and keep energy levels up
Socialization — Being with family/friends, doing hobbies/travel, and affording pain care (insurance)

PITS Sample Worksheets (page 4) — PITS Treatment Timeline

PITS "Acute" Pain Care Transition to PITS "Chronic" Pain Care

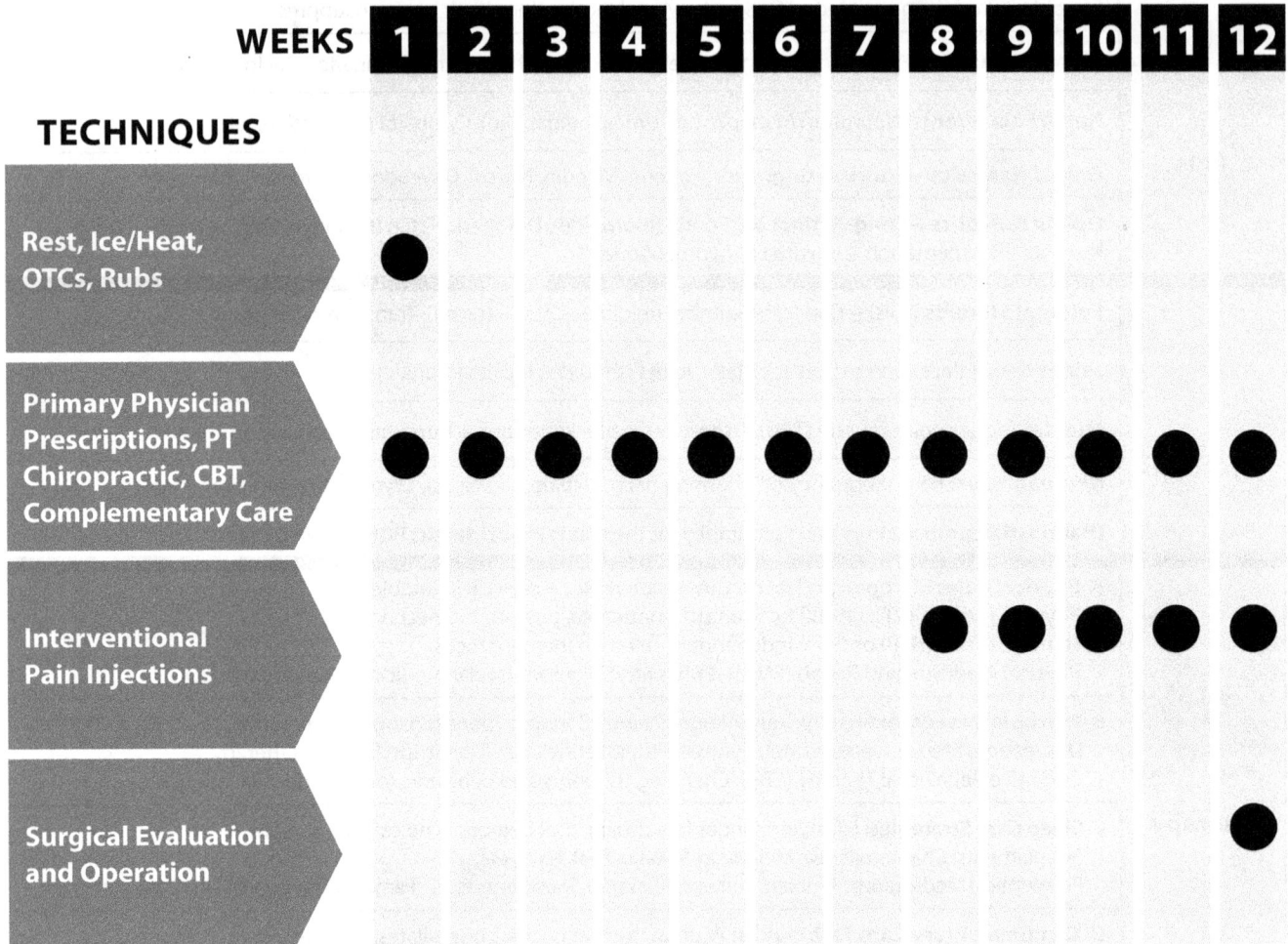

TECHNIQUES	WEEKS 1	2	3	4	5	6	7	8	9	10	11	12
Rest, Ice/Heat, OTCs, Rubs	●											
Primary Physician Prescriptions, PT Chiropractic, CBT, Complementary Care	●	●	●	●	●	●	●	●	●	●	●	●
Interventional Pain Injections								●	●	●	●	●
Surgical Evaluation and Operation												●

NOTES

- The first 12 weeks above represents "PITS Acute" care, and then the next 12 weeks (considered the Sub-Acute pain period) patients transition to "PITS Chronic" care (defined as any treatment beyond a 6 month period in the Pain is the PITS Program).

- The timeline is designed to move patients through a continuum of care from Medical pain management options (rest-medications-therapy), to Interventional pain management options (injections), and then to Surgical (operation) pain management options.

- Note that conservative treatment is maintained as more aggressive approaches are taken along the timeline of recovery.

- Depending on the severity of pain, patients may need to start interventional pain management or seek a Surgical pain management consult earlier in the timeline.

PITS Sample Worksheets (page 5) — **Patient Notes & Questions**

Notes and Reminders

Questions and Concerns

PITS Opioid Narcotic Comparison Dosing Chart

DRUG CHOICES: The PITS Program vs. CDC Patient Treatment Levels for Opioid Narcotics				
Dosing (daily mg)	Low	Moderate	High	
Morphine CDC Levels	30	50	90	CDC Potency Ratio Relative to Morphine
Drugs	Corresponding PITS Program Treatment Levels			
Morphine	60	100	180	1.0
Oxycodone	40	60	120	1.5
Hydrocodone	60	100	150 max	1.0
Hydromorphone	12	24	50	4.0
Oxymorphone	20	30	60	3.0
Tapentadol	150	250	500 max	0.4
Tramadol	200–400 max	N/A	N/A	0.1
Buprenorphine	10–20 max (patch)	N/A	N/A	1.8
Fentanyl patch	25	50	75	2.4
Methadone	10	20	40	3.0
Levorphanol	4	8	12	11.0
Butorphanol	2x2	N/A	N/A	7.0
Codeine	120–360 max	N/A	N/A	0.15

NOTES

- Morphine Milligram Equivalents (MME/Day) and Morphine Equivalent Dose (MED/Day) are the same
- CDC = Centers for Disease Control and Prevention
- Opioid Rotation Rule: when switching drugs use 25–50% less (Methadone 75% less)…then go 10–20% up or down depending on clinical variables (frail, elderly, respiratory disease, severity of pain condition, etc.)

PITS Opioid Risk Screening Assessment

PITS Opioid Risk Screening (PORS) Categories

1

Patient History of Abuse:
- Opioids, Illegal Drugs, Alcohol = **HIGH RISK**

2

Any Psychological Disorder:
- Anxiety/Depression, PTSD, ADD, Bipolar = **MODERATE RISK**

3

Use of Sedative/Hypnotic Medications:
- Valium and Ambien type drugs, Soma = **MODERATE RISK**

4

Any Other Risk Factor Issues:
- Age < 50 years, sleep apnea, lung disease, social alcohol use, smoker, multiple car accidents = **LOW RISK**

Overall PITS Opioid Risk Screening (PORS) Level

Category 1	High Risk
Category 2+3 or 2+4 or 3+4	High Risk
Only Category 2	Moderate Risk
Only Category 3	Moderate Risk
Only Category 4	Low Risk
If No Category	Low Risk

PITS Program Motto: **Feel Better and Live Your Life, Because Pain is the PITS!**

PITS Depression Screening Assessment

PITS Depression Screening (PDS) Score
Using the M-E-E-S-I-C acronym

Directions: For each screening question, indicate how much you **Agree** or **Disagree** (**on average,** *in the* *last week*), by circling a number from 0–10, where **"0" = Totally Disagree** and **"10" = Totally Agree**.

M Mood	**Disagree**	**Is your mood down all the time?**	**Agree**
		0 1 2 3 4 5 6 7 8 9 10	

E Energy	**Disagree**	**Are your energy levels low all the time?**	**Agree**
		0 1 2 3 4 5 6 7 8 9 10	

E Eating	**Disagree**	**Are you eating too much or too little?**	**Agree**
		0 1 2 3 4 5 6 7 8 9 10	

S Sleeping	**Disagree**	**Are you sleeping too much or too little?**	**Agree**
		0 1 2 3 4 5 6 7 8 9 10	

I Interest	**Disagree**	**Is your interest in life lacking?**	**Agree**
		0 1 2 3 4 5 6 7 8 9 10	

C Concentrating	**Disagree**	**Do you have difficulty concentrating?**	**Agree**
		0 1 2 3 4 5 6 7 8 9 10	

SCORING: Add up all the individual question scores to determine your PDS Score

Total Score

0–20 = Not depressed

21–40 = Probably depressed

41–60 = Definitely depressed

PITS Clinical Pathway and Protocol for the Assessment and Treatment of Chronic Pain

Guidelines for Structured Multidisciplinary Integrative Chronic Pain Care	
1. Assessment	**PAIN!** Comprehensive Medical Care Evaluation (including PITS Score): History, Physical Exam, and Studies used to formulate an Assessment + Plan
2. Plan	**A Standardized Plan for Chronic Pain Care** • PITS Program Worksheets • Anesthesiology, Psysiatry (PM&R), Neurology + Psychiatry • Spinal Surgery, Rheumatology, Palliative Care + Oncology • Internal Medicine + Family Practice, Pediatrics + OBGYN, ER
3. Implementation	**P-I-T-S Protocol Treatment Options**
	P = Pills (Medications)—Pharmacological Choices
	• Anti-inflammatory (NSAIDs + Steroids), Immunosuppressants • Tylenol (Acetaminophen) + Topical pain creams • Muscle relaxants + Nerve Pain Agents • Opioid Narcotic Analgesics (short and long acting)
	I = Injections—Interventional Pain Techniques
	• Epidural steroid injections, nerve blocks, joint injections • Muscle (trigger point injections), tendon + bursa injections • Radiofrequency (burning) + Cryoablation (freezing) of nerves • Diagnostic Discography of the spine, Botox for migraines
	Need to break the pain cycle to better rehabilitate
	T = Therapy—Therapeutic Choices

	• Physical Care: Chiropractic, Traction/Inversion Table
	  Physical Therapy, Occupational Therapy, Home exercise/Gym
	  Physician Care—Neuromuscular-Osteopathic, Physical Medicine & Rehabilitation
	• Psychological Care: Anxiety + Depression, Cognitive Behavioral Therapy
	• Sleep Strategies: Lifestyle changes, Herbals/Supplements, Prescriptions
	• Complementary Care: Acupuncture, Massage, Yoga/Pilates, Reiki, Herbals

	Need to stay functional and decrease recurrent pain
	S = Surgery—Surgical Interventions
	• Minimally invasive (spine, joint, nerve, tendon, bursa, abdomen, foot) • Laminectomy – Discectomy – Spinal Fusion – Joint replacement • Diagnostic Laparoscopy – Laparotomy – Hysterectomy • Implantable Devices—spinal cord stimulation (SCS), spinal narcotic pump
	If intractable pain persists and conservative treatments have failed
4. Evaluation	Reassessment—Are Pain Goals being met?
	• Staying functional and resuming productivity at home and work • Improved comfort and duration of pain control; minimizing side effects • Control of anxiety and depression; improved socialization Focus on **Pain and Quality-of-Life Score (PITS SCORE)**

PITS Treatment Timeline

PITS "Acute" Pain Care Transition to PITS "Chronic" Pain Care

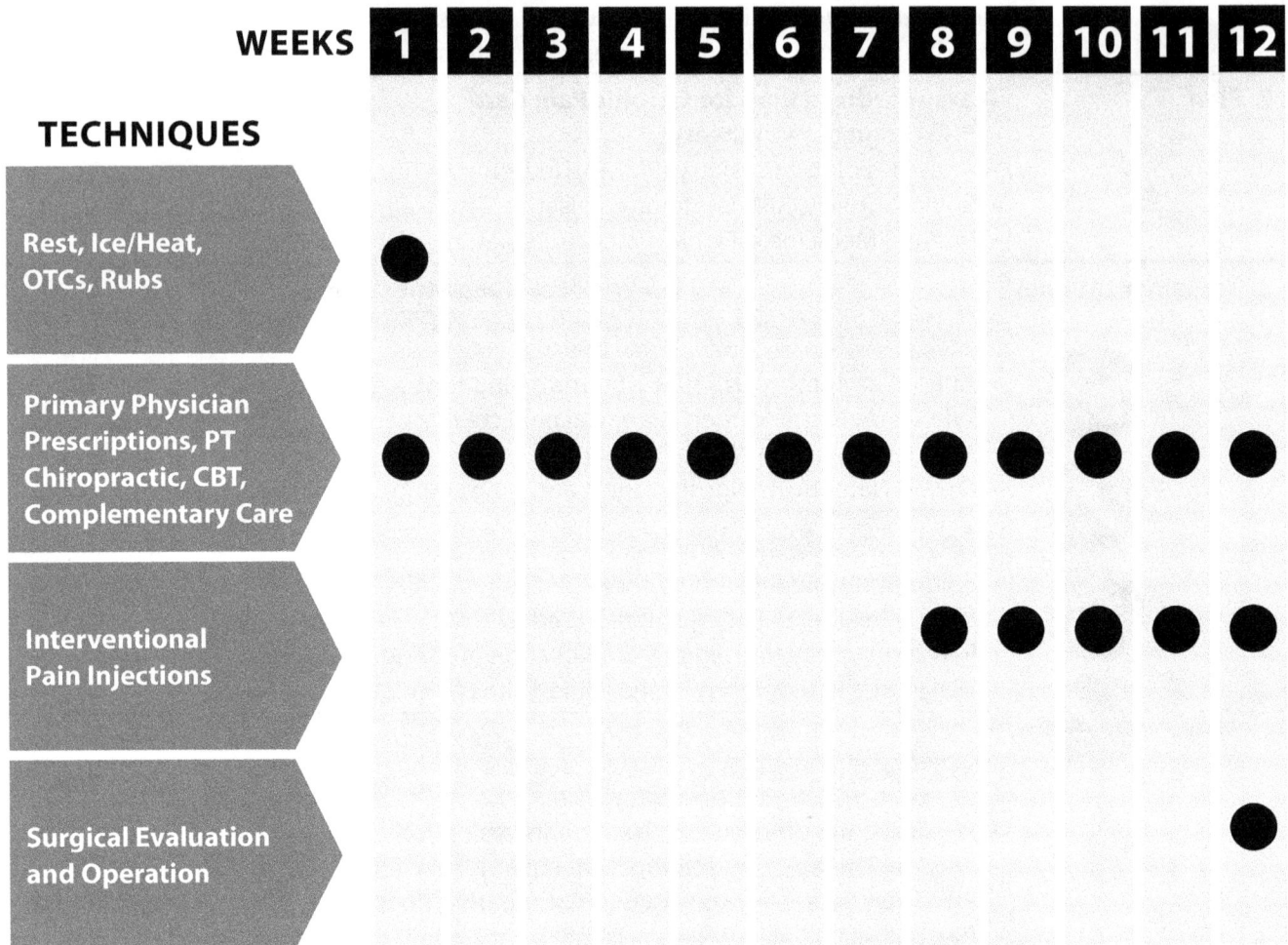

WEEKS	1	2	3	4	5	6	7	8	9	10	11	12

TECHNIQUES

Rest, Ice/Heat, OTCs, Rubs	●											
Primary Physician Prescriptions, PT Chiropractic, CBT, Complementary Care	●	●	●	●	●	●	●	●	●	●	●	●
Interventional Pain Injections								●	●	●	●	●
Surgical Evaluation and Operation												●

NOTES

- The first 12 weeks above represents "PITS Acute" care, and then the next 12 weeks (considered the Sub-Acute pain period) patients transition to "PITS Chronic" care (defined as any treatment beyond a 6 month period in the Pain is the PITS Program).

- The timeline is designed to move patients through a continuum of care from Medical pain management options (rest-medications-therapy), to Interventional pain management options (injections), and then to Surgical (operation) pain management options.

- Note that conservative treatment is maintained as more aggressive approaches are taken along the timeline of recovery.

- Depending on the severity of pain, patients may need to start interventional pain management or seek a Surgical pain management consult earlier in the timeline.

PITS Treatment of Opioid-Induced Constipation

Treatment of Opioid Induced Constipation (OIC)
FIRST ▶ Use Stimulants and Softeners
Senokot: 1–2 tablets, twice/day **Colace:** 100mg twice/day **Ducolax:** 1–3 (5mg tabs) everyday
SECOND ▶ Try Laxatives
Miralax (Polyethelene Glycol—PEG): 1 teaspoon in 7 ounces of fluid daily **Milk of Magnesia:** 30 mls every day
THIRD ▶ Start Opioid Antagonist or Chloride Channel Agents

Movantik (naloxegol): 12.5–25 mg orally every morning, one hour before meal or two hours after meal
    An oral opioid antagonist that offsets decreased GI motility at the enteric (gastric) opioid receptor as a "peripherally acting mu-opioid receptor antagonist" (PAMORA)…**or**
 	
Symproic (naldemedine): 0.2 mg orally once daily any time of day (PAMORA) **or**
 	
Relistor (methylnaltrexone): 8 mg (weight < 62kg); 12 mg (weight > 62kg)
    Subcutaneous everyday or every other day in upper arm, abdomen, thigh (prefilled syringes); an injectable opioid antagonist (PAMORA)…**or**
 	
Amitiza (lubiprostone): 24 mcg oral capsule twice/day; an oral chloride channel agent that increases fluid inside intestines by activating the chloride receptor

FOURTH ▶ Do an Opioid Rotation
Change to a different opioid and adjust dosing

Feel Better and Live Your Life, Because Pain is the PITS!

PITS Treatment Priority Table

Category	Priority	Treatments
P = Pills (medications)	**2**	• Anti-inflammatory (NSAIDs and steroids) • Muscle relaxants, Nerve pain agents • Opioids (short acting and long acting)
I = Injections	**3**	• Trigger point (muscle) injections (TPIs) • Joint injections, Epidural steroid injections (ESIs) • Nerve blocks with local anesthetic
T = Therapy	**1**	**Physical** • Physical therapy, Chiropractor, Gym, Home exercise, Rehab—osteopathic doctor **Psychological** • Psychiatrist, Talk therapy, Cognitive behavioral therapy, Mindfulness **Sleep** • Sleep hygiene, Herbals/supplements, Prescription meds **Complementary** • Acupuncture, Massage, Yoga, Meditation, Reiki, Aromatherapy—essential oils, Naturopathic doctor (ND) therapy
S = Surgery	**4**	• Minimally invasive procedures, Joint replacement • Spine: Laminectomy/discectomy—fusion • Implantable devices: Spinal narcotic pump and Spinal cord stimulation (SCS)

Feel Better and Live Your Life, Because Pain is the PITS!

PITS Diagnostic Categories of Pain

Six Different Types of Pain Conditions	
1. Biomechanical	**known as a "nociceptive" pain** Affects: vertebra, spinal discs, bones, ligaments, joints, cartilage
2. Soft Tissue	**known as a "nociceptive" pain** Affects: skin, fascia, muscles, tendons, visceral organs, vascular structures
3. Inflammatory	**an "inflammation-related" pain** • Joints—acute flare of osteoarthritis (OA) • Autoimmune—Active rheumatoid arthritis (RA) • Soft Tissue—Trauma and postoperative • Organs—Appendicitis and pancreatitis • Nerves—Herpes zoster (shingles)
4: Neuropathic	**a "peripheral or central nerve" pain** • Sympathetic and peripheral nerves • Complex Regional Pain Syndrome (CRPS)—previously known as Reflex Sympathetic Dystrophy (RSD), and diabetic neuropathy • Spinal cord and brain: spinal cord injury (SCI) and stroke
5. Dysfunctional	**an "undetermined" pain** • Migraine, fibromyalgia • Irritable bowel syndrome (IBS) • Temporomandibular joint (TMJ) pain
6. Psychogenic	**a "psychiatric-related" pain** • Anxiety and depression related • Somatoform pain disorder • Hypochondriac, pain adjustment disorder, catastrophizing, childhood abuse, substance abuse

Feel Better and Live Your Life, Because Pain is the PITS!

PITS GLOSSARY OF PAIN TERMS

Ablative Procedure   This is the term that describes interventional pain techniques that are typically performed on the peripheral or central nervous system to help alleviate chronic pain. An example is radiofrequency lesioning (RFL) of facet joint nerves in the spine, or RFL of the sacroiliac joint nerves, utilizing special needles that can be *heated* at their tips to control pain. Palliative care surgical ablative procedures on the spinal cord in the central nervous system can be performed in certain chronic intractable cancer pain states, typically performed by a neurosurgeon.

Abstinence Syndrome   A syndrome that occurs when a drug is abruptly or rapidly discontinued. Patients typically feel ill when their drug blood level drops too fast, which can occur when discontinuing high dose narcotics, antidepressants, or even anticonvulsant medications too quickly. These types of medications, depending on their levels and duration of usage, need to be weaned off slowly in order to avoid an abstinence syndrome situation.

Acetaminophen   A non-narcotic, non-anti-inflammatory, centrally-acting analgesic pain reliever that is commonly used to treat acute and chronic pain. Acetaminophen (APAP) relieves pain by a central effect in the brain allowing patients to handle a greater amount of pain. Acetaminophen also reduces fever and is not a blood thinner.

Acupuncture   A complementary medicine technique using small needles inserted in the skin and soft tissues at certain anatomical points in the body, commonly used to control pain and other symptoms in a wellness program. It is an ancient Chinese healing technique that is thousands of years old. Researchers still do not fully understand how acupuncture works, but it seems to exert its effect through a *counter irritant mechanism* that helps increase the body's natural narcotic-like substances, like endorphins and encephalins. This integrative care strategy is often used in conjunction with conventional **P-I-T-S treatment protocol** pain relief options.

Acute Pain   This is pain that has a known cause and typically occurs for a limited time of days to weeks or up to three months. If pain persists for three-to-six months, then it can be considered *subacute*. If pain continues beyond six months, it is then considered *chronic* in nature. Acute pain is a protective type of pain that warns the body to take care of the problem. Acute pain usually responds to treatment with analgesic medications and specific treatments known to cure the specific cause of the pain. As an example, for the common condition of appendicitis, removal of the appendix almost always leads to full healing with complete resolution of the previous pain. This contrasts with a chronic pain state, which occurs well after full healing, which occurs repeatedly over three to six months and longer, or that is due to a medical condition that is not expected to ever heal. Chronic pain has no long-term benefit to the body and is considered pathological. As an example, diabetic peripheral neuropathy is a type of pain that patients can battle for a lifetime, with persistent progressive burning and sharp neuropathic chronic pain afflicting their hands and feet.

Addiction   A chronic disease condition that leads patients to crave a drug or other addictive substance. With addiction, patients show a compulsive drug-seeking behavior that involves a pattern of self-destructive overuse. Addiction is a primary, chronic neurobiological disease with genetic, psychosocial, and environmental factors influencing its development and manifestations. Addiction is the same irrespective of whether the drug is an opioid narcotic, alcohol, amphetamine, cocaine, heroin, marijuana or even nicotine. It is important to note that sometimes addiction is called *dependence*, but this is not to be confused with the normal physical dependence that can occur with taking a drug, such as an opiate medication, for an extended period—typically for a week or more. If chronic pain patients stop taking high dose opioids abruptly, they can have a *withdrawal syndrome* that is unlike addiction itself.

Adjustments   A chiropractic manipulation technique involving the application of pressure to specific bones to correct *subluxations*—or misalignments. Adjustments use a gentle yet firm thrust, which is meant to help relieve pressure from spinal nerves in the neck and back and restore bone, joints, and soft tissues back to their normal anatomical position. Adjustments are often done in conjunction with physical therapy or massage or acupuncture techniques to optimize a patient's rehabilitation progress.

Adjuvant Analgesic   A scientific name given to a medication that is not primarily an analgesic drug pain reliever but has independent or additive pain-relieving effects, like the drug Elavil, for example. Elavil is an antidepressant medication that has adjuvant analgesic effects, especially for nerve pain. Adjuvant medication can offer a *"booster"* drug relief effect, which works alongside the main analgesic pain killer a patient may be taking, whether it be an opioid narcotic, an anti-inflammatory medication, or other medication, like a muscle relaxant.

Adverse Effects   A term used to describe any negative or unwanted side effects, typically from effects of analgesics and adjuvant medications, like sedation, nausea, upset stomach and constipation. Adverse

effects can also apply to injection and surgical procedures, like resultant bleeding, infection, or nerve injury that can occur after invasive treatments.

Algology   The science and study of pain, focusing on its causes and treatment. An *algologist* is the fancy name for a pain management doctor who diagnoses and treats chronic pain conditions.

Allodynia   A scientific name given to pain that is caused by something that does not normally cause pain, such as lightly touching the skin with your fingers, or clothing that touches the skin. This can be very distressing to patients and needs to be treated aggressively with *desensitization* **P-I-T-S treatment protocol** options, so patients can better rehabilitate when using hands-on therapy techniques in their care program.

Analgesic   A medication used to relieve pain, also generally known as a *"pain killer"*—but not necessarily an opioid narcotic medication. It could be in the form of a pill or medication, injectable agent, a skin patch, a gel or cream, and other delivery forms. Pills could include anti-inflammatories, muscle relaxants, anti-neuropathic medications, and of course, opioid narcotics.

Analgesic Ceiling   A scientific name for a dose of an analgesic pain killer that has limited pain relief effects as the dose is raised to a certain point. An example would be the anti-inflammatory medication ibuprofen, the generic form of Motrin and Advil. Continuing to take high doses of ibuprofen of more than 800 mg three times-per-day does not offer increased pain relief, but rather causes increased side effects, such as gastric upset and bleeding, as well as potential kidney and blood pressure problems. This is unlike certain powerful opioid narcotic medications, such as morphine for example. With increasing doses of morphine, added pain relief is potentially obtained rather than reaching a ceiling effect or therapeutic limit. What typically limits strong opioid narcotic dosing increases in patient care is really the development of side effects, like excessive grogginess, nausea, constipation, dizziness, and so forth.

Anesthesia   The loss of a patient's sense of feeling using an injectable local anesthetic drug, like lidocaine, or the loss of a patient's awareness using an intravenous drug, like propofol. A *general anesthetic* puts a person into unconsciousness, typically with an inhaled anesthetic gas. *Conscious sedation* or *monitored anesthesia care (MAC)* puts a patient into varying degrees of twilight sleep, commonly using IV propofol. A *local anesthetic*, like lidocaine or bupivacaine (Marcaine), causes loss of feeling in the part of the body that is injected without making a person lose consciousness. *Regional anesthesia* numbs a part of the body, such as the leg or arm, through an injectable local anesthetic technique, again without affecting consciousness.

Anesthesiologist A medical doctor (M.D. or D.O.) who provides unconsciousness and pain relief in a variety of care settings. Scenarios include, providing general anesthesia during a major operation, IV monitored anesthesia care (MAC) sedation for a pain management procedure or outpatient endoscopy/colonoscopy, and regional anesthesia with local anesthetic nerve blocks for certain procedures or operations. Minimally invasive outpatient interventional pain management procedures are performed more comfortably, especially for very anxious patients or for the more painful procedures, when anesthesiologists or *certified registered nurse anesthetists (CRNAs)* administer IV sedation to keep patients in a twilight sleep to minimize procedure discomfort.

Antidepressants Medications that are typically used to treat symptoms of depression. They also help manage chronic pain and some of its symptoms, such as insomnia or difficulty sleeping. There are different types of antidepressants, some of which in addition to treating depression can serve as adjuvant analgesics helping to treat different pain states—like bio-mechanical, soft tissue, nerve pain types, psychogenic, and other pain conditions.

Anti-Inflammatory A medication type that reduces inflammation, and often a first choice when patients experience an acute pain episode, whether it be an over-the-counter (OTC) medication or by prescription. Basically, there are two groups of anti-inflammatories—the *nonsteroidal forms*, like aspirin, ibuprofen, and naproxen, and the *steroid forms*, like oral

prednisone and injectable Kenalog (triamcinolone), for example. *Steroids are stronger than nonsteroidal anti-inflammatory drugs (NSAIDs)*, and caution needs to be taken for potential side effects if these medications are to be used for an extended period of time to treat patients.

Anxiolytics Medications that help manage anxiety. Anti-anxiety pills reduce pain-related anxiety that can lead to worsening psychological and physical pain symptoms. Many anxiolytics are drugs known as *benzodiazepines*, like the drugs Xanax, Valium, Klonopin, and Ativan, all of which are addictive to different degrees. They can also interact negatively with opioid narcotics and alcohol. Short-term anti-anxiety medication, along with longer-term talk or behavioral therapy, can help patients cope better and stay more functional with their chronic pain condition.

Arachnoiditis A medical term given to painful inflammation and thickening of spinal nerve root membranes that can occur after infection or trauma in the spine, or after a prolonged complicated spine surgery. Arachnoiditis can produce progressive disabling pain, and in some cases result in permanent pain. This is a difficult neuropathic pain state to treat where patients typically end up trying a spinal cord stimulator (SCS), especially if their pain remains intractable.

Arthritis A general term for painful inflammation, swelling, and stiffness of joints. There are many different types of arthritic conditions that involve hands and feet, arms and legs, and the spine. Osteoarthritis, rheumatoid arthritis, gouty arthritis, ankylosing spondylitis, and other types are typically quite painful for patients during times of flare-ups. Patients may complain of swelling and redness and warmth and tenderness in the affected joints. When X-rays are taken, there may be loss of the joint space or formation of spurs, erosions, or cysts in the bone. Millions of Americans suffer from arthritic conditions where there is a gradual breakdown and deterioration of the joint spaces through time, many times due to natural aging, from recreational activities, or from accidents and injuries.

Arthroscopy An outpatient orthopedic procedure involving the insertion of a *lighted endoscope* within a joint for both diagnostic and treatment purposes for painful conditions. This is a surgical procedure that is performed percutaneously through the skin and is not considered an open wound procedure like a total knee replacement.

Aspirin   A nonsteroidal anti-inflammatory medication used to treat pain and inflammation. It is also known as acetylsalicylic acid (ASA). It is an *over-the-counter (OTC) medication*, like Tylenol (acetaminophen). Aspirin also has anti-platelet effects and therefore can thin the blood, unlike Tylenol.

Assessment   In a general medical sense, an assessment is an initial consultation involving history, physical exam, review of tests, and so forth, or as part of an ongoing evaluation, like an office follow up reevaluation—all focused on reaching a diagnosis and developing a treatment plan for a painful condition. Patients are typically assessed monthly for chronic opioid narcotic management, after interventional (injection) procedures, with ongoing physical therapy, after surgical procedures, and so forth. When it comes to assessment in the **PITS Program**, as it relates to a patient's **PITS Pain and Quality-of-Life Score**, this is the all-important 12 categorical question **PITS Score** (see **APPENDIX A**).

Atrophy   A medical term that means wasting or decreased size of a muscle, whether the cause is from a long period of disuse or a muscle that has damage to its nerve supply. Atrophy can happen in patients who have casts or splints for weeks to months and, as mentioned, in patients who have had permanent nerve damage in their arms or legs that is responsible for muscle size and strength.

Aura   A visual disturbance, such as flashing lights or blind spots, which can signal the onset of a migraine headache.

Autoimmune   An abnormal immune response in the body that occurs when the body attacks itself, due to disease or other abnormal circumstances. Examples of autoimmune conditions include lupus, multiple sclerosis, rheumatoid arthritis, scleroderma, and many other medical conditions. These disease states can be very painful at times, especially with flare ups, and are typically treated with multiple medications and therapies by rheumatology specialists.

B

Back Pain   A nonspecific term used to describe pain below the cervical spine, typically in the low back lumbar area, but also in the middle midback thoracic region. There are many sources of back pain that arise from problems in discs, joints, nerves, bones, muscles, and ligaments. Low back pain is the single largest chronic pain condition in America that affects millions of patients, and is typically due to work-related accidents, motor vehicle accidents, sports injuries, slips and falls, or chronic aging from being upright weight-bearing humans. There are many different **P-I-T-S treatment protocol** options for back pain, all tailored for specific patient clinical cases, to help patients meet their specific pain and quality-of-life goals—in other words, to maximize their **PITS Score**.

Behavioral Therapy   Therapy that can be taught to patients to help them control chronic pain symptoms through a psychological approach. This can be an important psychological strategy where patients learn different methods to better cope and deal with all their pain disease symptoms. Patients can acquire skill in monitoring and evaluating their own behavior, and ultimately learn to modify their reactions to pain, so they can remain more functional in their everyday tasks.

Benign   A medical term meaning non-cancerous. Benign lesions or conditions do not invade nearby tissues or spread to other parts of the body in any malignant manner. An example is a fatty lipoma tumor under a patient's skin that you can feel as a lump when your roll your fingers over the area.

Benzodiazepines   A class of drugs that work as tranquilizers and anti-anxiety medications like Xanax (alprazolam), Valium (diazepam), Klonopin (clonazepam), and Ativan (lorazepam). These medications have a place in psychological and psychiatric care, but patients should not be mixing benzodiazepines with opioid narcotics and alcohol because of the real potential of drug interaction and death. Many patients in America unfortunately die every year from this fatal *drug triad* adverse reaction.

Beta Blockers A class of drugs that inhibit the sympathetic nervous system of the body. By reducing sympathetic activity, certain physical responses and symptoms of pain can be better controlled. Beta blockers, like the medication Inderal (propranolol), although most common for high blood pressure and cardiac conditions, are also used in pain management as prophylactic medical therapy to help prevent migraine attacks and to help control certain anxiety states.

Biofeedback A complementary medicine technique that trains patients to control the body's unconscious processes. It has been demonstrated that if patients can learn to regulate breathing, heart rate, and muscle tension, then they can apply this skill to alleviate chronic pain. Biofeedback often goes along with other complementary techniques, like behavioral therapy and relaxation training, among others.

Biopsychosocial This is a key term used in chronic pain management relating to the biological, psychological, and social aspects of pain assessment and care. This is opposed to focusing on just the biomedical aspect of a disease process, like for most acute pain states. The biopsychosocial approach looks at the mind-body-social connection of a patient as three important overlapping systems that all need to be addressed for best long-term care. These three aspects command varying importance during a patient's clinical care course, so that patients can make their best gains at getting well and staying well. This approach is best accomplished using a multidisciplinary care plan looking at causes of organic disease or injury, psychological conditions that develop, like depression, and society's influences, such as secondary gain or catastrophizing—internalizing and showing outward ill behavior. All of these play a part in the actual development of different chronic pain conditions. The **PITS Program** strives to maximize a patient's **PITS Score**, which incorporates *bio-psycho-social focused goals* (see **APPENDIX A**).

Botulinum Toxin Type A (Botox) A purified onobotulinum toxin that is used for injection for a variety of medical conditions, but commonly for pain management purposes to treat chronic migraines and chronic muscle spasms. Botox acts by blocking the neurotransmitter acetylcholine responsible for transmission of nerve impulses to muscles and can last for up to three months duration. It is very safe and effective when used by properly trained medical professionals—doctors, nurse practitioners, and so forth.

Brachial Plexus This is a collection of peripheral nerves that arise primarily from the cervical spine that course through the shoulder and into the arm. When injury or disease affects these nerves, patients can develop painful brachial plexopathy, a difficult neuropathic pain syndrome to treat.

Breakthrough Pain Pain that occurs suddenly or because of a particular activity. This can happen even when patients are taking medication on a regular basis. Patients can frequently have *breakthrough pain* due to weather changes, doing too much activity on a given day, their previous pain relief is wearing off from previous successful treatments, or when patients unfortunately reinjure themselves from an accident. Therefore, patients taking a long-acting pain medication, whether it is an opioid or not, frequently need a second pain medication that is fast-acting, to use as rescue relief when breakthrough pain arises. Breakthrough medication choices can include an opioid, anti-inflammatory, muscle relaxant, or other medication that is fast-acting. You do not take a long-acting drug for breakthrough pain because it takes too long to work effectively. Long-acting opiate pain medication, on the other hand, works best when taken at regular fixed times during the day to maintain blood levels, whether it is once, twice, or three times a day depending on the specific medication.

Breathing Therapy This is the type of complementary therapy involving a rhythmic pattern of inhalation and exhalation of air through the lungs. Through this exercise, many chronic pain patients can promote physical, mental, and spiritual well-being in their bodies. Conscious attention to breathing is common in many forms of relaxa tion and meditation, such as yoga.

Bulging Disc A common condition and source of pain in the spine that occurs when disc material bulges through the back or sides of the spinal disc, resulting in compression and irritation of spinal nerves and other surrounding tissue. This pathologic condition typically leads to an intense inflammation that causes severe back pain and radiating leg symptoms or sciatica. Like bulging discs, actual *herniated discs* impinging on nerve roots and compressing the spinal sac have even more of a tendency to create back and radiating leg pain, with can then lead to varying degrees of numbness and tingling neurologic symptoms in patients.

Buprenorphine This is a semisynthetic opioid narcotic used as an analgesic for moderate-to-severe pain that is formulated for sublingual use under the tongue and as a skin patch, with both forms used as around-the-clock delivery of opioid to control pain. The patch form is for patients to wear once a week as a long-acting, controlled-release pain medication to treat chronic pain, and the sublingual film form is typically dosed twice a day for similar treatment. Patch and sublingual forms of opioids are especially useful if patients do not tolerate oral narcotic medication. Buprenorphine is also commonly used in *addictionology medicine* care, with the medications Suboxone and Subutex, to help keep patients from craving other opioids.

Bursitis A painful inflammation of a bursa or a small fluid filled sac that can lie between a bone or a joint or a muscle. There are many bursae in the shoulders, elbows, hips, knees, heels, and even the spine, which cause pain when they flare.

C

Cancer Pain Pain due to a cancerous condition that may be acute, chronic, or intermittent in nature. Cancer pain often has a definable cause, usually related to an initial tumor or recurrence of a tumor that was once in remission. Unfortunately, cancer pain can sometimes be due to the actual treatment a patient receives, like radiation therapy or certain chemotherapy agents. Tumor invasion can involve organs, bone, muscle, or nerves and often leads to a state of continuous pain with periodic episodes of breakthrough pain.

Cannabis Cannabis, commonly known as marijuana, is a plant that is well known to almost everyone for its illegal and abuse status in this country at the federal level, but now being used by most states for medical purposes as an *analgesic pain killer* and for antianxiety and relaxing effects—different states cover different conditions for use. Recreational-use marijuana is also rapidly expanding in this country, and we will see how that plays out in the coming years. From a medical pain management standpoint, there are different types of cannabinoid pain receptors in the body and science and research support cannabis use for treatment of many conditions like neuropathies, chronic pain, myofascial pain with spasticity, irritable bowel disease (IBD), cancer pain, HIV-AIDS pain, multiple sclerosis (MS) pain, spinal cord injury (SCI), and other conditions like post-traumatic stress disorder (PTSD). *Cannabidiol (CBD)* and *tetrahydrocannabinol (THC)* are the two active ingredients in medical cannabis, where the CBD component has been best shown to have analgesic pain relief effects and the THC psychoactive component is best for muscle relaxation and sedative and calming effects. Many chronic pain sufferers are continuing to explore this relief therapy, feeling it is a safer option compared to opioids and overdose risk. The downside is that it is expensive to maintain treatment monthly, as many insurances do not cover the medical prescription cost. A lot of patients just try the CBD oil or other formulations itself, without the THC, which can be purchased OTC in smoke shops.

Capsaicin Capsaicin is a compound in certain *hot pepper plants* and is used topically as a cream or patch to relief minor arthritis and neuralgia pain. When capsaicin is applied to the skin, it causes a burning sensation which is tolerable to most patients. The science behind the relief is that capsaicin has been shown to deplete the nerve cells of a chemical called substance P, which plays a key role in transmission of pain signals and messages from the skin, through peripheral nerves, and on to the central nerves of the spinal cord.

Carpal Tunnel Syndrome (CTS) A painful neuropathic condition which occurs when the median nerve, which is a large peripheral nerve that runs from the forearm into the hand, becomes compressed at the wrist. Patients typically experience symptoms of pain and numbness into the hand and fingers, and typically seek out an orthopedic hand specialist for care options at some point, as the condition worsens through time. Medications, injections, and therapy can help with treatment relief, but surgery must be considered if patients start to experience weakness of the hand before irreversible atrophy and weakness develops.

Cartilage Tissue that cushions bones and joints in the shoulders, knees, hips, spine, and other body locations. Cartilage can be gradually worn down through time or injured traumatically, and this can lead to a frequent source of chronic pain.

Catastrophize This is a psychiatric term that describes the tendency of patients to constantly focus on their pain and to experience constant worry, like *doom and gloom*. When patients catastrophize, they tend to underestimate their ability to control the pain they experience on a daily basis, and this leads to a lack of effective coping skill development.

Cauda Equina Syndrome Cauda equina syndrome is a dangerous condition caused by excessive compression and narrowing of spinal canal nerves at the end of the spinal cord. Causes of this syndrome include spinal stenosis, traumatic injury, a large disc herniation, spinal tumors, inflammatory conditions like arachnoiditis, and infectious conditions like an abscess. Acute cauda equina symptoms, especially if associated with high impact spine injury, are considered a surgical emergency, because if left untreated it could lead to permanent loss of bowel and bladder control, numbness, and leg paralysis. Typically, a lumbar laminectomy and/or discectomy is needed to relieve the compression on the spinal nerves.

Caudal This is the anatomic area where the end of the sacral spine joins the upper tailbone area. Caudal epidural steroid injections (ESIs), also known as lumbosacral level injections, can be performed in this part of the spine to treat lower spinal inflammatory pain conditions. These minimally invasive injections are typically performed outpatient under fluoroscopic X-ray guidance, similar to patients who undergo neck and lumbar back ESI procedures.

Celiac Plexus This is an anatomic network of nerve fibers in the back of the abdomen that conduct pain sensations from abdominal organs, including the lower esophagus, liver, stomach, pancreas, and certain parts of the intestines. If certain chronic and severe conditions cause pain within this plexus coverage area, then local anesthetic and/or neurolytic agents such as *medical alcohol* preparations can be injected percutaneously through the skin under radiology guidance around these nerves to control intractable abdominal pain symptoms—as in the case of pancreatic cancer pain.

Central Pain Syndrome The name given to a type of chronic neuropathic pain condition that is caused by a disease process or injury in the central nervous system that involves the brain and/or spinal cord. This could be due to a spinal cord injury, a medical disease such as multiple sclerosis, an amputee patient experiencing phantom limb pain, or a post-stroke victim who develops chronic central pain. Most central pain conditions are very difficult to treat and demand a comprehensive multidisciplinary approach to chronic treatment—frequently with periods of inpatient medical care—to optimize a patient's overall comfort and functional status.

Central Sensitization A medical term that describes the gradual process of an increase in neuron nerve excitability within the central nervous system, that results in the creation of chronic and sometimes permanent changes that lead to abnormal nerve transmission. This sensitization often leads to the start of many chronic painful disease states, especially if not suppressed aggressively early in the course of pain treatment. A classic setup for central sensitization and chronic pain is uncontrolled severe acute post-operative pain, where the spinal cord central nervous system gets continually bombarded by all the constant post-op pain stimuli in the periphery—from skin, soft tissue, muscle, bone, and so forth. This, in turn, leads to permanent inflammatory and ischemic-related cell death changes in spinal and brain nerves and their connections. Current research has revealed that this pathological process is real, with evidence of *glial cell death* in the central nervous system (CNS). These glial cells play a vital role in CNS nerve transmission.

Centrally-Acting Analgesic This is a medical term of a pain medication that works primarily at a brain receptor site, like acetaminophen (Tylenol) and tramadol (Ultram and Ultracet) to relieve pain. This contrasts with nonsteroidal anti-inflammatory medications, like ibuprofen (Motrin) and naproxen (Aleve), which work primarily out in the peripheral nerve and tissue receptors in the extremities and trunk to inhibit inflammatory prostaglandin substances.

Chiropractor (Doctor of Chiropractic or D.C.) These practitioners are involved with the medical practice of diagnosis and treatment of physical conditions that cause pain and discomfort in the musculoskeletal and nervous systems of the body. Chiropractic care is a professional, noninvasive, safe, manipulation-type of approach for acute and chronic pain problems. Chiropractors are trained very much like medical doctors in anatomy and physiology and pathologic states, but not with all the medication prescribing. Chiropractic therapy is typically a repeatable program care process over many weeks duration to get patients back to improved comfort and activity levels. Chiropractic care is considered mainstream medical care in the **PITS Program philosophy** of treatment, and is not just considered a complementary and alternative technique or approach. Chiropractors often have as their task to relieve the pressure of joint subluxations and compressed nerves for pain relief of the spine, and to improve a patient's overall health. Chiropractic care is often used in conjunction with physical therapy to optimize a patient's rehabilitation potential, where *chiropractic care straightens* and *physical therapy care strengthens* painful areas of the body.

Chronic Fatigue Syndrome A condition of prolonged and severe fatigue or excessive tiredness that can occur after an injury or illness. It is not relieved by rest or sleep itself, and the syndrome is not directly caused by other medical conditions. Chronic fatigue syndrome is often seen in patients suffering with fibromyalgia and other dysfunctional pain states. Fibromyalgia typically causes chronic widespread soft tissue pain, chronic fatigue, irritable bowel, and memory and sleep disturbances.

Chronic Pain Pain that can be defined as persisting for six months or greater, pain that persists beyond the normal healing of a traumatic injury, or pain that persists beyond the normal treatment and healing process of an acute medical illness. Chronic pain negatively affects a patient's well-being and quality of life. Chronic pain is a biopsychosocial phenomenon that can persist for years, which can be considered the opposite of a classic acute pain, which is typically just a biomedical pain that heals fully in just weeks to months. Long-term chronic pain is considered pathological and serves no biologic or protective purpose, like touching a hot stove and immediately jerking your hand away serves a bio-protective purpose. Chronic pain persists over time and is often resistant to medical treatments because chronic pain often damages the central nervous system which can lead to ongoing persistent inflammation flares. With the resultant central nervous system damage, the pain itself starts to persist as a disease state, and not just as a symptom of an illness. Because of these changes in the central nervous system, treatment requires a specialized care approach, and in certain cases involves putting patients on opioid narcotic therapy at some point for severe-level pain problems that fail non-opioid therapy care. It turns out that chronic pain can be minor or severe in nature, and can go away for many months and then return with a vengeance, and can be caused by something that is not expected to ever heal. The **Pain is the PITS Program** provides an answer for what to do about all the ongoing chronic pain in America, especially considering America's ongoing opioid crisis that developed along the way.

Chronic Pain Syndrome (CPS) A general term given to a biopsychosocial chronic pain disorder that involves a lot of symptoms and signs of pain that consumes the attention of the patient and can become incapacitating. Examples include, complex regional pain syndrome, fibromyalgia pain syndrome, post-surgery pain syndrome, myofascial pain syndrome, and many others.

Claudication   Pain in the calf and leg that occurs after patients walk a certain distance, typically related to either vascular reasons, like atherosclerotic plaques that block arteries in the legs from peripheral vascular disease, or from spinal neurogenic claudication reasons, like spinal nerve compression in the low back from progressive lumbar spinal stenosis.

Clinical Pathway   This is the medical term used in the **PITS Program** to represent the multidisciplinary integrative protocol guideline used for pain management for all the pain sufferers in America. The **PITS Clinical Pathway** is based on both evidence-based medicine practice showing what works and what does not work in medical practice based on *science and research*, as well as expert *medical provider opinion* from all the healthcare pain management professionals who perform the clinical treatments. The **PITS Clinical Pathway** provides repetitive optimal diagnosis, treatment, and reevaluation pain management steps for anybody who complains of persistent *PAIN*, which will then allow the healthcare pain team to maximize an individual's comfort and quality-of-life goals moving forward.

Clinical Trials   These are medically planned and monitored experiments to test a new drug or treatment. These trials are carefully constructed by a team of researchers to establish the science behind treatment effectiveness, and to help determine risk-and-benefit of different drugs and treatments. In America, the *Food and Drug Administration (FDA)* oversees human clinical trial regulations and conduct.

Cluster Headache   A type of headache that that can be episodic in nature or repeat in a more chronic pattern. These headaches are typically severe, and are characterized by one or more short attacks occurring behind the eye, which occur on a daily for a period of weeks to months. After the attack period is over, cluster headaches can go into remission for six months to a year. They tend to be seasonal-type headaches, usually in the spring and fall. Other common headaches include tension-type and migraine.

Coccydynia   This is the medical term given to nerve and ligament pain in and around the coccyx joint area.

This pain, which can be both acute and chronic, is typically caused by trauma to the area, most commonly through a hard fall on the tailbone. If medical pain management fails to offer enough relief with pain medication, heat, and soft donut-cushion to sit on, then interventional pain management can be offered with injection of steroid and local anesthetic in the coccyx ligament and nerve area, to treat persistent symptoms and to help with further healing.

Cognitive-Behavioral Therapy (CBT)   A type of psychological therapy for patients to learn to control painful thoughts and feelings and behaviors. Science and research have shown CBT to be very helpful and effective for the treatment of chronic pain disorders, especially when combined with other medication and talk therapies, so patients can start changing *negative* aspects of their pain and quality of life into *positive* ones. There are professionals trained in this field of care in the country that motivated patients can seek out and gain the knowledge necessary to make CBT a proactive treatment in their **PITS Program**.

Comparative Effectiveness Research   this is the scientific process of doing research comparing different interventions and strategies to diagnose and treat pain. The purpose of the research is to determine which interventions are most effective for patients under specific conditions. This information is important to inform patients and doctors, and even insurance companies, as to effective pain management strategies. This is important in the development of evidence-based pain management—*what works and what does not work*.

Complementary Care Medicine   Approaches to medical treatment that are typically outside of mainstream medical training and conventional pain care strategies—medications, injections, physical therapy, and surgery—that can make a difference in a patient's overall successful pain management wellness program. Complementary medicine treatments used for pain include acupuncture, meditation, Reiki, aromatherapy and essential oils, Chinese medicine, dance and music therapy, herbal medicines and supplements, massage and therapeutic touch, yoga and Tai Chi, naturopathy using alternative medicine approach using natural products, low level laser therapy (LLLT), diet and other lifestyle changes to improve homeostasis in the body, and homeopathy using alternative medicine approach using remedies of dilute natural substances—*"like cures like"* philosophy. In the **P-I-T-S treatment protocol**, I put chiropractic treatments in with mainstream therapy care options, like physical therapy, because of their medical importance in straightening patients for proper alignment, as patients continue to pursue formal physical therapy for strengthening their painful body areas. Complementary medicine techniques are used in conjunction with conventional standard ones to give patients their best comprehensive *"integrative"* pain management care. Conventional medicine is practiced by a medical doctor (M.D.) or doctor of osteopathy (D.O.) or chiropractor (D.C.), along with all the allied health professionals, like nurse practitioners (NPs), physician assistants (PAs), registered nurses (RNs), medical assistants (MAs), physical therapists (PTs), and psychologists.

Complex Regional Pain Syndrome (CRPS)   CRPS, also still referred to in the pain management world as Reflex Sympathetic Dystrophy (RSD), is a mixed nociceptive and neuropathic pain condition that afflicts many patients, and has a specific diagnostic criterion to follow involving sensory, motor, and autonomic nervous system findings and changes. Many patients with CRPS continue to suffer for months to years without a diagnosis, well after the initial precipitating incident is gone and full healing has occurred. When diagnosed early, typically within three months, CRPS has the best chance to be controlled and *put into remission*, without persistent longer-term subjective pain symptoms— what the patient feels—and physical signs—what the doctor finds on examination. When pain is present chronically, from six months to a year, many patients will need longer-term multidisciplinary pain care strategies to optimize their relief. Without trying to get too scientific, CRPS—or RSD, as a lot of patients and physicians still refer to it as—can have both sympathetic nervous system-maintained pain due to *sympathetic nerve* involvement and sympathetic-independent nervous system-maintained pain due to *peripheral nerve* component involvement. Not all patients experience all the signs and symptoms, which again, can include

skin sensitivity to touch, out-of-the ordinary pain response to a minor painful stimulus, excessive sweating, hot or cold changes, skin color mottling, swelling in hands and feet, stiffness and tremor, and nail bed and hair growth changes. Therefore, treatments are individualized to each presenting clinical situation and modified through time depending on a patient's clinical response course. Patients typically follow the various **P-I-T-S treatment protocol** options for best care, as revealed through ongoing clinical research and previous patient positive outcomes.

Complication   This a general medical term given to a clinical problem that arises in patient care, whether it comes from a drug treatment, procedure, or a pain illness. Complications are not anticipated but always possible and can happen at any point during pain management, due to the nature of medical science and care which is not an exact science.

Computerized Axial Tomography (CAT) Scan   A diagnostic radiology procedure, commonly referred to as a CT scan, involving computer-generated radiation X-ray technology pictures that are helpful in diagnosing a patient's source of pain. A CT scan can provide cross section images of soft tissue and bone, and especially helpful in diagnosing spine and organ abnormalities. CT scan technology—when needed for diagnosis and treatment decisions by your healthcare providers—uses ionizing radiation that takes image slices of the body's organs, bones, the brain, and other tissues offering a more detailed picture than what a regular black and white X-ray can reveal. CT scan images are sometimes used as guidance for certain diagnostic and therapeutic interventional pain procedures, like discography and celiac plexus block.

Congenital   The general medical term that describes a disease or structural condition that is present at birth. Congenital conditions stay with patients throughout life and can worsen through time, until corrected if ever corrected, like *congenital spinal stenosis* that results in patients having a premature narrowed spinal canal area.

Conscious Sedation   An anesthesia medical term that means light sedation, also known as twilight sleep. This anesthetic is typically given intravenously (IV) by an anesthesiologist for outpatient minimally invasive interventional pain management procedures that are associated with moderate-to-severe level procedure pain. IV sedation is also offered to those patients who are excessively nervous during procedures. During IV sedation, patients can still respond to verbal stimuli and can maintain control of their protective airway reflexes to minimize the risk of aspiration—the passage of liquid and solid stomach contents into the lung.

Constipation The common term that describes difficulty having a bowel movement. This could be due to a medical condition or treatment, especially for patients on chronic opioid narcotic pain medication. When opioid narcotics are deemed responsible for a patient's symptoms, this is known as *opioid-induced constipation (OIC)*. Patients often consider taking stool softeners or stimulants, or other prescription medications, if they cannot have a bowel movement at a frequency of every two days or less.

Contraindication A medical term that describes a treatment (medication, injection, therapy, or surgery) that is inappropriate and could result in an adverse outcome for a patient. An example would be a patient who continues to take Coumadin (a blood thinner) and has an epidural steroid injection (ESI), which could result in bleeding in the spine leading to paralysis from excessive spinal nerve compression from the blood accumulation (hematoma) in the limited epidural nerve space.

Costochondritis A painful inflammatory and arthritic nociceptive pain condition that causes irritation in the chest wall where the bony ribs meet the cartilage connection of the sternum or breastbone. Pain and discomfort in this area typically arises from repetitive activity or injury. This type of musculoskeletal chest pain frequently mimics symptoms of pain that patients confuse as having a real heart attack.

Counterirritant A term given to a drug (like capsaicin), a procedure (like acupuncture), or medical device (like a transcutaneous electrical nerve stimulator or TENS unit) that produces irritation or stimulation at one site in the body—typically on the skin—to obtain pain relief through a decreased perception of

pain locally or to achieve relief at a distant pain site. It is thought that pain relief from counterirritant treatments is due in part to a change in the body's natural *endorphin and encephalin* pain killer activation, and other chemical changes at the pain receptor level, that in turn lessens the transmission of these pain impulses through the spinal cord that would otherwise be perceived by our brains full force.

Cranial Nerves There are twelve cranial nerves that affect the face and head in patients. If there are any abnormalities of these nerves, whether it is from a disease or traumatic cause, then neurologic symptoms can afflict a patient like numbness, sharp shooting pain, or burning pain. Certain cranial nerves are often implicated as being involved in the chronic mechanism that creates recurrent headache like a migraine and facial pain like trigeminal neuralgia.

Cryoanalgesia A safe and minimally invasive outpatient interventional pain procedure that involves deactivation of peripheral nerves using extreme cold therapy to achieve prolonged pain relief that can last for weeks to months. Cryoanalgesia can be applied to intercostal nerves for persistent chest wall and rib pain after fractures or chest operation, certain neuromas that can form after an inguinal hernia operation, a Morton's neuroma in the foot, and other conditions.

Cryotherapy The therapeutic use of cold to reduce discomfort locally where applied creating a local anesthetic-like effect and to decrease swelling or edema in injured tissues. By breaking the pain cycle with this commonly repeated outpatient physical therapy modality, along with the counter use of heat as needed, patients can attempt to speed up their rehabilitation process.

Cyclooxygenase-1 (COX-1) A medical enzyme involved with certain body functions and organs—stomach, kidney, platelets, and so forth—that is produced in normal physiological amounts to protect patients. For example, COX-1 produced in the stomach serves a protective role for the lining of the stomach to prevent ulcers. Nonsteroidal anti-inflammatory drugs (NSAIDs) like Aleve and Motrin inhibit COX-1 (as well as Cyclooxygenase-2 or COX-2—the actual undesirable inflammatory enzyme form) in a non-selective fashion and can result in ulcer formation in susceptible patients. Other NSAIDs that inhibit the enzyme form like Celebrex, are more selective in their inhibition and do not affect the protective COX-1 form, only the pain-causing COX-2 form, and thus do not tend to harm the stomach lining as much.

Cyclooxygenase-2 (COX-2)   A form of cyclooxygenase enzyme (unlike COX-1) that arises at sites of pathologic inflammation, especially in joints. COX-2 enzyme formation is undesirable and harms the body when not controlled. If COX-2 is produced in joints by inflammation, then a COX-2 inhibitor, like a non-steroidal anti-inflammatory drug (NSAID), can block the enzyme resulting in reduced inflammation and pain relief. COX-2 inhibitors that are selective like Celebrex can be used to treat pain and are less likely to cause gastrointestinal bleeding than other nonselective NSAIDs (like Motrin and Aleve), which inhibit both COX-1 and COX-2 enzyme forms (the COX-1 enzyme is the desirable form that normally protects the body). Recent research studies uncovered evidence that COX-2 inhibitors may increase risk of heart attack and stroke, so two out of the three common COX-2 inhibitors—Vioxx and Bextra—were removed from the U.S. market years ago. Celebrex remains available by prescription, and in lower doses has been considered safe in patients who do not have an active cardiac disease history.

D

D.C.   An abbreviation for *Doctor of Chiropractic* for those professionals practicing chiropractic medical care. This is different than the letters M.D. which stands for *Medical Doctor* and different from D.O. which stands for *Doctor of Osteopathy*.

Deafferentation Pain   A difficult type of neuropathic pain that is due to the loss of normal sensory input into the central nervous system. This can occur when there is an injury to the brachial plexus nerves (plexopathy) that run from the neck through the shoulder and into the arm, or from a traumatic amputation of a leg, where the normal sensory input from the leg nerves to the

spinal cord is now lost. This can also occur if there are lesions of peripheral nerves, such as the sciatic nerve (buttock) or median nerve (wrist). Deafferentation pain typically leaves the skin with exquisite sensitivity and can be difficult to treat.

Decompression   A term used to typically describe a form of chiropractic traction using a device or table that stretches and *releases the spine* while the patient lies face down. This form of treatment is often used to treat arthritis, herniated and bulging discs, and soft tissue conditions, while improving circulation. A *surgical decompression* often refers to many surgical procedures—spine, shoulder, wrist/elbow—where physical bone and tissue are removed to relieve pain.

Deep Tissues   Tissues including bone, muscle, tendon, joint capsules, and fasciae. This is the opposite of superficial tissue, like the skin.

Degenerative Disc Disease (DDD)   A progressive condition involving the vertebral discs, particularly in the lumbar spine, in which the inner core of the disc, called the nucleus pulposis, leaks proteins that can inflame and scar the nerves around the outside of the disc, called the annulus fibrosis. As discs lose a lot of their height—also through loss of hydration with time—patients start to feel variable amounts of *discogenic pain* in their back or neck. This process typically leads to a chronic pain state, especially in patients whose job involves a lot of physical labor.

Dependence (Physical Dependence)   This is a medical physiologic state or phenomenon that typically results when patients take an opioid narcotic pain medication for over a week. When physical dependence occurs, then patients are at risk of developing withdrawal symptoms that can be produced by a number of factors, including abrupt cessation of a drug when patients stop the drug cold turkey, rapid dose reduction when a drug is weaned too fast, decreasing blood level of the medication for patients on short-acting narcotic as opposed to long-acting narcotic to keep blood levels from dipping, or the administration of a reversal agent opioid antagonist, like the drug naloxone given to heroin overdose victims, for example. What can happen to a patient when their body gets use too dependent on a narcotic and then the narcotic is suddenly taken away, is that they start to feel horrible from the withdrawal effects of rapidly decreasing blood levels of drug in their system. The stronger the narcotic, the sicker a patient typically feels. Patients experience an abstinence syndrome where they feel flu-like symptoms of tremulousness, nervousness, palpitations, sweating, muscle cramps, and nausea. Physical dependence is different from addiction—addiction is an actual psychiatric disease state. It turns out that if patients are given back the opioid narcotic, then all the withdrawal symptoms promptly disappear.

Depression This is an underappreciated and treatable medical illness that affects the mind, body, and mood of many chronic pain patients. Medications, talk therapy, and other cognitive-behavioral therapies (CBTs) are common treatment options to help patients understand and treat their symptoms of depression. Uncontrolled depression leads to a negative emotional experience of pain—remember pain is both a physical and emotional experience. If depression is left untreated through time, then a patient's physical pain complaints can worsen. We now know, through recent research and science using functional-MRI imaging techniques and chemical nerve pathway analysis in the brain, that the physical pain and emotional pain pathways are intermingled as they lead to final pain perception and interpretation in the brain. Patients cannot fully recover their quality of life unless both pain and depression are addressed and controlled during treatment. A psychogenic pain state exists if only a patient's depression is the cause of all their pain and no physical organic condition or disease is identifiable.

Dermatomes The medical term given to the cutaneous (skin) sensory pathways that are defined by sensation. Each dermatome corresponds to the area of skin that is supplied by the spinal root of a sensory nerve, from the cervical spine right down to the sacral spine dermatomes. Dermatomal wall charts are often seen in neurology, spine surgery, and pain management offices.

Diabetic Neuropathy A medical condition leading to numbness, weakness, and pain in the hands and feet, caused by the effects of diabetes on nerve function and transmission. Medical pain management if the mainstay of treatment for this often progressive and often difficult to treat disease. Diabetics who control their blood sugar well typically do the best with slowing down the neuropathy progression.

Disability A legal term given to a state of patient functioning that arises when a physical impairment limits an individual's capacity for work and independent living. Most slip-and-fall victims, motor vehicle victims, and workers' compensation (WC) patients, must go through the disability evaluation process at some point in their acute and chronic pain treatment process. Keep in mind that pain alone is typically not considered a disability. Pain alone is too subjective, so you need objective physical evidence of impairment causing a chronic pain condition with formal diagnosis and treatment of that painful condition, to support a claim of a certain level of disability.

Disc A round cartilage and gel-like cushion between the bones (vertebrae) of the spinal cord. These spinal discs are subjected to different forces—crush, shear, and so forth—over many decades of life and therefore are susceptible to painful injury and chronic disease states. Common painful disc conditions are degenerative disc disease (DDD) and bulging or herniated discs.

Discectomy The name given to the surgical removal of part or an entire intervertebral disc. Removal of disc material that is compressing and inflaming spinal nerves and tissue is a common orthopedic and neurosurgical specialty procedure. This procedure is considered safe and minimally invasive spine surgery. Immediate relief of leg pain symptoms, for example, typically results from this decompression process where a lumbar spinal nerve is freed from a piece of compressive lumbar disc material.

Distraction A psychological cognitive strategy of focusing a patient's attention on something other than the pain itself, like playing music played through a set of headphones or playing solitaire with a deck of cards, and so forth.

E

Efficacy This a general medical term describing the ability of a drug, injection, or surgical procedure to produce a desired therapeutic effect in a patient. For example, after research and clinical use in patients, it was found that anti-inflammatory medications were efficacious in controlling signs and symptoms of acute and chronic inflammatory pain conditions like arthritis pain—as opposed to a placebo or sugar pill which has no meaningful anti-inflammatory benefit.

Electrotherapy A pain management physical therapy modality technique that applies electrical stimulation to affected nerves and muscles to encourage the body to release pain-killing chemicals, such as endorphins and enkephalins, which can then block pain signals from being transmitted to the brain. Electrotherapy is often done in conjunction with heat and ice, and other modalities for symptomatic relief of musculoskeletal disorders, like back pain and arthritis.

Electromyogram (EMG) This is a medical diagnostic test to determine neuromuscular activity and health of peripheral nerves and muscles using needles and electrical stimulation—a NCS (nerve conduction study) is often performed in conjunction with an EMG. This outpatient test is typically for patients suffering with pain and numbness and/or weakness symptoms in the arms and legs. It can test nerve function and motor function and is administered under the medical direction of either a neurologist or physiatrist—rehabilitative physician. EMG/NCS tests are often utilized in combination with other imaging tests, such as CT scan or MRI, to diagnose painful conditions which can then lead to better directed treatment options for patient care moving forward. Interventional and surgical procedures can be more successful when patients undergo a *full workup* to confirm the most likely pain-generating source, so that the pain management and surgical team care plans have the best chance at producing a desired relief outcome.

EMLA (Eutectic mixture of local anesthetic) An ointment that contains a mixture of two local anesthetics, namely lidocaine and prilocaine. It is placed through a topical application and it results in a local anesthetic effect that lasts for a short period of time. This process avoids the need for injection, especially in the pediatric population. EMLA is often used in children prior to painful injection procedures, like placing an intravenous catheter through the skin.

Endocrine System This is the organ system in the body that involves glands that produce hormones. Hormones, like testosterone and estrogen, help to control normal metabolic activity in patients. Examples of these glands are the hypothalamus, pituitary, thyroid, adrenal glands above the kidneys, ovaries, and testes. There a body of research showing that taking long-term, high-dose opioid narcotic pain medications can suppress the endocrine system and lead to opioid-induced endocrinopathy, which includes negative patient effects on the stress response, mood, sleep patterns, fatigue, weight gain, sex hormones and libido, osteoporosis, and other bodily effects.

End-Of-Life Care This is a general care term for patients who are expected to die within weeks to months. It can be considered the same as *hospice care*, where a dedicated team of physicians, nurses and caregivers provide care to patients primarily focusing on quality-of-life issues. Comfort, psychological care, and spiritual support are the patient's most important goals with this focus of care—but support for the patient's family, as well, should not be ignored or undervalued.

Energy Medicine A type of complementary medicine offered by holistic practitioners based on the concept that patients possess a *vital energy chi form* that needs to be maintained for good health. If this energy form is disturbed, especially when patients are ill or in pain, then they use certain learned techniques to restore and rebalance the flow of the body's energy—resulting in return of pain relief and overall improved health. Examples of energy medicine include Reiki, Qi Gong, and healing touch.

Epicondylitis A medical term given to a type of inflammation or damage around the epicondyle bone, typically in the elbow. Tennis elbow is the common name for lateral epicondylitis and golfer's elbow is the same as medial epicondylitis in the elbow. Overuse injury to the elbow is the typical clinical course and leads to damage and inflammation arising to pain. If medical pain management with medication and therapy results in limited relief, then interventional pain management injections can be offered to break the pain cycle and speed the rehabilitative process.

Epidural Medication This refers to medication—local anesthetic, opioid narcotic, steroid, or other medication—that is injected into the epidural region of the spine, often to treat labor pain in pregnancy, for surgical operations, or to treat chronic pain due to inflammatory and nerve-related spine conditions. Anatomically, the epidural space is the outer layer that surrounds the brain and spinal cord. It is situated outside of the *dura matter*, which is an inner layer that contains the cerebrospinal fluid (CSF) in the center of the spinal canal.

Epidural Steroid Injection (ESI) This is one of the most common interventional pain management procedures performed for back and neck pain, and for radiating leg and arm numbness and tingling symptoms. It is a safe outpatient fluoroscopic-guided needle injection of steroid—typically a depot-steroid particulate steroid—delivered into the cervical, thoracic, lumbar, or lumbosacral (caudal) level areas of the spine, with the goal of relieving inflammatory and nerve-related spinal pain conditions. These injections are for patients with typical pain and radicular symptoms due to bulging or herniated discs resulting in a *pinched nerve*, spinal stenosis or spinal space *narrowing*, spinal listhesis or *slippage* of one vertebral spine bone over another, or other spinal disease reasons. Lumbar and cervical radiculopathy are the most common pain conditions treated with ESIs. Most ESIs are performed by board-certified, pain-fellowship trained physicians—typically an anesthesiologist, physiatrist, or neurologist. Relief from ESIs can last for weeks-to-months or longer, depending on an individual patient's overall clinical situation, and they are repeatable as needed for future flares of pain.

Equianalgesic This is a medical term that describes the potency of different opioid narcotic medications as having an equivalent analgesic relief effect when doses are compared to each other, like *this much* oxycodone gives the same narcotic pain relief effect as *that much* morphine. Equianalgesic also describes the different drug routes of administration like oral (PO) compared to intravenous (IV)—for example, *this much* IV Dilaudid (hydromorphone) is equivalent to *that much* PO Dilaudid conversion to achieve the same narcotic relief effect in a patient. In terms of opioid narcotic, morphine is generally used for opioid analgesic standard comparison—it has always been this way. An *equianalgesic dose table* is a chart that converts from one analgesic or root of administration to another. Such a chart typically describes the dose of an opioid required to produce the same degree of pain relief provided by a standard oral or injectable dose of morphine. Again, equianalgesic dose tables help pain providers answer the question of converting patients from one type of opioid to an equivalent dose of another opioid, should the case arise during different patient pain care situations. Refer to the **PITS Opioid Narcotic Comparison Dosing Chart** (see **APPENDIX D**).

Ergonomics The common term that typically applies to a work or home environment, specifically addressing the type of work that is done and how a person would perform that work. Ergonomics focuses on the goal of finding the best fit between a patient and his or her job conditions, with the typical aim being to minimize pain and disability. An example is sitting at a computer desk where the chair is upright, the arms are flexed 90 degrees for typing, and the neck is in neutral position—not looking up or down too much on a computer screen. Another example is manual labor work, such as doing heavy lifting, with a focus on keeping your back straight and bending at the legs—not bending the back forward too much.

Ergotamine Ergotamine is a type of abortive headache medication, whether taken PO at home or IV in an emergency room, for treating severe patient symptoms. It reduces pain symptoms by narrowing blood vessels through vasoconstriction, and is often used for relief of cluster or migraine headaches. For safety reasons, patients are not to take ergotamine products and triptan headache products at the same time because of potentially dangerous side effects.

Ethics A discipline of medicine and science that involves a system of *moral principles and rules* that are used as standards for professional conduct. Both doctors and patients are generally aware of basic ethical care, which is the usual common sense, straight forward decision-making process, but many hospitals for example, have created ethics committees that can help doctors and patients and family members in making more difficult decisions regarding medical and pain management care—like issues surrounding end-of-life care.

Evidence Based Healthcare It is a combination of best research evidence through medical studies, clinical experience with a physician's expertise, and the patient's preference or wishes and desires, all combined to make final treatment decisions. From a pain management perspective, evidence-based pain care all comes down to picking the right pain management treatment option, for the right pain patient, at the right time in a protocol. The **Pain is the PITS Program** protocol options for treatment provide a *universal treatment guideline* for all patients who suffer with any type of pain, whether acute, chronic, or cancer related.

Extremities A medical term that pertains to the arms and legs. The upper extremities include the upper limbs, the shoulders, arms, forearms, wrists, and hands. The lower extremities include the lower limbs, the hip, thighs, legs, ankles, and feet.

F

Facet This is the medical term for the joints in the back of the spine that connect one vertebral level to the next level—one facet joint on each side of a particular vertebral level. Facets exist in the cervical, thoracic, and lumbar spine, and allow for the normal range of motion between spinal segments like bending and twisting. These joints are susceptible, not only to injury, but also progressive degeneration and inflammation over the course of time, leading to a painful biomechanical and inflammatory back and neck condition commonly known as *facet pain syndrome*.

Facet Joint Injection A common and safe minimally invasive interventional pain management procedure involving the injection of steroid, with or without the addition of local anesthetic, into suspected painful facet joints of the spine, whether they be in the cervical, thoracic, or lumbar region. These injections can be performed for both diagnostic and therapeutic pain relief reasons. They are performed in an outpatient setting under fluoroscopic (X-ray) guidance, with or without IV sedation for comfort and anxiety. When facet injections are performed solely for diagnostic reasons for facet radiofrequency ablation (RA) nerve burning or for surgical planning, then the *facet joint nerves* themselves can be blocked by injecting local anesthetic just outside the joints around targeted facet nerve areas, to diagnostically determine if these joint levels are a patient's suspected painful source—which would then be further treated with a follow-up RF procedure if the patient felt pain relief in this specific pain area for a certain duration of time.

Facetectomy The surgical term given for a procedure involving excision or surgical removal of a facet joint. This may be necessary if patients have intractable mechanical facet pain syndrome that was not responsive to steroid and local anesthetic injections or radiofrequency lesioning (RFL) facet nerve burn procedures. Facetectomy is often performed in combination with other spinal surgical procedures, like laminectomy involving removal of a particular piece of bone, discectomy involving removal of a piece of spinal disc, or with a spinal fusion involving joining vertebral segments together with spinal hardware fixation.

Failed Back Surgery Syndrome (FBSS) An unfortunate chronic back pain condition characterized by a persistent back and often leg pain following one or more spinal surgery operations. Other names for such a clinical situation are post-lumbar laminectomy pain syndrome, failed spinal surgery syndrome, and post-spinal surgery pain syndrome. There are many reasons why back surgery fails to relieve pain symptom, including a retained disc fragment or new disc process, epidural fibrosis and scarring, slippage of one vertebral body over another—listhesis, previous known degenerative discs that were not included in the site of surgery, possible technical error on the part of the surgeon, the development of painful hardware syndrome, and other reasons.

Fasciitis The medical term meaning inflammation of the body's fascia, which is a tissue lining under the skin that covers the surface of tissues and muscles. Anatomically, the fascia can extend beyond muscle to become the tendon that attaches muscles to bone. Anything that irritates fascia, like repetitive motion or injury, can cause pain and inflammation. Classic pain in the fascia of the foot is commonly known as *plantar fasciitis*.

Food & Drug Administration (FDA) A governmental agency, within the U.S. Public Health Service, which is part of the Department of Health and Human Services. The FDA overlooks medications and medical devices, among other things, to regulate their safety and efficacy in the United States. In comparison, Europe has agencies that often-set different rules and regulations for release of medications and medical devices to the public.

Femoral Nerve A large sensory and motor nerve responsible for sensation and muscle control in the upper front thigh. Anesthesiologists can offer patients a femoral nerve local anesthetic block when they undergo knee surgery procedures, to better control postoperative pain. In comparison, the nerve in the buttock and back of the leg is the sciatic nerve—*of sciatica fame.*

Fibromyalgia The most common chronic, widespread pain syndrome, characterized by tenderness in the muscles and soft tissues, including multiple tender points in the body above and below the waist. Fibromyalgia can be caused by a traumatic or very stressful event, or from a severe infection or from other causes, and is associated with irritable bowel, sleep problems, chronic fatigue, memory problems, and a variety of other symptoms. The exact cause of fibromyalgia is still unknown, but it results in muscles, tendons, and joints being stiff and painful, even in the absence of any primary inflammatory disease process. *Fibromyalgia pain syndrome* is a type of dysfunctional pain that does not cause body damage or deformity—but can be very

disabling for many patients if left untreated. The current diagnosis of fibromyalgia is based entirely on a patient's history, not on a blood test or a physical exam. Medications, cognitive-behavioral therapy, and aerobic exercise are the mainstay of pain care.

Fibrosis The medical term given to replacement of normal tissue with scar tissue. This can happen after spinal surgery if there is epidural fibrosis and scarring. This may be a reason why some spinal surgery patients continue to have pain, especially if epidural fibrosis creates scar tissue that wraps around spinal nerves.

Fluoroscopy A type of radiological imaging that shows a continuous black and white X-ray image of the patient on a monitor screen, for diagnostic and interventional pain management procedures, as well as, for certain surgical procedures. Fluoroscopic guidance for interventional pain management is considered a *standard of care*, and makes injection procedures more accurate, safe, and comfortable.

Foramen A medical term meaning an *opening*. For example, foramina exist in the spine where bony openings allow spinal nerve roots to travel from the spinal cord to the rest of the body. If these spinal nerves are compressed and inflamed in the spinal foramen, then a transforaminal epidural steroid injection (TF ESI) can be directed in this area to treat pain and inflammation that causes sciatica symptoms. If, on the other hand, there was excessive physical compression as opposed to mostly inflammation—where the attempted TF ESI did not result in relief—then a spine surgeon can offer a patient a foraminotomy, which is a surgical procedure to directly remove the spinal compression source(s)— typically due to a disc, facet joint, or bony spur issue. This would then reopen the foramen to release the pressure on the targeted spinal nerve and hence relieve the sciatica symptoms.

Fracture A common medical term describing a break in bone or cartilage usually because of trauma, but it can happen in patients with severe osteoporosis and brittle bones, especially in the spine. Common fractures in the upper and lower spine are known as vertebral compression fractures, where part of the vertebral body collapses and creates a lot of immediate pain.

G

Gait his is the term that relates to how a patient ambulates or walks. With patients who experience painful sciatica or painful osteoarthritis in the knees or hips, they may have an abnormal gait and may limp to avoid weight-bearing on the affected side, secondary to the pain in their legs or joints—known in medical terms as an *antalgic gait*.

Gastrointestinal (GI) This is the human body system involving the mouth, esophagus, stomach, small and large intestines, and the rectum. The upper GI consists of the esophagus to the end of the small intestine and the lower GI consists of the large intestine to the rectum. There are several chronic pain conditions such as stomach ulcer disease, irritable bowel syndrome, Crohn's disease, ulcerative colitis, and diverticulitis that can cause chronic gastrointestinal pain. Besides specific dietary care and restrictions, medications and surgical options are the mainstay of treatment for persistent chronic pain symptoms.

Gate Control Theory This is the name given to a pain management theory that explains how the spinal cord can regulate a high intensity pain sensation that starts in the peripheral nerves, travels through modulation nerve interconnections in the spinal cord, then ultimately to the brain where the pain is finally recognized as not as intense. For example, if a patient hits his head on the corner of a kitchen cabinet, then rubs the spot on his head that hurts, this reduces the final pain sensation felt in the brain—the touch nerve fibers that are stimulated by the rubbing of the head *"block"* the pain fiber transmission that goes from the spinal cord, where the pain is adjusted, to the brain where the pain is finally experienced. The activation, conduction, adjustment, and final experience of pain are shown in the **PITS Pain Diagram—Mind/Body Relationship** (see **APPENDIX B**).

General Anesthesia A state of unconsciousness induced by anesthetic agents that also eliminates pain perception. Use of IV medication and inhaled anesthetic gas, along with close monitoring under the care of an anesthesiologist or Certified Registered Nurse Anesthetist (CRNA), enable patients to undergo many different types of surgical procedures.

Generic This common term relates to the chemical name of a drug, as opposed to its marketed brand name. For example, ibuprofen is the generic name for Advil, which is a brand name. The brand name is the pharmaceutical company name for a drug, for marketing and selling purposes.

Glutamate An excitatory amino acid transmitter, which after much scientific research and study, was found to be responsible for much of the excitatory transmission in the central nervous system for various painful conditions. Treatments that can decrease or inhibit this glutamate transmitter, like opioid narcotics and other medications, can hope to offer patients improved comfort from acute and chronic pain.

Greater and Lesser Occipital Nerves—These are names of peripheral nerves that arise from the upper cervical spinal segments which affect the back of the head and neck when injured or irritated. Patients who suffer from *occipital neuralgia* typically experience sharp, shooting headache sensations that originate from the base of the back of the head and radiate up to the top of the head. If patients fail to obtain relief with medication and therapy, then injection therapy with steroid and local anesthetic can break the pain cycle and aide in the rehabilitative process. Also, Botox injections, pulsed radiofrequency ablation with heat lesioning, or cryoanalgesia with cold lesioning, can offer longer-term relief if needed in selected patients.

Guided Imagery This is a relaxation and stress reduction complementary technique used by patients, both on an outpatient and inpatient basis, involving the use of positive thoughts and images to relieve acute and chronic pain states. Guided imagery can slow the heart rate and stimulate the body's healing responses.

H

Headache A common term for head pain that patients typically feel from anywhere between the back or occipital part of their head to the front or frontal area of their eyes. All headaches are grouped into primary headaches and secondary headaches. Primary headaches, which are not associated with other diseases, include migraine, tension-type, and cluster headaches. For complicated headaches, most internists and family physicians will refer patients to a headache-trained neurologist for comprehensive specialty evaluation and treatment. Secondary headaches are caused by other diseases, like an aneurysm, tumor, or infection, albeit uncommon, are obviously very serious conditions that require immediate attention in an emergency room.

Herniated Disc The common term that describes a rupture in one of the gel-filled, shock-absorbing discs between the spinal vertebrae. Whether it be from an injury or progressive disc degeneration, when the internal disc viscous material leaks out, these substances irritate nerve roots and tissue in the spine and cause patients to experience radiating pain with numbness and tingling down their arms, in the case of a cervical disc, or legs when a lumbar disc is involved. If medical pain management with medications and therapy fails to relief symptoms, then interventional pain management with epidural steroid injections (ESIs) are the next step in treatment. Surgical intervention considering a discectomy for ongoing herniated disc disease is left for those patients who remain in intractable pain, despite aggressive medical and interventional pain management, or for patients who experience ongoing and progressive neurologic symptoms.

Herpes Zoster Virus (Shingles) An acute viral inflammation that afflicts the spinal and cranial head and face nerves of patients due to reactivation of the virus causing chickenpox. Herpes zoster can result in vesicular eruptions and neurologic pain along the dermatomes or skin sensation patterns on one side of the body. It can affect the face, upper limbs, chest, and back and lower limbs. The pain that patients feel after a herpes zoster breakout usually goes away in weeks, but if moderate-to-severe pain persists for months with a lot of skin sensitivity in the area, then *post-herpetic neuralgia (PHN)* can set in—a more difficult pain disease state to treat chronically.

Homeopathy A medical system based on the principle that *"like heals like."* Homeopathic practitioners use highly diluted solutions of natural substances from plants, animals, and minerals as remedies. They are used to stimulate the body's natural healing responses. Although not regulated by the Food and Drug Administration (FDA) as medical treatment—only regulated for safety issues—patients who subscribe to this philosophy of care elect to use homeopathic treatments as part of a complementary and alternative approach to treating their pain.

Hospice This is an outpatient or inpatient care service offered for patients with terminal illnesses, whether it is from cancer or non-cancer reasons. It is a specialized treatment option for total end-of-life consideration, not only at the individual patient level, but also for addressing the needs of the patient's family. The patient's physical, emotional, social, and spiritual needs are the primary focus, as they live out the remaining weeks-to-months of life in the most compassionate way possible. So, the primary goal of hospice is to keep the patient as comfortable as possible as they prepare for death. The average stay in a hospice situation is two weeks before the patient eventually passes away.

Hyaluronic Acid The medical term for the substance that normally exists in the synovial fluid of joints providing viscosity and cushioning support. It is important in the lubrication and protection process of joints in general, especially in weight-bearing joints, like the hips and knees. When hyaluronic acid levels decrease in a joint—whether it be in the shoulder, knee, or hip—patients will often start to feel joint grinding pain sensations. When this occurs, patients become eligible for *viscosupplement replacements* that can be injected directly into joints, in a safe outpatient office setting, usually with an orthopedist, rheumatologist, or pain management physician. Synvisc, Hyalgan, Euflexxa, and Supartz are some of the current FDA-approved viscosupplements available for injection. Patients often refer to these injections as rooster comb or chicken cartilage shots.

Hyperpathia   A scientific name given to a pain syndrome that is characterized by an exaggerated abnormal pain response that follows from a less intense painful stimulus. In patients that have a hyperpathic pain state, a pinprick to their painful area causes much more intense and expanded pain that would have normally been expected—the usual minimal short-lived pain that a needle would have caused in patients. This abnormal pain sensation is often seen in central pain syndromes, often along with *allodynia* or skin sensitivity to touch, when patients undergo central-sensitization pathological nervous system changes in the spinal cord.

Hypnotherapy   This is a complementary technique that uses hypnosis strategies to change a patient's conscious mind to an altered mental state. The aim of the altered mental state is to change a patient's negative and abnormal behavioral and emotional state to a more positive and healthier one. Hopefully, the hypnotic state will help treat stress and promote healing.

Hypochondriac   This a common term to describe a patient who is obsessed with feeling sick or complaining of different pains all the time, even though no signs or evidence of disease exists on medical or pain management examination. Psychological care approaches for these patients work best to help patients get more functional.

I

Ilioinguinal Nerve   This is a peripheral nerve that controls sensation in the groin area that can be irritated or injured after inguinal hernia operations. If neuromas or nerve entrapment develop in the scar after an operation, then injection of steroid and local anesthetic can be offered to desensitize the painful sensations and promote further healing.

Iliotibial Band (IT) Syndrome   A painful thigh condition usually associated with the repetitive motion associated with running and cycling or lifting weights. This condition involves tightness of the fascia and muscle that runs from the side of the hip down to the outside knee area. When inflamed or injured, the IT band can refer radiating pain down the outside of the upper thigh. The mainstay of treatment is medication, rest/ice, therapy, and injection management, as needed.

Immediate-Release (IR) Medication   Medication that takes effect over a short period of time as measured in minutes, like the opioid MSIR (morphine sulfate immediate release), for example. This contrasts with a controlled-release (CR) or sustained-release (SR) medication, which is medication that is formulated to release over many hours, like MS Contin and OxyContin, or over several days, like the Duragesic fentanyl patch.

Immune System   This is the body's complex self-defense system that is responsible for warding off diseases, foreign bodies, and infection. When the immune system weakens, mostly as patient's naturally age, it can leave the patient susceptible to illness, like cancer, shingles, autoimmune diseases, and so forth. Although uncommon, sometimes patients reject medical devices that are inserted in the body, like a spinal cord stimulator or an intrathecal infusion pump, because they are perceived as foreign bodies by the immune system.

Impairment   An objective limitation to normal physical functioning, such as strength, sensation, or range of motion. Impairment does not necessarily result in disability or handicap. For example, an impaired ability to lift heavy objects is not disabling if it does not affect a patient's ability to function independently—cook, clean, use the toilet, wash, shop, and so forth. So, in a sense, impairment is more of a medical term, whereas disability is more of a legal term.

Incident Pain   This is a term that represents a type of *breakthrough pain* related to a patient's specific activity—also referred to as movement related pain. Patients often develop rescue strategies in anticipation of this kind of pain which can include, resting, using ice or heat, taking quick acting pain medication, using breathing and relaxation techniques, and so forth.

Informed Consent   This is the term given to the process of making decisions about medical care that are based on open communication of the risks and benefits and alternatives of treatments—typically between the healthcare provider and the patient. Sometimes a patient's family is also involved with the informed consent process, especially if a patient is incapacitated. If a patient is offered an interventional pain management procedure, as an example, then the pain physician would typically discuss the possibility of procedure pain, nerve damage, infection, bleeding, lack of relief response, and so forth—the common and uncommon risks associated with such procedures—versus the benefit of breaking the pain cycle and obtaining prolonged pain relief.

Intercostal Nerves These are peripheral nerves that run underneath each rib. When patients sustain trauma to the ribs with resultant rib fractures or undergo a surgical procedure like an open chest wall operation, then these intercostal nerves can become irritated or scarred and result in a painful condition known as *intercostal neuralgia*. If medical management with medications and therapy fails to give relief, then patients can be offered intercostal nerve blocks with steroid and local anesthetic as an attempt to desensitize the affected painful areas.

Interventional Pain Management This is a subspecialty of medicine in the U.S. designated *Interventional Pain Management* and the general name of the pain management treatment option that encompasses both diagnostic and therapeutic injection techniques. When controlling pain from a spinal source, for example, patients first attempt medical pain management options of medications and therapy—the subspecialty deemed *Pain Medicine*, then they consider injection options—the subspecialty deemed *Interventional Pain Management*, then they turn to surgical pain management options, if necessary—the surgery subspecialties of orthopedics and neurosurgery involved with surgical correction techniques. Diagnostic procedures include local anesthetic blocks of spinal facet joint nerves to determine if facet joints are a source of pain, discography to determine if spinal discs are a source of pain, and many others. Common examples of therapeutic procedures include, epidural steroid injections, facet and sacroiliac joint injections, trigger point and bursa injections, radiofrequency and cryoablation procedures, knee and hip joint injections, sympathetic and peripheral nerve injections, spinal cord stimulation and intrathecal infusion device implantation, and many others. By blocking the body's transmission of pain signals to the brain, this allows patients to break an intractable pain cycle to achieve an improved functional activity level and a decrease in pain medication usage.

Intractable Pain This is a severe pain state that is beyond the usual intermittent and manageable chronic pain that one third of adult Americans experience. Intractable pain is very intense, chronic, and unremitting pain that is considered incurable, particularly when patients fail aggressive medical high dose opioid narcotics, interventional approaches with multiple injection procedures, and multiple surgical operation attempts at controlling the recurrent pain. This is the unfortunate pain patient population that represents around 10% of all the pain sufferers with *high-impact pain* states in America, and who subsequently suffer the highest levels of disability. A longer-term, compassionate, integrative pain management system and program of care is a must for these patients.

Intrathecal An anatomical term meaning within the *subarachnoid cerebrospinal fluid (CSF)* space in the spinal column, or more simply referred to as the spinal fluid space. Intrathecal infusion devices have spinal fluid catheters that deliver small amounts of continuous pain medication –mostly morphine—directly to the spinal pain relief receptors. These spinal morphine pumps are typically needed for the more intractable pain patients, including those patients who have failed multiple surgical operations, for those patients who have failed the spinal cord stimulation device, for cancer patients who have failed relief on high dose oral opioid narcotics, and for other indications.

Ischemia A medical term for the reduction in local blood flow due to obstruction or injury to the blood supply, usually an artery, which eventually leads to tissue breakdown and pain. This is typical in *peripheral vascular disease (PVD)* patients who develop painful ischemic legs.

J

Joint   A common term that describes an area where two bones are attached, thereby providing mobility between different body areas, from the head to the toes. A joint is usually formed of fibrous connective tissue and cartilage. There are three structural types of joints in patients, which include *fibrous*—connective tissue, like in the wrists and ankles, *cartilaginous*—cartilage, like between vertebral bodies, and *synovial*—cavities, like the hips and knees. When joints become inflamed or degenerated, whether it is from medical diseases, injury, or normal aging, they can cause varying amounts of pain. **The P-I-T-S treatment protocol** offers a full range of treatment options for acute and chronic pain relief for joint problems. For example, taking medications—like anti-inflammatory and opioid narcotics, receiving injections—like local anesthetic combined with steroid or viscosupplementation, performing therapies—like physical therapy with modalities, and undergoing surgical options—like arthroscopy and total joint replacement, are all available treatment options depending on a patient's particular clinical situation.

K

Ketamine   This is an injectable anesthetic and analgesic agent that can produce profound pain relief effects in small doses, and in higher doses, can induce a general anesthetic effect. In terms of pain control, it is often used to treat burn victims for wound dressing changes, in the emergency room for opioid-tolerant patients with severe pain, for intractable pain due to complex regional pain syndrome (CRPS, or RSD), and for other painful conditions. Ketamine comes in a topical cream that patients can apply as needed and in an IV form that anesthesiologists can administer as an outpatient continuous IV infusion in a monitored healthcare setting. Dosing of ketamine is based on a certain milligram (mg) amount of ketamine per kilogram (kg) of patient body weight, infused over a time period—typically several hours per day over a five-day period. The duration of significant relief can last for weeks to months, whereby breaking the pain cycle

can allow patients to better rehabilitate to achieve longer-term comfort and functional goals.

Kyphoplasty   This is a minimally invasive spinal surgical technique to correct thoraco-lumbar vertebral fractures, whether they occur from osteoporosis, a traumatic event, or secondary to cancerous vertebral bony invasion. This process basically involves putting *medical cement* into the area of fracture after balloon stenting to increase the height of the vertebral fracture, thus offering mechanical relief for patients. Many patients report pain relief in as little of 24 hours after cementing. Both orthopedic and neurosurgical spine specialists perform this procedure, as well as certain trained interventional pain management physicians, typically with the use of local anesthetic injection and under IV sedation. The procedure called Vertebroplasty, also for correcting thoraco-lumbar vertebral fractures, is similar but without balloon stenting.

L

Lamina   This is the anatomical term for the part of the vertebral body in the back of the spine. If this bony area becomes a source of compressive pain in the spine, and if conservative treatment fails to give relief of sciatica like symptoms and back pain symptoms, then spinal surgeons can perform a laminectomy with removal of the portion of the involved offending bony lamina to control pain. This is often done in conjunction with a discectomy, involving the removal of a piece of disc, for additional decompression of the painful nerve space area.

Lancinating Pain   A type of neuropathic pain quality that manifests as an episodic shooting, stabbing, or knife-like pain. This is typical of *trigeminal neuralgia*, where sharp pain can shoot through the face, and be very disabling to patients. This is compared to burning neuropathic pain, which is typical of diabetic neuropathy.

Low-Level Laser Therapy (LLLT)   A therapeutic medical device that uses a focused beam of light of varying wavelengths to treat painful conditions. *"L-a-s-e-r"* stands for *light amplified by stimulated emission of radiation*. Low-level laser therapy can be used to treat acute and chronic conditions in both musculo-skeletal and neuropathic pain states. Patients typically undergo outpatient treatments of two-to-three times a week, for two-four weeks, whether it is in an orthopedic, podiatry, rehabilitative, or pain management office setting. This is an FDA-approved device that often serves as a complementary technique alongside conventional medical pain care.

Lateral An anatomical term that refers to being situated away from the midline of the body, and toward one side or the other. This is opposed to the term *medial* which refers to the midline of the body.

Lateral Epicondylitis This is the medical term for the common condition known as *tennis elbow* where there is painful inflammation on the outside of the elbow due to trauma or overuse activity. Patients who swing a hammer for a living, or play sports like tennis and racquetball, are most susceptible to irritating a particular arm tendon—the common extensor tendon that originates on the lateral epicondyle—that leads to this painful condition. If medical pain management with medication, ice and rest, and therapy gives limited relief, then interventional pain management with a local anesthetic and steroid injection can be offered for longer relief.

Lateral Femoral Cutaneous Nerve This is a peripheral nerve that supplies normal sensation to the outer portion of the thigh. When this nerve becomes inflamed or compressed, usually in the outer groin area of obese patients or in patients who wear tight belts, the pain that develops leads to a condition known as *meralgia paresthetica*. Patients often feel a lot of skin sensitivity in the outer thigh that can be desensitized by injection therapy with combination of local anesthetic and steroid around the painful nerve area. This procedure is performed in an outpatient pain management setting. It can take two to three injections, a week-or-two apart, for full desensitization relief.

Lidocaine This is a common short-acting local anesthetic that produces pain relief by blocking the transmission of nerve signals. This is in contrast to bupivacaine (Marcaine), which is a long-acting local anesthetic. Lidocaine is prepared in a patch form as 5% Lidoderm or 4% cream formulation, is added to topical pain creams in conjunction with other therapeutic anti-inflammatory, muscle relaxant, or neuropathic medications, and is most frequently used in its injectable form for general medical care procedures. Lidocaine uses include local application over a painful skin area to treat post-herpetic neuralgia, injection around peripheral nerves, like the median nerve in the wrist to treat carpel tunnel syndrome, injection in muscle spasm trigger points for relief, or injection into the epidural/spinal fluid space to block spinal nerves for pain management procedures, labor and delivery, or surgical operations—and so forth.

Ligaments This is an anatomical term for the fibrous tissue that connects bones to other bones. This is opposed to tendons, which connect muscles to bones. Ligaments can undergo *sprain injury*, like an ankle sprain, when they are overused or with direct injury. When tendons and muscles are injured, this is called a *strain injury*, like a biceps tendon strain.

Living Will A legal document, also known as an advanced health care directive, which outlines the kinds of medical care a patient wants and does not want. It is used only if the patient is unable to communicate his or her own wishes, and cannot make decisions on their own. Typically, a power of attorney or health care proxy will carry out the patient's wishes. A living will document is especially important when a patient faces an end-of-life situation.

Loading Dose This is a term that represents an *initial dose* of medication administered for an acute pain episode to reach therapeutic blood levels, which is typically accomplished in an inpatient, surgical, or emergency room pain control situation. After a loading dose of pain medication, a *maintenance dose* of medication can be continued for ongoing control of pain, for as long as needed to keep pain scores at improved levels.

Long-Acting Medication This is the general term for medication that is released over a period of time, *delayed-release* or *sustained-release*, and is taken on a regular basis to maintain therapeutic blood levels in the body to achieve a continuous drug effect. This is the opposite of an *immediate-release* medication, which typically only lasts for a three-to-six-hour range. There are many long-acting medication classes and preparations for all types of medical conditions, but one of the most common are the opioid narcotics for the treatment of pain, including long-acting morphine (MS Contin, Kadian, and others), oxycodone (OxyContin), hydromorphone (Exalgo), fentanyl patch (Duragesic), and others.

Lordosis   This is the medical name that refers to the normal curvature of the cervical and lumbar spine. With injury however, the normal lordosis can become abnormally increased or decreased and lead to painful post-traumatic conditions, especially in the presence of permanent ligament damage and persistent muscle spasm pain.

Lumbar Spine   This is an anatomical term given to the *low back area*. The lumbar spine is the most common area in the spine susceptible to the development of pain because of its weight-bearing nature, among other reasons. Vertebral bodies, spinal discs, facet joints, ligaments and muscles, and other bony structures are all part of the lumbar spine that are vulnerable to different forces that can precipitate pain.

M

Magnetic Resonance Imaging (MRI)   This is a common diagnostic radiological procedure using magnetic fields and a computerized image to help determine the source of pain in a patient's body. There is no radiation exposure involved with an MRI, as opposed to a CT scan. For example, with spine pain, MRIs are often used in patients with persistent mechanical and radiating neck and arm pain, or back and leg pain, to determine a specific *pain generator*, like a disc problem that may be amenable to treatment with interventional pain management. MRIs give excellent resolution best imaging of soft tissues and joints and excellent resolution of different degrees of spinal disc pathology, including fissure, bulge, herniation, or a free disc fragment. CT scans, in contrast, are better at visualizing bony structures, in general, and the chest and abdomen structures—especially for discovering certain internal organ conditions.

Maintenance Dose   The medication dosage required to produce a given level of pain relief or analgesia. It typically follows a loading dose of medication to keep blood level therapeutic, so patients can be comfortable. Maintenance dosing is important in acute postoperative and trauma situations, where patients can self-dose medication using an intravenous patient control analgesia (IV-PCA) pump device. Also, for certain chronic persistent pain conditions, chronic oral maintenance dose medication is often utilized for maintaining comfort and function for an extended period of time.

Manipulation   Is commonly referred to as a form of chiropractic treatment applying gentle yet firm pressure to bones and soft tissues for the purpose of correcting subluxations or dysfunctional spinal segments in the spine. In this sense, manipulation serves to realign bones and spinal joints to take pressure off spinal nerves, leading to restored normal range of motion and a restored functional status, for the many patients who opt for this safe outpatient therapeutic procedure. Many Osteopathic physicians also perform a type of manipulation therapy known as *OMT—osteopathic manipulative therapy*—which can make all the difference in the world for patients who are candidates for this medical therapy.

Meditation   This is a common term that refers to a complementary technique that focuses the mind on a state of calmness. Through the meditation process patients achieve wellness by integrating the mind and body into one thus facilitating healing.

Methadone   This is a type of long-acting synthetic opioid narcotic medication. The most common medical use for methadone is a legal substitute for heroin in treatment programs for drug addiction, but also trialed sometimes to treat chronic pain. Many patients get anxious when they hear about methadone used for pain management because of its reputation as an *"addiction"* drug, but the reality is that methadone becomes a potential medication to use in selected patients who have failed many other opioid narcotics. Methadone can be helpful in both nociceptive and in certain neuropathic pain states because of its multiple mechanisms of action and is very inexpensive.

Methadone is not used in patients who suffer from prolonged QT-interval cardiac arrhythmia because of risk of death from precipitating a fatal arrhythmia. Physician experience in the use of methadone is very important, especially if methadone is to be used for long-term pain control.

Migraine The common term for a complex neurovascular periodic headache, usually unilateral over the temporal and eye area, is very severe in nature, and associated with either aura or without aura. An *aura* is a set of neurologic symptoms, often visual in nature, that patients can experience right before a migraine starts. Migraine is associated with nausea and vomiting and sensitivity to light, and a lot of general irritability. Patients often need to be in a dark quiet place until the migraine passes. A migraine typically lasts 24–72 hours and is aggravated by excessive activity. It can be disabling to patients and often patients seek migraine neurology experts for chronic care. *Lifestyle adjustments* are the mainstay of prevention and treatment of migraines including trying to avoid excessive stress in your life—as hard as that is, avoiding disruptive sleep patterns because of the importance of regular restful sleep, and avoiding certain trigger foods like wines, cheeses, and so forth. Medications for *abortive treatment* of acute intermittent attacks, include use of simple analgesics like ibuprofen and Tylenol, short-acting opiate narcotics like oxycodone, triptans like Imitrex, ergotamine preparations like dihydroergotamine-DHE or Cafergot, and barbiturate compounds like Fioricet. Patients are encouraged to limit abortive, quick-acting rescue effect, migraine medication to maximum recommended doses to avoid medication overuse headache (MOH) or rebound headache. For patients who continue to experience many attacks per month, *prophylactic treatment* strategies can be offered which can accomplish long-acting baseline relief treatment for between acute attacks, and include Topamax, Elavil, valproic acid, Inderal, and many others. For headaches that are referred to as *chronic migraine*—as defined by migraine and tension-type attacks for fifteen or more days per month—Botox injections are an FDA approved option administered every three months as safe outpatient office-based prophylactic therapy. Also,

new *calcitonin gene-related peptide receptor* prophylactic migraine medications and electric stimulation devices for migraine prophylaxis are FDA-approved in America. Again, for most Americans it is very difficult to deal with chronic migraines—and other types of headaches—as many of us lead busy, difficult, and stressful lives. After all, headaches and low back pain are the two most common pain reasons for patients to seek medical care in our country.

Mind-Body Medicine Mind-body medicine is a complementary medical approach that focuses on the interactions between the brain and body to empower patients to take active control of their pain care, thus promoting healing and wellness. This medical focus considers, in a holistic approach, the ways in which the emotional, mental, social, spiritual, and behavioral factors directly affect health—besides the primary physical factors. Patients are taught techniques that include relaxation, hypnosis, visual imagery, meditation, yoga, biofeedback, and spirituality and prayer. This kind of *integrative pain management*—conventional and complementary combined treatment philosophy—is especially important in patients suffering from cancer-related pain conditions and complicated life issues.

Minimally Invasive Surgery (MIS) This is general term given for a surgical technique that typically requires just small incisions, often involving the use of endoscopic visualization, to correct a painful condition. A common spine procedure for example, is minimally invasive discectomy to relieve herniated disc nerve sciatica pain. A common abdominal procedure is minimally invasive laser laparoscopy for endometriosis-related pelvic pain. Also, many hernia repairs and appendix or gallbladder surgeries can be done minimally invasive in select patients. Another common procedure is knee arthroscopy for a torn meniscus repair.

Modalities This is a term that often refers to therapeutic methods used in physical therapy as part of an inpatient or outpatient rehabilitative program. Modalities include hot packs for spasm and restored circulation, cold packs for pain and swelling, electric stimulation for spasm and muscle strengthening, ultrasound for spasm and restored circulation, TENS (transcutaneous electrical nerve stimulation) units, and other devices for pain control. Therapists typically start patients off with modalities to relief pain and spasm and help restore circulation, and then get into the active exercise routine –stretching, strengthening, conditioning, posture and biomechanics training, and so forth.

Morphine This is the principle naturally occurring opioid narcotic used in the treatment of moderate-to-severe pain due to acute, chronic, and cancer conditions. All other opioid narcotics are traditionally compared to morphine—considered the *gold standard*—in terms of their analgesic potency or the potential pain-relieving effects as measured in MME=morphine milligram equivalent or MED=morphine equivalent dose (see the **PITS Opioid Narcotic Comparison Dosing Chart** in **APPENDIX D**). Also, potential side effect profiles of nausea, vomiting, itching, constipation, sedation and mental clouding, respiratory depression, and so forth, can also be compared among different opioid analgesics. Morphine acts in the central nervous system to control pain through specific receptor activity. It is available in different preparations, like other pain medications—oral, rectal, and injectable, and others. Research has shown that there is not one opioid narcotic that is superior to another, rather it is typically a trial-and-error basis when using different opioid narcotics in different patients to find the right dose and frequency to maximize relief and minimize side effects. Genetic testing for opioid response potential in patients is still being developed and is not routinely used. Oral morphine comes in both an immediate-release and extended-release form, like other opioid narcotic formulations.

Morphine Milligram Equivalent (MME) This is a medication term—similar to MED or morphine equivalent dose—that compares all the strengths of other opioids to that of morphine, where 1 milligram (mg) of morphine = 1 MME. The MME is added up daily for any opioid a patient may be taking, as many patients are on more than one daily opioid. Now, as an example, oxycodone—the opioid in Percocet—is 50% stronger than morphine, and therefore 1 mg of oxycodone is 1.5 MME comparison. Hydrocodone—the opioid in Vicodin and Norco—is equal to morphine, and therefore 1 mg of hydrocodone is 1 MME comparison. Get it? The Centers for Disease Control and Prevention (CDC) want physicians in general to be more aware of MME levels and the risk of patients having an adverse event on opioid therapy, where the higher the daily MME of opioid the greater the potential risk. The CDC wants MME levels not to exceed 90 MME for patients, especially for new patients starting out on opioid therapy, or else strongly consider referring the patient to a pain specialist or try a different approach to treating the pain. Now, the **PITS Program** considers for a *pain management specialist* an upper dosing MME is 180, with sometimes up to 10–20% more if needed, especially for *legacy patients* who historically have been on much higher doses of opioid therapy for years and doing well. In the **PITS Program**, daily levels of opioid therapy are individualized to a patient based on opioid-tolerant severe pain, their **PITS Opioid Risk Screening (PORS) Assessment** (see **APPENDIX E**), their **PITS Score Assessment** status, and previous response to non-opioid therapies in the **PITS treatment protocol** like non-opioids, injections, therapies, and even surgery attempts at comfort.

Multidisciplinary Pain Center This is the highest level of a pain management organization, typically associated with a medical school or teaching hospital, which encompasses many different disciplines of healthcare professionals and scientists. This interdisciplinary pain team consists of physicians—interventional anesthesiologists, physiatrists, psychiatrists, and neurologists—physical therapists, clinical psychologists, nurse educators, and others—all working in a coordinated interactive manner and involved with research, teaching, and direct patient care, as it relates to acute, chronic, and cancer pain conditions and illnesses. This is the premier level of comprehensive pain care, where all the diagnostic and treatment options are under the same roof, and all patients have full access to care options. Otherwise, the clear majority of chronic pain patients are managed in their local communities with different physicians and allied health professionals performing different aspects of care. For example, one pain physician may be responsible for monthly narcotic pain medications for patients on chronic opioid therapy, another may be involved for certain interventional pain management injections, another may do surgery evaluations and may operate on patients when needed, the physical therapist and chiropractor may do the outpatient therapies for rehabilitation, and so forth. Certain patients with persistent intractable pain states, who fail outpatient pain management, may be candidates to enter an inpatient multidisciplinary pain center—as a next step in their progressive care plan. Although the number of these centers has decreased in the United States, both in academic institutions and privately owned and operated centers, a well-motivated chronic pain patient can still find this level of care if needed, to obtain access to the latest and greatest cutting-edge research and medical care—in major institutions, like Johns Hopkins, Mayo Clinic, Cleveland Clinic, Massachusetts General Hospital, and others.

Multimodal Analgesia   This is the scientific name for treating pain with a balanced analgesia approach, where using multiple methods to control pain is thought to work better at controlling symptoms, rather than just one method. For example, using two classes of drugs, like an anti-inflammatory and a muscle relaxant, will achieve better relief through the advantage of two medications that work by different pain relief mechanisms. Taking smaller amounts of two different analgesics often work better than taking larger amounts of just one medication. In addition, patients tend to have more side effects with using higher and higher doses of just one medication, especially when it comes to taking opioid narcotics. Other examples of multimodal analgesia are combining pain medication with physical therapy modalities and exercise, using minimally invasive interventional pain management procedures in combination with medication and therapy, or even a surgical pain management procedure to control pain along with medication, therapy, and injections. The ultimate purpose of the multimodal approach is to obtain additive beneficial effects of different approaches that work through different mechanisms of effect to maximize pain relief for patients and reduce overall side effects of treatment.

Music Therapy   A complementary technique that uses music as a form of distraction to aid in relaxing patients, which in turn will promote health and wellness.

Myelogram   This is a radiology (CT scan) test using contrast dye that is placed in the spinal fluid space through a spinal needle, with the purpose of diagnosing spinal nerve compression caused by a herniated disc, spinal fracture, or a slippage of the vertebral bodies. It is often ordered by spine surgeons in preparation of surgery to better determine which specific spinal nerve root levels—right side, left side, or both sides—need to be decompressed.

Myelopathy   This medical term refers to pathology of the spinal cord due to compressive physical changes on the spinal cord, typically from severe spinal stenosis, degenerative disc disease, or herniated disc material. The diagnosis of myelopathy is often confirmed on an MRI study and is considered a severe diagnostic condition. It is often treated by spinal surgeons to keep the patient's sensation, strength, and reflexes from deteriorating to a permanently damaged state. Surgeons will typically do a decompressive spinal fusion procedure in this situation to relieve the pressure on the spinal cord.

Myofascial Pain Syndrome (MPS)   An acute and chronic condition that describes pain, soreness, and spasm in muscles. This is a type of nociceptive pain state. Hopefully, acute muscle spasm is treated early and completely for best outcome. But, if persistent muscle spasms continue for weeks-to-months, this may result in the formation of active long-lasting *trigger points* or tight muscle bands, and the subsequent development of a chronic pain syndrome. MPS can cause patients varying levels of pain that can last for years or even a lifetime. The mainstay of treatment is anti-inflammatory and muscle relaxant medications, trigger point injections of local anesthetic, and therapy-based approaches—physical therapy followed by an active home exercise program. All these treatments are aimed at keeping trigger points in a less active state or in remission. The key is to find a balance of daily activity where a patient tries not to be too inactive but also not too active with stressing the particular muscle(s) that are prone to spasm flares.

N

Narcotic This is a common term that legally applies to many different controlled substances like, opioids, benzodiazepines, and barbiturates, which are overseen by the federal government—the Drug Enforcement Agency (DEA). However, in pain management circles, we use the term narcotic to refer to *opioid narcotics*, which are pain-relieving drugs derived from opium, like morphine and codeine. These medications produce varying amounts and durations of pain relief by depressing the central nervous system through specific receptor binding in the brain and spinal cord. Opioid narcotics are effective in controlling most types of pain in patients, especially in acute and cancer-pain situations. However, its continued high-dose use in chronic non-cancer pain becomes increasingly concerning and controversial, because of the potentially severe negative effects on the body through time. Nearly all pain patients realize at some point in their opioid narcotic treatment varying degrees of negative effects, including tolerance to opioid medication or getting use to a drug where it becomes less effective in its relief, negative endocrine system effects leading to a decrease in sex hormones and libido, and addiction development due to psychiatric disease manifestations. These negative opioid effects are three commonly talked about mainstream concerns among pain patients and their pain providers. With the advancement of science and research in the field of pain management, the *development of opioid-induced endocrine syndrome* is now quite concerning. This endocrine syndrome is caused by high-dose opioid narcotic lowering critical hormone levels in the body which can lead to a host of poor outcomes, including fatigue, anxiety, depression, insomnia, loss of muscle strength, decreased libido, and osteoporosis and vertebral fracture. *Treatment of opioid-induced endocrine syndrome is threefold*: First, slowly decrease existing high levels to more moderate levels of opioid as tolerated; secondly, attempt an opioid rotation where an equivalent dose of a different opioid takes the place of the previous regimen; thirdly, consider sex hormone replacement to bring the levels back to normal—this is becoming more popular as education and training advance and protocols become more

mainstream. Other opioid concerns include *decreasing immune system function*, *potential drug interactions* with valium-type drugs and alcohol intake, *aberrant (misuse) use of prescription opioids* with patients sharing their narcotic with family and friends who have pain, an *association with increased traffic accidents and decreased return-to-work potential*, an *increased risk of falls* especially in older patients, and the *development of what is called opioid-induced hyperalgesia* which is a condition where patients actually experience increased pain as their opioids are increased to higher and higher levels—this a paradoxical or opposite response that can happen in susceptible patients. As a last note, research indicates that true addiction to opioid narcotics is relatively uncommon in chronic pain patients who are followed closely by narcotic contract and urinary drug testing where adjustments can be made sooner-than-later in a patent's opioid care.

Nerve Blocks This is a general term that refers to an interventional pain management technique that involves injecting a local anesthetic—with or without steroid or other substances—around nerves to *numb or block the area* to help diagnose a painful condition or to treat and relieve a known source of pain. Nerve blocks are common in patients undergoing both surgical and interventional pain management procedures.

Nerve Root This is an anatomical term for the paired nerves that leave the spinal cord on the right and left sides and pass out of the spinal canal through the intervertebral foramen, where they then branch out and form motor, sensory, and sympathetic nerves that carry out all the body's normal functions. When patients suffer from a *pinched nerve root(s)* due to a herniated disc, they can feel different amounts of numbness and weakness in their extremities. The sympathetic nerve branches run along the sides of the vertebral column and are often involved in abnormal pain states like reflex sympathetic dystrophy (RSD), where patients can feel a lot of increased hot and burning sensitivity in their extremities.

Neuralgia The medical term that describes pain in the distribution of a nerve or nerves, with *"algo"* meaning pain in Greek. For example, trigeminal neuralgia derives from pathology in the trigeminal cranial nerve distribution in the face, resulting in shooting pain.

Neuritis The medical term that describes inflammation of a nerve or nerves, with *"itis"* meaning inflammation. For example, a flare of systemic lupus can cause neuritis, resulting in varying degrees of pain.

Neuroablative Therapy This term describes a type of interventional and surgical pain management therapy whose aim is to stop nervous system transmission of pain for many months, especially in patients with chronic persistent pain conditions. Neuroablation literally means *nerve destruction*. Some of these techniques include using various injectable substances around nerves, like *medical alcohol or a drug called phenol* to block pain signals, or using controlled heat ablation (radiofrequency) and cold ablation (cryoablation) for joint and nerve pain, or using neurosurgical destruction of specific targeted nerves as in the case of cervical spinal cord ablation to help control pain for certain cancer pain patients. Neuroablative strategies are often tried after failed attempts at relief using local anesthetic and steroid interventional pain management techniques. Nerve destruction is typically not permanent since the ablated nerves often slowly regenerate with time to varying degrees. Again, neuroablative therapy is used when more conservative therapies have failed, such as medications, physical therapy, and injections of local anesthetic and steroid, and patients continue to experience high degrees of ongoing pain.

Neurologist This is a medical doctor (M.D. or D.O.) who diagnoses and treats problems related to the nervous system including peripheral nerves, spinal cord, and brain, as well as chronic pain conditions. Most neurologists diagnose and treat patients who are afflicted with general neurology conditions, including stroke and spinal cord injury, Alzheimer's and Parkinson's disease, epilepsy and seizure disorders, traumatic brain injury (TBI), dizziness and restless leg syndrome, multiple sclerosis, and many other conditions. Neurologists also aid in the diagnosis and treatment of different neuropathic pain diseases, including acute and chronic headache syndromes—like migraines, concussions, and so forth—trigeminal neuralgia, diabetic and HIV neuropathy, post-herpetic neuralgia (shingles), phantom limb pain from amputations, and other pains of a chronic neuropathic nature. Some neurologists are fellowship-trained in interventional pain management, like fellowship-trained anesthesiologists and physiatrists. Many neurologists perform diagnostic electromyograms (EMGs) and nerve conduction studies (NCSs) to help direct future pain management and surgical treatments—physiatrists are the other group of physicians that frequently do EMG/NCS. A neurologist is often an important component of the multidisciplinary team that represents a best-care patient model for chronic pain management, along with a physiatrist, psychiatrist/psychologist, interventional pain physician, and surgeon.

Neurolytic Block This is a specialized type of nerve block that involves injection of a chemical agent, such as medical-grade alcohol or phenol agent, which can cause longer-term destruction of nerves—but often not permanent—to offer extended periods of relief in certain chronic pain conditions. For example, injecting 100% alcohol around the celiac plexus of nerves in the abdomen for pancreatic cancer patients suffering with severe pain can hopefully offer an extended period of relief for 3–6 months duration.

Neuroma This is a bundle of nerves or nerve endings that form a painful benign tumor-like structure, which typically arises in nerve cells due to trauma to an area of the body, or because of repetitive motion injury like running, or after an operation. As examples, a *Morton's neuroma* is a painful neuroma that can form in the foot, an ilioinguinal neuroma in the groin can arise after a hernia operation resulting in a lot of mechanical sensitivity over the scar, and neuromas from nerve resection can arise in the end of the residual limb of an amputation patient.

Neuropathic Pain This is one of the main categories of types of pain—besides nociceptive, inflammatory, dysfunctional, and psychogenic types of pain—that arises from a damaged nerve, a peripheral or sympathetic nerve, or from the central nervous system involving the spinal cord and brain. Symptoms may include, burning, tingling, sharp shooting pain, hypersensitivity to cold or touch, or excessive sweating and swelling. Peripheral neuropathic pain conditions are many and include different sensory neuropathies, like HIV neuralgia, post-herpetic neuralgia (PHN), complex regional pain syndrome (CRPS), diabetic neuropathy, and others. Central neuropathic pain includes, post-stroke pain, spinal cord injury (SCI) pain, trigeminal neuralgia, multiple sclerosis, and others. There are mixed neuropathic pain states, combining peripheral and central mechanisms for the propagation of constant pain, like patients with phantom limb pain often experience. Neuropathic pain can be very difficult to treat because it tends to be less responsive to just traditional anti-inflammatory and opioid narcotic therapy. It usually requires a multimodal analgesic approach using different FDA-approved and off-label *anti-neuropathic medications*. These neuropathic medications that are used off-label and not FDA-approved have been used clinically in pain management programs for many years with a high degree of success, and are generally considered safe and reliable in selected patients.

Neuropathy   This is the general medical term for nerves in the body that change in an abnormal way, typically due to a disease or traumatic injury. Neuropathy can affect one nerve (mononeuropathy) or several nerves (polyneuropathy) at a time and it can affect different types of nerves—sympathetic versus peripheral nerves. There are also small-fiber and large-fiber neuropathy distinctions. Technically speaking, small-fiber neuropathy involves what are called C-fibers and Delta nerve fibers associated with burning and sharp shooting pain. Large-fiber neuropathy affects what are called Beta and Alpha nerves associated with sensory numbness and motor imbalance. When neuropathy is associated with pain, it is often referred to as *neuralgia*. An example is diabetic neuropathy that can occur through time in diabetic patients with poor blood sugar control and high A1c numbers, leaving them with intermittent or constant pain and burning or sharp pains in the hands and feet.

Neurosurgeon   This is a surgeon that specializes in diseases and conditions of the central nervous system, including the brain and spine. They can operate for tumors, bleeding, and infection in the brain and spine,

as well as for many painful conditions including kyphoplasty and vertebroplasty for repair of spinal vertebral fractures, discectomy for removing a piece of spinal disc material to relieve pain and pressure, laminectomy for removing an area of spinal bone to relieve pain and pressure, and spinal fusion for the placement of stabilizing hardware in the spine. The orthopedic spine expert is the other equally-qualified surgical discipline that is fellowship-trained in spinal surgery. Neurosurgeons and orthopedic spine surgeons often operate together on more complex spinal surgery cases to optimize both skill sets for better patient outcomes, where the neurosurgeon will typically focus on the nerve decompression component and the orthopedist will focus on the bone and hardware insertion part of the procedure.

Neurotransmitter   his is the term given to our body's own natural chemical compounds that are involved with normal nerve transmission, both of an *excitatory* nature and an *inhibitory* nature. Some of the main neurotransmitters include acetylcholine which is involved with muscle contraction, serotonin which is involved with mood and sleep cycles, norepinephrine which is involved in arousal and the reward center in the brain, dopamine which is involved in motor, cognition, and the major reward center in the brain, glutamate which is a modifiable excitatory chemical that in excess can lead to CNS cell death, GABA or gamma-amino butyric acid which is an inhibitory chemical leading to sedation and tranquilizing effects, Substance P which is responsible for pain transmission into the CNS, opioid peptides which are involved in pain analgesia relief and emotional euphoria, and many others. Any disruption or major change in the levels of these neurotransmitters and any changes in synaptic connections between nerves from illness or injury can lead to pathologic disease states and chronic painful conditions. There is a lot of ongoing pain research in neurotransmitters to design drugs that are more targeted for specific neurotransmitter receptors. This will help to maximize the beneficial effect of a medication and minimize the potential side effects.

NMDA (N-Methyl-D-Aspartate) Receptors   It is a type of glutamate receptor in patients that is involved in mediating excitatory neurotransmission between nerves, and hence an important receptor for pain medication to target for controlling many neuropathic pain problems. These receptors are thought to play an important role in the development of central sensitization pain, where glutamate levels are excessively high resulting in receptor overstimulation. Methadone is a synthetic opioid narcotic that can block the NMDA receptor and reverse some of its negative pain-causing actions. Glutamate receptors are different than the classic opioid narcotic receptors, anti-inflammatory receptors, and other neurotransmitter receptors in the body.

Nociceptive Pain This is one of the main categories of types of pain—besides inflammatory, neuropathic, dysfunctional, and psychogenic types of pain—that arises from damage to soft tissue or biomechanical structures including skin, subcutaneous tissue, muscle, fascia, tendons, ligaments, bones, internal organs, vascular structures, and vertebral discs. This type of pain involves what are called *nociceptors*, which are specialized sensory receptors in these tissues and structures. Somatic and visceral pains are two broad subtypes of nociceptive pain. Symptoms may include a dull ache, sharp pain, gnawing and squeezing sensations, hot and cold sensations, cramping, and prickling. Examples of nociceptive pain include, postoperative pain involving skin, muscles, bones, and organs, arthritis joint pain, mechanical low back pain, sickle cell crisis pain involving bones, chest, and internal organs, sports and exercise injuries—like sprain and strain—gallbladder and pancreatitis attacks, heart attack pain, cancer pain from bone and internal organ involvement, and many others. This is different than neuropathic pain which is pain that arises from specific nerve injury and disease.

Non-Opioid This is any medication that does not contain an opioid and may be available over-the-counter (OTC) or by prescription, including acetaminophen (Tylenol), anti-inflammatory medications (NSAIDs and steroids), muscle relaxants, anti-neuropathic agents, and others.

Non-Pharmacologic Therapy A general term given to any pain management strategy, other than typical oral pain medications, especially for patients who prefer not to be on medications. Non-pharmacologic therapy includes interventional or injection pain management options, physical therapy exercises and chiropractic manipulation, surgical operation techniques, psychological approaches like stress management and cognitive behavioral therapy, and complementary and alternative pain management approaches—like acupuncture, massage, biofeedback, herbals, and others.

Nonsteroidal Anti-Inflammatory Drugs (NSAIDs) This is a major class of anti-inflammatory medication—the other being steroid—that is used to relieve pain and reduce inflammation including aspirin (acetylsalicylic acid-ASA), ibuprofen (Motrin, Advil), naproxen (Aleve, Naprosyn), celecoxib (Celebrex), meloxicam (Mobic), Voltaren gel (diclofenac), Relafen (nabumetone), Indocin (indomethacin), and many others. This is opposed to corticosteroid-based medications, such as prednisone, Decadron (dexamethasone), triamcinolone (Kenalog), methylprednisolone (Medrol), and Celestone (betamethasone). NSAIDs are often used in the treatment of pain and inflammation for conditions, including headache, menstrual cramps, minor musculoskeletal aches and pains, arthritis, tendinitis and bursitis, and others. NSAIDs work by blocking the production of certain body chemicals called *prostaglandins* that are involved in the process of inflammation and pain. There are nonselective NSAIDs and selective NSAIDs. Nonselective NSAIDs—like ibuprofen and naproxen—block both COX-1 and COX-2 forms of the enzyme cyclooxygenase (COX). COX-2 selective NSAIDs, for example Celebrex, just inhibit the COX-2 form, and not the COX-1 form. The advantage here is that the COX-2 selective anti-inflammatory can block inflammation, which is the primary goal of therapy, and not block the protective stomach lining action of the COX-1 form that minimizes the chance of gastritis and bleeding.

Nucleoplasty This is the name of a minimally invasive interventional pain management procedure used for decompressing a previously diagnosed painful vertebral disc bulge—typically after diagnostic discography. By using a special wand and a specific heating technology to reduce the inner disc gel contents of the nucleus pulposus, patients can be offered back and leg pain relief from these compressive discs. Nucleoplasty has the effect of *taking air out of an overinflated tire*, therefore offering relief from not having the disc exert as much pressure on spinal tissues and spinal nerve roots. This technique can be offered in carefully selected patients when surgery is not an option.

Nucleus Pulposus   This is the medical term for the gel-like tissue substance in the center of intervertebral discs that acts as a *shock absorber*. The nucleus pulposus is contained by the annulus fibrosis or fibro-cartilaginous portion of the disc. The annulus fibrosis prevents this nucleus pulposus material from protruding outside of the disc. However, with trauma or progressive wear-and-tear, the nucleus pulposus can bulge out resulting in a bulging disc, or herniate out of the nucleus fibrosis resulting in a herniated nucleus pulposus (HNP)—thus allowing this substance to leak onto spinal tissue and nerve roots. When this happens, a highly irritating and chemical inflammatory condition starts which then leads to back pain and sciatica pain—or pain in the neck and arms when this occurs in a cervical disc. Therefore, epidural steroid injections (ESIs) can be very successful in treating this type of inflammatory pain in the spine due to a bulging or herniated disc.

O

Opioid   This is the term for a morphine-like narcotic medication that produces pain relief. As related to pain management, the terms opioid and narcotic are often used interchangeably. There are different types of opioids including naturally occurring, semisynthetic, and totally synthetic medications. Opioids relieve pain in patients by binding to opioid receptors in the nervous system within the brain and spinal cord. Now the word *opiate*, which refers to drugs that are directly derived from opium and are considered the naturally occurring opiates, include morphine and codeine and thebaine. *Semisynthetic opioids* which are part natural and part synthetically altered, include oxycodone, hydrocodone, and hydromorphone, among others. *Totally synthetic opioids* include methadone, fentanyl (IV, oral buccal tablet-Fentora, lozenge lollipop-Actiq, and patch-Duragesic forms), and tapentadol (Nucynta),

among others. Opioids come in short-acting and long-acting forms. For example, plain oxycodone is a short-acting opioid and OxyContin is the long-acting or controlled-release form of oxycodone. Opioids are the most effective drugs for moderate-to-severe pain states utilized in acute, chronic, and cancer patient care settings. As effective as opioids are, they can have a lot of negative side effects, such as sedation, nausea, itching, constipation, respiratory depression, physical dependence, and addiction. Statistically, up to one-third of patients cannot tolerate opioid narcotics and another one-third do not achieve enough meaningful relief from them. So, there is always a balance between positives and negatives of any type of opioid drug used in pain management. If patients get in trouble with respiratory depression in emergency situations, there is an *opioid reversible agent known as naloxone*, commonly marketed as *Narcan*, which can be administered nasally to restore a normal breathing pattern.

Opioid (Narcotic) Agreement   This is a written contract or promise between the patient and a healthcare provider, mostly a pain specialist but frequently a primary care physician, intended to set up a system of rules, regulations, and restrictions when managing opioid medications, especially on a long-term, monthly basis. This kind of agreement typically focuses on the safe and effective use of opioids in chronic pain management, and protects both the patient and the physician's medical practice. These agreements typically require patients to follow certain rules, regulations, and restrictions, including taking their opioid narcotic(s) as prescribed with directions on dose and frequency, not escalating dose without approval from the pain doctor, obtaining monthly prescriptions for a 30-day supply from the same pain doctor or pain management group, filling the narcotic prescriptions at the same pharmacy when possible, letting the pain doctor know all the other mood altering medications that you are prescribed by other doctors, securing their medication at home in a lock box for example, not sharing their medication with family and friends, undergoing periodic urinary drug testing to check for expected and illegal drugs in their system, receiving only a 3-day supply of narcotic medication in an emergency room situation or 7-day supply of pain medication in a postoperative discharge situation, and other provisions. Opioid agreements are strongly recommended by governmental narcotic regulatory agencies for medical-legal purposes, along with urinary drug testing to check compliance, as mentioned above. In a strict sense, many pain providers will wean or discontinue opioid narcotics altogether in favor of other treatment avenues in patients who fail to improve their pain control and physical functioning on narcotics or to improve their **PITS Pain and Quality-of-Life Score (PITS Score)**. Discontinuation can also be triggered in patients who develop too many opioid side effects, like opioid-induced endocrine syndrome for example, develop excessive tolerance to the narcotic and it loses its overall treatment benefit, receive narcotic from another physician without a prior discussion as to why, refuse the urinary drug monitoring testing, misuse the pain medication by *giving it away* or actually abuse it and *"get high"* on the narcotic drug, or for any patient who cannot continue the required monthly office reevaluation and prescribing process.

Opioid Rotation   This is the name given to *a strategy of switching opioids in patients* whose pain becomes resistant to the current pain medication levels, or in patients who start to develop toxicity and side effects with their current regimen. The switch allows the previous opioid, which may have been causing toxicity or no longer helping to manage pain, to be eliminated and washed out of the patient while substituting with a trial of a new opioid to still maintain the desired analgesic pain-relieving effect. The optimal new trial dose should avoid underdosing or overdosing patients, so an opioid rotation often requires the use of an *equianalgesic dose table* to determine the equivalent dosage for the new opioid to help ensure that pain will be well controlled.

Orthopedist—This is a surgeon that specializes in diseases and conditions of the musculoskeletal system, including the spine. They operate on acute fractures of bones throughout the body, on torn ligaments, tendons, and muscles, on degenerative joints with arthroscopy and replacement, and the spine with discectomy, laminectomy, and spinal fusion. The other

surgical discipline that is fellowship-trained in spinal surgery is the neurosurgeon spine expert.

Osteoarthritis (OA)   This is a type of arthritis caused by inflammation breakdown and eventual loss of cartilage in a patient's joints. It is also known as degenerative arthritis or wear-and-tear arthritis, and is the most common type of arthritis. Osteoarthritis is accompanied by pain and stiffness usually after prolonged activity or inactivity. Patients complain a lot about pain and stiffness in the morning, and then eventually feel better as they get more active and their joints *warm up*, so to speak, typically within an hour. Common joints areas that are affected include, knees and hips, shoulders, wrists and ankles, neck and back spinal facet joints, and fingers and toes. The pain of osteoarthritis is one of the most common reasons why patients are evaluated by their primary physician—besides back pain and headaches—and the full **P-I-T-S treatment protocol** options are available for care, including medications, injections, therapy, surgery, supplements, yoga, and so forth.

Osteopath   This is the short name given to a doctor of osteopathy (D.O.). Osteopaths are medical doctors that diagnose and treat illness much like medical doctors (M.D.), but also train in the field of manual medicine using musculoskeletal system manipulative techniques to aid in diagnosis and treatment. Patients that suffer from musculoskeletal dysfunction can do well with *osteopathic manipulative therapy (OMT)*, especially if they fail to get enough from traditional physical therapy.

Osteoporosis   This is a common term for a disorder that occurs in a patient's aging bones, especially in postmenopausal women, where bones become thin and brittle and susceptible to fracture due mainly to depletion of calcium in the body. Older patients who are on prolonged oral steroids are even more at risk of osteoporosis fracture. Besides common hip fractures when older osteoporotic patients fall, compression fractures of the vertebral bones can also be very disabling leading to painful kyphotic curvature of the spine. If caught earlier enough, fractures of the vertebral bones can be treated by a minimally invasive procedure called *kyphoplasty*, which involves a special medical cement being injected into compression fractures to support them—with subsequent pain relief.

P

Pain   The official international definition of pain as of this year according to the International Association for the Study of Pain (IASP), a worldwide pain management organization, is: *"An unpleasant sensory and emotional experience associated with, or resembling that associated with, actual or potential tissue damage."* This is very much a worldwide academic definition of pain and encompasses not only real tissue damage, but also psychological reasons for real pain if a person feels threatened and feels that they are about to get hurt. In other words, if a person was being held at gun point, and they felt that they could be shot at any point, then their nervous system and pain pathways can be activated biochemically—and consequently feel real pain! The definition of pain according to the **Pain is the PITS Program**, is: *"Any physical, psychological, or social hurt that affects quality of life."* This is a simplified clinical definition and real-life multidimensional perspective of pain. This speaks to the critical importance of improving a patient's **PITS Pain and Quality-of-Life Score** (see **APPENDIX A**) with the guidance of the integrative **PITS Program**. Pain still cannot be directly measured by all our advanced science, so if a patient says, *"It hurts and it's affecting my life,"* then *it hurts and it's affecting their life*, and all healthcare professionals should believe that the pain complaint is real and start addressing it by asking questions and initiating an assessment. Pain is complex and differs from person to person. Unpleasant sensations can range from mild and localized discomfort to agony in different patients, which has both physical and emotional consequences in the body and brain of patients. Pain is processed by specific nerve receptors and fibers that carry the pain impulses from the peripheral and spinal nerves to the brain, where they are modified and eventually perceived. Some modifying factors involve cognitive intellectual judgments on the part of patients, emotional reactions that are shaped by psychological anxiety and depression, social contexts at home or work in which the pain occurs, and even culturally and spiritually modifiable factors in stoic and very religious patients. All these factors account for the vast variations in patient's pain complaints—or lack of them—so one patient's *"2 out of 10"* pain may be another patient's *"8 out of 10"* pain, where *0 is no pain* and *10 is the worst pain imaginable.*

Pain Management   This is the general name of the medical specialty and the term given to the process of providing medical, interventional, and complementary care that alleviates or reduces pain of any type. In the United States, pain management providers can designate themselves within the American Board of Medical Specialties, as either *Pain Medicine* specialists, dealing mostly with pain medications and various therapies, or as *Interventional Pain Management* specialists, dealing mostly with injection-type pain procedures. Providing pain relief is an extremely important part of healthcare, both medically and ethically, because if patients are remaining in a continuous moderate-to-severe pain state, then they will often suffer a quality-of-life crisis. Patients will cease to function normally, be depressed and exhausted, and be withdrawn socially from family and friends. For any kind of pain, whether it is acute, chronic, or related to cancer, it can be treated using a multidisciplinary approach with appropriate and indicated medications, injections, therapies, and surgical techniques to control that pain. The multidisciplinary disease-like integrative **P-I-T-S Protocol** model for chronic pain assessment and treatment is likened to other disease models of medical care, including diabetes and high blood pressure. So, if patients are in need of great long-term pain management care, then the **PITS Program** is the way to go—I am just saying!

Pain Medicine   This is a specialty of medicine designated by the American Board of Medical Specialties (ABMS), also known as *algiatry*, with an *algologist* being a physician specialist that treats pain. Algiatry is a fancy word for the medical discipline that is concerned with not only the prevention of pain, but also the evaluation and treatment of pain when it flares, so that patients can better rehabilitate and continue to live their lives. A pain management specialist can have different levels of training in the United States. Physicians who are multidisciplinary fellowship-trained have experience with interventional anesthesia pain management techniques, rehabilitation pain management approaches, and neurology and psychiatry pain management methods. The top trained pain specialists learn about all the different types of pain including postoperative and trauma nociceptive pain, cancer malignancy pain, non-cancer chronic biomechanical pain, chronic neuropathic pain, dysfunctional pain states, and psychogenic pain conditions. The pain specialists often work closely with primary care doctors and other specialists to help coordinate optimal care and best treatment outcomes.

Pain Scale   This is a universal system of rating pain on a scale for patients, to not only report how much pain they are experiencing at any given time, but also to track trends in their pain scores through time, to help determine if a particular condition is improving. There are different types of pain rating scales. The most common pain score rating is based on a verbal or written scale of 0 to 10, with *0 being no pain* and *10 being the worst pain imaginable*. There is a descriptive scale using *"mild, moderate, and severe"* as pain level choices. There is also a faces pain scale, especially for younger pediatric patients who do not fully understand a 0-through-10 scale until they are older. The faces scale shows a series of progressive happy faces to more crying faces to represent different levels of pain.

Palliative Care   This is the discipline of medical care that is provided by an interdisciplinary team that promotes quality of life and relieves suffering, especially in terminally-ill patients. The goal is to promote the best possible quality of life for patients who are facing serious, life-threatening illness, with a primary focus that is typically on supportive medical care rather than on a cure itself.

Paradoxical Reaction   This is the medical term given to a response, typically to a medication, which is opposite of the usual expected response, such as agitation produced in an individual patient by a drug that would normally be considered a sedative. For example, Benadryl which is usually sedating, can make some patients hyperactive.

Paresthesia   This is the medical term for an abnormal nerve sensation that patients feel. For example, *when a nerve is "bumped,"* like the funny bone in the elbow, this can activate the ulnar nerve that courses under the elbow and cause an electric feeling. Another example is a radiation sensation in the leg(s) that a patient can feel when they undergo an epidural steroid injection (ESI), due to the gentle pressure around the spinal nerve(s) as the volume of the shot spreads in the epidural space. Yet another example, is the sensation that a patient would feel when they get a nerve block for an operation, where the procedure needle may contact a targeted nerve.

Patient's Rights   As a patient, you do have certain rights guaranteed by law concerning your medical records and care and the right to keep that care private. You have rights to informed consent for your treatment by your healthcare professionals. There is even a movement in this country to have pain management added to the patient Bill of Rights. It has not yet appeared on the Bill of Rights for patients, but again, there is a push by many pain management organizations to treat pain as a human right, not only in this country but in the international pain community, as well.

Patient-Controlled Analgesia (PCA)   This term for pain relief refers to patient self-administration of analgesics, typically opioid narcotics like morphine and Dilaudid, usually for intravenous or epidural use after surgery, trauma, or for cancer pain management. PCA pumps are programmable, with several built-in safety features, and represent a common modality of pain relief for patients of all ages, as long as they can understand how the pump works. There are limits preset on these pumps to keep patients safe with total usage, and patients are in a monitored environment when inpatient care is needed. PCAs can also be used for outpatient pain relief, especially for cancer patients who require frequent high dosing of IV-opioid narcotics for comfort. The main advantage of this medical device is that patients have immediate access to pain medication, and do not have to wait for a nurse to assess them and then bring them the medication, which can take a significant amount of time.

Percutaneous This is the medical term for a minimally-invasive approach to pain management that accesses body structures and cavities, such as spinal discs, joints, nerves, or the abdominal cavity—*through needle puncture of the skin*—as opposed to a full open surgical approach.

Periosteum This is a fibrous membrane that surrounds the surface of bones. The periosteum has periosteal nerves that are responsible for severe pain that patients feel when they break a bone, or the brief pain a patient feels when an injection needle contacts bone during an interventional pain management procedure.

Peripheral Sensitization A medical term that describes the process of increased skin sensitivity to touch, pressure, and low-level pain stimuli, which occurs at the site of tissue damage and inflammation in an acute pain state. Typically, there is an increase in nerve impulse firing and hyperexcitability in tissue damage and inflammation at the peripheral nervous system level, like in patients who suffer with severe osteoarthritis of the knee. If this process continues without adequate pain treatment, then peripheral sensitization can lead to a central sensitization over a period of weeks to months, resulting in the development of a chronic persistent pain state.

Phantom Limb Pain This a pain condition that a patient experiences in a body part that is no longer present, such as an arm and a leg after amputation. This is due to a combination of a peripheral neuropathic pain state and a central nervous system pain state. Phantom pain is typically difficult to treat, and requires many of the **P-I-T-S treatment protocol** options to put the typically severe pain into remission. Many patients find themselves needing a repeat operation for neuroma formation at the residual limb site, or may need a spinal cord stimulator if intractable symptoms persist.

Pharmacy This is the common term for a location where prescription drugs are sold, and other medical supplies. According to the law, a pharmacy is constantly supervised by a licensed pharmacist. There are a lot of rules, regulations, and restrictions at the state and federal level that are put on pharmacies, especially when it comes to chronic opioid narcotic prescription dispensing. As a rule, patients who are on chronic monthly opioid prescriptions should go to the same physician or pain management group for the prescription, and not doctor shop. They should go to the same pharmacy for dispensing of the opioid and not jump around to different pharmacies. Patients should also closely follow the monthly refill plan to renew the prescription of opioid medication, typically on a thirty-day frequency.

Phonophobia This is the medical term for an abnormal or painful intolerance of sound. Phonophobia and photophobia or light disturbances are symptoms that can occur in migraine headache pain patients.

Photophobia This is the medical term for an abnormal or painful visual intolerance of light. Photophobia and phonophobia or sound disturbances are symptoms that can occur in migraine headache pain patients.

Physiatrist This is a medical doctor (M.D. or D.O.), also known as a *physical medicine and rehabilitation (PM&R) physician*, whose specialty of medicine is the diagnosis and treatment of musculoskeletal disorders and chronic pain conditions. Most physiatrists diagnose and treat patients afflicted with general rehabilitative conditions, including stroke and spinal cord injury, traumatic brain injury (TBI), sports injuries of the shoulder rotator cuff, knee ACL, and Achilles tendon, multiple sclerosis and Parkinson's disease, and many other conditions. Many physiatrists are fellowship-trained in interventional pain management and treat various pain conditions, including chronic low back pain, painful osteoarthritis, complex regional pain syndrome (CRPS), carpel tunnel syndrome, fibromyalgia, and myofascial pain syndrome (MPS), and others. Many physiatrists perform diagnostic electromyograms (EMGs) and nerve conduction studies (NCSs) to help direct future pain management and surgical treatments. A physiatrist is often an important component of the multidisciplinary team that represents a best-care patient model for chronic pain management, along with a neurologist, psychiatrist or psychologist, interventional pain physician, and a surgeon.

Physical Therapy This is the general term for the method of treating injuries, diseases, or other bodily derangements, both internal and external, by employing physical methods, such as using modalities—heat, ice, TENS, ultrasound, and electric stimulation—and exercise, as opposed to medications, injections, or surgical techniques. Physical therapies, along with other **P-I-T-S treatment protocol** therapy options, are a critical component to patient treatment for achieving strengthening and conditioning, flexibility and range-of-motion, and body mechanics and posture outcomes. Along the way, patients are taught self-directed techniques at home or in a gym setting, for long-lasting care.

Pilates This is a type of mind-body complementary care exercise—like yoga to improve strengthening and conditioning, posture and body mechanics, and flexibility—to help optimize a patient's functional status. There is a helpful mindfulness component to Pilates to help with mental conditioning, and has a breathing component, as well. This system of exercise can be challenging to learn but many patients benefit from this philosophy of rehabilitation and maintenance therapy when they can handle the difficulty level. Pilates was named after its inventor, Joseph Pilates.

Piriformis Syndrome This is a pain condition in which the piriformis muscle, which lies deep in the buttock from the lower spine to the hip, starts to contract with spasms and resultant pressure on the sciatic nerve passing under this muscle, with subsequent pain in the buttocks and down the back of the leg. This is a common condition, both in physically active individuals, as well as those whose jobs or activities involve prolonged sitting, and especially in men who sit on their wallets all day. This referred muscle pain is very similar to true sciatica pain, which is typically caused by a herniated spinal disc, and is often underdiagnosed. If medical management of medication and therapy fails, then guided injection of the piriformis muscle with steroid and local anesthetic can be considered, to break the spasm pain cycle and hopefully speed up the rehabilitative process.

Placebo Effect This is a common term for a treatment that is not medically known to help patients, but nonetheless, results in a short-lived beneficial effect in patients, due to the strong positive patient expectations that a treatment will work. This could be a sugar pill or chemically inert substance, or an injection of neutral (non-active) medication, or any other treatment that is not medically known to have a benefit in patients. Placebo effects also commonly occur in one third of patients who receive an actual known medical treatment for their pain.

Plantar Fasciitis This is a pain condition due to inflammation of the plantar fascia in the sole of the foot, extending from the heel to the front of the foot, where excessive pressure and inflammation can lead to chronic pain. Podiatrists or foot surgeons treat this common pain condition with medications, injections, orthotics, and physical therapy. Treatment with surgery is reserved for the most intractable pain cases, but this is not common.

Polypharmacy This is a term that describes when patients take multiple drugs that have the potential for resulting in excessive medication interactions and adverse reactions. Patients who mix an opioid narcotic with a benzodiazepine, like Valium or Xanax, and alcohol—*"the perfect storm"*—have a much higher risk of adverse reaction, and even death in certain circumstances. Unfortunately, scores of people die each day in this country from opioid-related polypharmacy drug interactions.

Post-Herpetic Neuralgia (PHN) This is a neuropathic pain state that involves a painful neurologic skin condition in an area of a specific body nerve site, whether it is the face, arms, chest, trunk, or legs, which occurs after an acute herpes zoster shingles attack. PHN usually manifests months after the vesicle skin rash has crusted over and healed. A case of herpes zoster pain should normally resolve with time, but in certain patient populations, especially older patients and immunocompromised patients, they are at risk of developing longer-term neuropathic pain which can be difficult to treat. Research shows that susceptible PHN patients do better when treated within three months of the pain presentation, compared to six months to a year from initial presentation.

Postoperative This is a term that describes the time period immediately following an operation. It encompasses the time a patient is in the recovery room until the rehabilitative healing process is completed in the future.

Post-Thoracotomy Pain Syndrome This is a post-surgical pain condition involving pain in the chest wall after an operation due to the disruption of muscles, ribs, and nerves. If medical pain management fails to offer sufficient relief, then interventional pain management using intercostal nerve injections of steroid and local anesthetic, or cryoanalgesia using a cold probe ablation to relieve pain, can be offered for additional relief.

Prophylaxis This is the medical term that represents an intervention that can help prevent the occurrence of a disease or severe pain. For example, taking an oral antibiotic during a spinal cord stimulation trial to prevent infection or taking a daily medication to keep from having a migraine headache attack.

Prostaglandins These are the hormone-like substances involved in the pain and inflammatory process due to tissue trauma or other medical condition that results in prostaglandin formation. Excessive prostaglandins sensitize pain receptors to mechanical and temperature stimulation, and cause blood vessels to dilate, all of which contribute to the development of peripheral sensitization. Anti-inflammatory medication, such as aspirin and Motrin, block the action of prostaglandins, thus inducing a pain-relief state.

Pruritus This is the medical term for *itching*. Pruritus is sometimes a bothersome side effect of opioid narcotic therapy when first started in patients. When it occurs, symptoms are usually treated symptomatically, otherwise the medication therapy can be changed altogether.

Pseudoaddiction This is a term used for a pattern of medication seeking behavior that a patient demonstrates when they are receiving inadequate pain management. This real pain behavior can be mistaken for addiction. An example is a patient with sickle cell crisis bone pain asking for medication on a regular basis that could be construed as addiction—but it is really due to not enough pain medication to relief the actual pain

intensity. True addiction involves more of a compulsive asking for pain medication despite excessive side effects and even bodily harm.

Psychiatrist This is a medical doctor (M.D. or D.O.), whose specialty of medicine is the diagnosis and treatment of mental and addictive illness. Psychiatrists understand the biologic, psychological, and social components of illness and are able to treat the whole person to decrease the overall *suffering experience*. In chronic pain management, psychiatrists—along with psychologists—are often part of the multidisciplinary pain management team, working in conjunction with interventional anesthesia pain management specialists, physical medicine and rehabilitation specialists, and neurologists. Statistically, dysfunctional psychological profiles can appear in half of all chronic pain patients who experience moderate-to-severe recurrent pain symptoms.

Psychogenic Pain This is a type of pain state that does not originate physiologically in a patient, but rather is believed to be caused by a patient's psychological factors. *Somatoform pain disorder* is an example of a psychogenic pain, where due to primarily psychiatric conditions, a patient manifests physical symptoms of a pain disease. This is a very real pain that patients feel and experience, yet the blood work, tests, and examination reveal no organic pathology. So, this condition is typically treated through psychiatry, rather than traditional interventional or surgical pain management. This is especially true if a patient's depression is the leading reason that they feel pain. With improvement of the patient's depression, typically comes improvement in whatever their pain complaints were manifested earlier. Fortunately, pure psychogenic pain states are not commonly seen in non-psychiatric pain management practices.

Psychosocial This is a term used to refer to a broad class of factors that may influence a patient's physical pain disorder and their pain behavior as it relates to psychological and societal influences, not just biological issues. Some examples of psychosocial factors include, depression, pain preoccupation, and monetary rewards for disability. Unfortunately, in certain patients, a lot of the biomedical treatment offered along the way of care is limited due to these potential negative psychosocial circumstances.

Q

Qi Gong This a type of complementary Chinese therapy involving combinations of movement, meditation, and regulated breathing to enhance the flow of Qi—also spelt Chi—vital energy in a patient's body. Qi Gong also can improve blood circulation and enhance immune function, much like acupuncture which activates or promotes chi energy flow enhancement along designated meridians in the body.

QT Interval This is one of the cardiac heart rate intervals that is measured on an electrocardiogram (EKG) that can be prolonged with the use of certain medications, such as higher dose methadone or tapentadol, among other medications. A prolonged QT interval can lead to arrhythmia and adverse reactions. A baseline EKG in patients with cardiac disease and who are on medications that can prolong the QT interval is advisable, and often obtained yearly.

R

Radiculopathy This is a common type of neurologic symptom that involves pain and frequent neurologic deficit caused by inflammation and injury to a spinal nerve root in the spinal canal. When radiculopathy is caused by compression, inflammation, or injury to a spinal nerve in the low back this is commonly known as *sciatica*. A pinched nerve from a herniated spinal disc is the classic cause of acute pain and eventually chronic lumbar and cervical radiculopathy. The full P-I-T-S *treatment protocol* options for care are available to get radiculopathy pain under control including medications of NSAIDs, muscle relaxants, anti-neuropathics, and opioids, along with injections (ESIs), therapy (PT), and surgery (discectomy) as needed.

Rebound Headache This is a term given to a headache experienced by patients who have built up a specific medication tolerance and occurs immediately after a medication wears off. This is classical for migraine

patients who take too much of their abortive pain medication –Fioricet, triptans, opioid narcotic—and later feel worse than before they took the medication. This can lead to a cycle of pain medication, followed by rebound headache, followed by repeat medication to help the headache, which leads to more rebound headache symptoms and more medication, and so forth. This viscous cycle creates the common pain condition known as *medication overuse headache (MOH)*.

Referred Pain This is a term that describes pain that a patient feels in a part of their body that originates from a different site—not from where they feel it. An example is sciatica where nerves can be compressed and inflamed in the lower spine, but the patient feels the pain in the buttock and lower leg, below the knee, or into the foot. The sciatic nerve is the largest peripheral nerve in the body originating from the lower spinal nerves and courses through the buttock down the back of the leg and all the way to the feet. Because of this anatomy, a pinched nerve in the spine can refer pain all the way into a patient's toe! So, you do not treat the toe in this case, you treat the pinched nerve in the spine to make a patient well again.

Reflex Sympathetic Dystrophy (RSD) Now known as Complex Regional Pain Syndrome (CRPS, renamed in 1994 by the International Association for the Study of Pain)—see Complex Regional Pain Syndrome in this glossary.

Refractory Pain this is a term for pain that is resistant to ordinary treatment, such as medications, injections, therapy, and surgery. This is a classic setup for a chronic pain state and these patients are typically treated by a pain specialist using a multidisciplinary approach with a lot of cognitive and behavioral care.

Regional Anesthesia This is the type of anesthetic technique for surgery that involves injecting a local anesthetic around a nerve(s) that results in blockade of pain, sensory and motor transmission and feeling. This is commonly called *nerve block anesthesia*. Regional anesthesia and general anesthesia are often performed together for orthopedic repair of major joints, such as shoulders and knees. Nerve blocks offer great immediate post-operative pain control and allow patients to adjust their oral pain medication, so by the time the nerve block fully wears off they have already had enough oral pain medication to maintain comfort.

Rehabilitation This is a general term for the process of restoring a patient's functional activity status and relieving pain through an exercised-based program. Rehabilitation can be offered as an inpatient, as outpatient care, or both, depending on the type and severity of the illness or injury. Physiatrists or Physical Medicine & Rehabilitation physicians typically evaluate and develop the overall care plan along with the rest of the healthcare rehabilitation team, including the physical therapists, occupational therapists, and so forth. For example, a patient who undergoes bilateral total knee replacement will often be discharged from the hospital and undergo several weeks of inpatient rehabilitation before being discharged home for their outpatient therapy.

Reiki This is a complementary medicine technique that uses gentle pressure from the hands to encourage healing energy and it is often used to treat acute and chronic pain in conjunction with conventional pain care.

Rescue Dose This is a term given to a bolus or extra dose of medication given as needed to relieve pain that breaks through, despite a regimen of medication that is given at regularly scheduled intervals. This is typical of patients who are on IV-patient controlled pain pumps after operations, where they need the nurse to give a rescue bolus dose of pain medication through the pump to get their blood levels of pain medication adjusted to get the pain back under control.

Resection This is a term that involves the surgical removal of part of a structure such as bone or organ. For example, patients who suffer from chronic recurrent diverticulitis abdominal pain sometimes undergo a surgical resection of the diseased bowel to get the pain symptoms under control.

Rheumatoid Arthritis (RA) This is a common chronic inflammatory painful condition in which the body's immune system attacks cartilage, bone, and sometimes internal organs, usually causing moderate-to-severe joint disease through time. Joints become inflamed which leads to swelling, pain, stiffness, deformity, and possible loss of function. RA is characterized by a symmetrical pattern of joint synovial fluid inflammation leading to progressive destruction especially in a patient's hands and fingers. It is very important that patients be followed by a rheumatologist for best treatment options, typically for periodic IV infusion disease-modifying medication treatments, like Enbrel, Remicade, Humira, and other choices.

Rheumatologist This is a medical doctor (M.D. or D.O.), whose specialty of medicine involves the diagnosis and treatment of inflammatory and autoimmune illnesses and chronic pain conditions affecting joints, muscles, bones, organs, and soft tissues. Medical condition examples include, rheumatoid arthritis, psoriatic arthritis, gout, fibromyalgia, lupus, osteoporosis, and many others. Many rheumatologists will treat chronic painful conditions, especially fibromyalgia and rheumatoid arthritis, along with a pain specialist as needed for co-management, to optimize a patient's comfort and functional status.

Rotator Cuff This is an anatomical term for the group of four muscles and their tendons that stabilize the shoulder. The rotator cuff is susceptible to traumatic injury and general wear-and-tear, especially in patients who do a lot of repetitive motion, who are active athletes, and whose job requires a lot of heavy lifting. Rotator cuff pain can come from tendonitis, bursitis, or tear in the muscle(s). Injury to the rotator cuff is a common workers' compensation reported case.

S

Sacroiliac Joint (SIJ) This is the anatomical name of the paired joints in the low back and buttock area formed by the sacrum and iliac bony pelvis. When these joints become inflamed or degenerated or unstable, they can become a source of low back and buttock pain. *Sacroiliitis* pain occurs when the joint is inflamed and *sacroiliac dysfunction* exits if the joint becomes mechanically deranged and disrupted. If medical management with medication and physical therapy fails to relieve symptoms, then the joint can be injected with steroid with or without local anesthetic to break the pain cycle.

For longer-term relief, lasting months, as opposed to weeks, radiofrequency (RF) lesioning of the joint nerves can be offered, where heat is used to safely disrupt nerve conduction to achieve pain relief. There are even minimally invasive surgery (MIS) fusion procedures with titanium implants to stabilize the SIJ if necessary, usually reserved for intractable pain cases due to progressive degenerative sacroiliitis or joint instability.

Sacrum This is the anatomical term for the large triangular bone at the base of the spine which is made up of fused sacral vertebrae. It begins after the lumbar spine and extends to the coccyx. Where the sacrum contacts the iliac bony pelvis on each side, these areas represent the anatomical sacroiliac joint (SIJ) location.

Sciatic Nerve The largest nerve in the body that begins from the lumbosacral nerve roots in the lower spine and extends through the buttock area and down the back of the leg to the foot. When the sciatic nerve is irritated from whatever reason—spine, pelvic or buttock causes—this is what is generally known as *sciatica*. When the specific reason for sciatica is due to a herniated spine disc, this is conventionally called *lumbar radiculopathy* in medical terms.

Sciatica This is the common term that describes nerve pain that runs down the back of the buttock and leg area. It indicates that pain along the course of the sciatic nerve where pain can run from the back of the thigh below the knee. The medical term for these sensations is *lumbar radiculopathy*. Sciatica can involve pressure on spinal nerves caused by herniated discs, lumbar stenosis and degenerative disc disease putting pressure on spinal nerves, lumbar facet joint spondylosis, or spondylolisthesis with slippage of one vertebral bone over another causing pressure on spinal nerves. Other conditions can also cause referred pain down the back of the leg, such as piriformis syndrome or sacroiliac joint dysfunction. Symptoms of sciatica that may constitute a medical emergency due to a large, herniated disc severely compressing spinal nerves, include progressive weakness in the legs and/or bowel and bladder incontinence. This is referred to as *cauda equina syndrome* and immediate surgical attention is necessary to avoid permanent nerve damage.

Scoliosis This is the medical condition that describes the lateral right or left-sided curvature of the spine. Scoliosis can be slowly progressive and stable, or it can be accelerated and severe and need major corrective spinal surgical correction with multilevel spinal hardware.

Secondary Gain This is a term that describes external factors that can influence a patient's psychological and behavioral wellness state. As an example, if there is a money incentive involved with a work-related accident or with a motor vehicle accident, then this can influence and encourage a patient not to get better for fear of negatively influencing a potential settlement. Secondary gain can result in ineffective treatments, continued high pain scores, and a chronic poor functional status, ultimately leading to permanent disability. Of course, the primary gain is to actually get better from the original physical pain condition, which is a much more common patient attitude, so secondary gain really hinders a patient's full recovery.

Semisynthetic Opioid This is the term used for an opioid compound derived from an original *"opiate"* such as morphine, codeine, or thebaine, that has been synthesized to have a functional modification of the original drug. For example, hydrocodone, oxycodone and oxymorphone are all semisynthetic derivatives of thebaine, the parent natural occurring opiate drug. Hydromorphone and heroin come from morphine, as does codeine. These are all slightly modified in the lab to produce different opioids each with different effects in different patients. Completely synthetic opioids are not at all related to morphine or codeine, including tramadol (Ultram), methadone, tapentadol (Nucynta), and fentanyl (Duragesic patch).

Shingles (Herpes Zoster) This is a medical condition due to an acute infection caused by the reactivation of the same virus which causes chicken pox. Shingles is most common after the age of fifty, and the risk rises with advancing age. This virus remains quiet in nerves for many years, and then can become reactivated in patients who are immunocompromised, overly stressed, or for other reasons. The neuropathic pain of shingles usually resolves with the crusting over of the skin vesicles that erupt from the infection. If patients suffer from longer-term shingles pain, then this is termed *Post-Herpetic Neuralgia (PHN)*.

Somatic Pain   This is one of the subtypes of the major category of nociceptive pain—the other subtype being visceral pain or pain that arises from organs in the body—and is derived from tissues such as skin, fascia, subcutaneous tissue, muscles, bones, tendons, joint capsules, or a bursa. Somatic pain includes both biomechanical and soft tissue sources of pain, excluding pain derived from organs. The other major types of pain include neuropathic pain, inflammatory pain, dysfunctional pain, and psychogenic pain (see the **PITS Diagnostic Categories of Pain** in **APPENDIX K**).

Somaticizing Pain Disorders   This is a term for psychiatric disorders that give rise to physical pain symptoms. These psychological processes that cause patients to feel pain differ from physiological pain diseases, in that there are no detectable organic changes to the body when these patients undergo examination and various tests. The pain is real to the patient, so the healthcare team has to address it and treat it accordingly. These disorders include somatoform pain disorder where patients complain of a lot of somatic bodily pains, factitious disorders where patients deliberately cause themselves pain symptoms and problems, and malingering where patients fake pain symptoms for personal gain. The focus of treatment is indeed psychiatric care, since there is no true physical illness, so most of these patients are best evaluated and treated by a psychiatrist to get better control of a patient's negative psychiatric pathology.

Spinal Cord   This is the common term for the major column of nerves in the vertebral canal in the back and neck that is connected to the brain. From the spinal cord come the spinal nerves that emerge from each side of the spine at different levels. There are thirty-one pairs of spinal nerves that originate in the spinal cord—8 cervical, 12 thoracic, 5 lumbar, 5 sacral, and 1 pair of coccygeal nerves. Both the brain and the spinal cord make up the *central nervous system (CNS)*. When the spinal cord and spinal nerves are diseased or injured, many acute and chronic neuropathic pain

conditions can arise, all with varying presentations and intensities.

Spinal Cord Stimulation (SCS)   This is a specialized pain management device using safe, minimally invasive implantable *"electrical"* spinal stimulation therapy, for patients with certain types of chronic neuromuscular and vascular pain conditions. SCS involves electrically stimulating the spinal cord to cause a new sensation—a gentle tingling feeling in many cases—that covers up the original painful sensation and blocks pain from being received in the brain. Patients usually have failed more conservative treatments before trialing SCS. Patients will undergo a period of spinal cord stimulation trial for a week or so, and if successful with more than 50% pain relief and a better quality of life, will then undergo outpatient permanent implantation of spinal lead wires and a pulse generator for longer-term use. It is likened to a *"pain pacemaker,"* like a heart pacemaker. Patients recharge the SCS typically on a weekly basis and can use different programs to cover different pains. Conditions where spinal cord stimulation has been shown to be efficacious include, failed back surgery syndrome (FBSS) where patients still feel a lot of back and leg pain after surgery, complex regional pain syndrome (CRPS, or RSD) where patients feel persistent burning pain and skin sensitivity in their arms or legs, peripheral vascular disease leg pain due to poor blood flow, and other conditions. There have been many advances in SCS therapy in recent years and can be performed without having to feel the tingling sensation, and with even wireless technology in selected patients.

Spinal Fluid (Cerebrospinal Fluid or CSF)   This is the term for the clear colorless fluid that bathes the spinal cord and brain and cushions it against shock and trauma. Some patients may experience a *spinal headache* after an epidural steroid injection from an inadvertent puncture into the spinal fluid sac, with subsequent leakage of CSF. A spinal headache arises from lower CSF pressure from the leak and usually improves with conservative treatment with lying flat, taking Tylenol and other analgesics as needed, and drinking a lot of caffeinated beverages. Sometimes an epidural blood patch is required to seal the leak and allow the spinal fluid to build up again to normal levels.

Spinal Fusion This is the term that describes a surgical procedure to permanently unite two or more vertebrae in the spine so that there is no longer abnormal painful motion occurring between them. This procedure is typically performed for patients who develop spinal instability and intractable back and sciatica pain that has previously failed to improve with both medical and interventional pain management—multiple medications, many therapy sessions, several epidural steroid injections, and so forth. There are many approaches and techniques for performing a spinal fusion operation, so patients typically have a detailed discussion with their spinal surgeon about risks and benefits and recovery time before proceeding. Many patients often seek out a second opinion before consenting. For example, if they see an orthopedic spine surgeon first, then their second opinion can be with a neurosurgeon spine specialist to get another discipline's viewpoint about the best approach to this option.

Spinal Stenosis This is the term that describes a *narrowing* of the vertebral canal, nerve root canal center, or intervertebral foramina side of the lumbar spine, usually resulting from soft tissue and bony encroachment of the spinal canal and nerve roots. This spinal narrowing process usually takes many years of normal aging, typically affects patients in their fifties, sixties, and seventies, but can also happen acutely at the time of an accident. Symptoms include pain, paresthesias or nerve sensations in the legs, and neurogenic claudication or pain in your legs, when patients walk for a while. Spinal stenosis pain is usually treated conservatively with medications, therapy, and epidural steroid injections (ESIs), but in severe cases, surgical spinal decompression, with or without a fusion, can be very successful in patients experiencing intractable pain.

Spondylolisthesis This is an anatomical term for an alignment abnormality of the spine, usually due to chronic degenerative changes of the spine or due to trauma in which one vertebra is displaced relatively to an adjacent vertebra. When the *slippage* is in front of the other level, this is referred to anterolisthesis, and

when in back, this is referred to as retrolisthesis. There are radiographic grades 1–4 depending on the severity of the slippage. With misalignment of vertebrae, spinal nerves can become compressed and facet joints can become disrupted, again leading to different mechanical and radicular pain states. If conservative measures fail with medications, therapy, and injections, then surgical options can be considered, such as spinal fusion. Spinal fusion is typically reserved for patients with intractable pain and/or severe ongoing neurologic symptoms, like bladder or fecal incontinence, or persistent numbness and weakness in the legs or feet.

Spondylosis This is a term for a degenerative disease of the spinal column that leads to immobilization of the vertebrae and spinal stenosis. It occurs in essentially the entire aging population to some degree, with some patients who have no pain and others that can develop severe pain. Conservative pain care is the rule, and only if patients experience intractable pain and ongoing neurologic symptoms, are surgical options necessary to decompress an excessively compressed spinal area.

Sprain This is the common term for excessive pressure or stretch that causes tearing of a ligament—as opposed to a muscle strain—caused by a movement beyond the ligament's *normal range of motion (ROM)*. This is a common type of injury when patients turn their ankle, for example, and develop varying degrees of ankle sprain.

Stellate Ganglion Block (SGB) This is the name of an interventional pain management procedure to relieve pain caused by overactivity of the sympathetic nervous system in the upper extremities, head, or neck. It involves a local anesthetic injection in the front of the neck that blocks the *sympathetic* nerves, while other sensory peripheral nerve pathways are not blocked. This is a common outpatient injection treatment procedure used to treat upper extremity pain caused by complex regional pain syndrome (CRPS), also known as RSD (reflex sympathetic dystrophy). When a local anesthetic is placed around this ganglion of nerves, it can desensitize pain and skin sensitivity in the arm and hand, resulting in subsequent relief and an improved functional status for patients. SGBs are typically performed under fluoroscopy X-ray guidance, once or twice a week, repeated for a total of 3–5 injections depending on the patient response, to fully treat the painful symptoms.

Steroids This is the common term given to a general class of anti-inflammatory chemical substances that are structurally related to one another, including prednisone, dexamethasone (Decadron), betamethasone (Celestone), triamcinolone (Kenalog), methylprednisolone (Depomedrol), and others. Steroids come in different treatment forms, including oral, injectable, and topical. Steroids are powerful anti-inflammatory medications that are different than nonsteroidal drug (NSAID) medications, like ibuprofen (Advil) and naproxen (Aleve).

Strain This is the common term for the overstretching of a muscle caused by overextension. This is a common type of injury when patients *"pull a muscle"*, like the hamstring muscle in the back of the leg or the low back muscles.

Substance P This is a neurotransmitter chemical involved in the transmission of painful nerve signals from peripheral receptors in the skin to the central nervous system spine and brain. Pain treatment drugs that can decrease the levels of Substance P can offer pain relief for patients, especially in inflammatory arthritis and neuropathic pain conditions. One such drug is called capsaicin—*hot pepper cream*—which comes in a topical formulation for application on a painful skin area, to alter C-fiber pain transmission activity and thus lessen painful sensations.

Sympathetic (Nervous System) Hyperactivity This is a term for symptoms and signs of sympathetic autonomic nervous system hyperactivity, which include increased heart rate, increased blood pressure, increased respiratory rate, increased sweating, dilated pupils, nausea and vomiting, dry mouth, and increased muscle tension. Uncontrolled pain in acute postoperative or acute traumatic pain patients gives rise to this classic sympathetic hyperactivity state, which can impede the overall healing process if it is prolonged and not treated sufficiently. Also, patients who acutely withdraw from opioid narcotics typically experience sympathetic hyperactivity.

Sympathetic Nerve Block This is a term for a procedure involving local anesthetic injection around sympathetic nerves on either side of the spine to treat pain that is of sympathetically-maintained pain (SMP) origin—as opposed to sympathetically-independent pain (SIP) from peripheral nerves. When placed in the front of the neck to block the stellate ganglion sympathetic nerves, this injection can give relief in patients suffering from complex regional pain syndrome (CRPS, or RSD) of the upper extremity and hand. When this injection is placed in the lumbar spine along the lumbar sympathetic chain, it can relieve similar pain in the lower extremity and foot. These safe minimally invasive injections are performed under fluoroscopic X-ray guidance, with or without IV sedation, typically in an outpatient setting. These sympathetic injections are typically performed once or twice a week, repeated for a total of 3–5 injections depending on the patient response, to desensitize painful extremities with the aim of having patients better rehabilitate moving forward with their overall care.

Symptom This is the term for any condition a patient may feel subjectively that may indicate a disease or abnormality. This can include patient complaints of pain, anxiety, fatigue, nausea, dizziness, and so forth. In contrast, a *sign* is objective evidence of disease found on physical examination by the medical staff, such as finding a muscular trigger point spasm, discovering weakness in the arms or legs on motor power testing, observing swelling in an extremity, discovering a rash or fever, and so forth. Different pain diseases have their usual signs and symptoms that go along with that pain condition, which helps the healthcare team formulate a pain diagnosis. Once a diagnosis is made, then a logical treatment plan can follow.

Syndrome This is a term for a set of pathologic signs and symptoms that tend to appear together in patients with certain conditions. Examples include, fibromyalgia pain syndrome, complex regional pain syndrome, myofascial pain syndrome, and others.

Synovitis This is the medical term for inflammation of the synovial lining of a joint as seen in inflammatory arthritic joint pain conditions of the hip, knee, or other afflicted joints.

T

Tapering (Weaning) This is a term that describes the process in which a medication is *gradually withdrawn* from a patient for whatever clinical reason, whether on a weekly or monthly basis. If tapering of a medication is done too fast, especially in patients who have been taking high doses of an opioid for a long period of time and who are more physically dependent on it, then uncomfortable withdrawal symptoms can occur.

Telemedicine This is the medical term for conducting patient care utilizing telecommunication technology where your healthcare provider may be in the office and the patient is at home. This type of remote location medical care is certainly applicable to chronic pain management and surgical consultation and follow up care, especially for patients who cannot make it into the office at times. Patients can undergo this type of evaluation through audio alone or in combination with video on a phone or computer. When the **PITS Program** offers this option of pain care, it will be known as **TelePITS**!

Temporomandibular Joint (TMJ) Syndrome This is a type of dysfunctional pain condition causing jaw joint muscle pain and dysfunction resulting in restriction of jaw movement, clicking, or popping sounds, muscle spasms, and grinding of teeth. There can be a history of trauma to the jaw, or no such history at all, as the exact cause of this condition goes unknown in many patient cases. Conservative care options are the norm—medication, therapy, injections—but surgical correction can be offered, if needed.

Tendonitis This is a common medical condition involving inflammation of a tendon that can cause pain. This is typically an overuse activity pain condition that can be both acute and chronic in nature. An example is bicipital tendonitis, where patients experience a lot of pain in the front of their shoulder area where the biceps muscle attaches.

Tendons These are structures that attach muscles to bone and are composed of fibrous-connective tissues which are densely packed collagen fibers. Injury to tendons can take a long time to heal, as they typically have a limited blood supply.

Tennis Elbow This is a common painful overuse injury condition of the common extensor tendon of the elbow, which runs from the outer elbow to the forearm muscle. This is due to repetitive twisting of the wrist or forearm which causes irritation and inflammation in this tendon. This is also known as *lateral epicondylitis*. This is the opposite of *golfer's elbow or medial epicondylitis*, which is inner elbow tendonitis pain due to a different tendon irritation.

Tension-Type Headache This is a common type of a *muscular contraction headache* of mild to moderate pain severity and of various duration affecting both sides of the head and neck area. Stress, fatigue, and neck muscle strain are typical causes of tension-type headache, and simple analgesics, like Tylenol and Motrin, are the usual medication choices. Heat, massaging the neck and scalp muscles, and relaxation techniques can also help. Other common primary headaches include migraine and cluster headaches.

Therapeutic Massage This is a complementary technique involving the manipulation of soft tissues of the body to treat various ailments including a specific active pain state, any ongoing musculoskeletal discomfort that impedes the progress of physical therapy, acute and chronic muscle spasm resistant to heat and ice and medication, or stress that is perpetuating a state of anxiety and depression in a patient.

Titration This is a term for the process of incremental adjustment of a medication in subsequent doses until a desired clinical effect is achieved. Medications are often titrated up slowly over days to weeks to achieve pain relief levels that are acceptable to patients, and which do not cause a lot of side effects. As a general principle, starting low and going slow with medications, helps the treating pain team find the optimal balance of maximum relief and minimal side effects.

Tolerance   This is a term that describes a common physiologic result of classic chronic long-term opioid use. It basically means that a larger dose of opioid narcotic medication is typically required to maintain the same pain relief level through time. Tolerance can sometimes be confused with the actual progression of the pain disease state itself, which could be the reason why a patient's previous pain relief level is lost. Patients could be on a stable dose of narcotic opioid pain medication for many months, and then suddenly feel a lot of breakthrough pain, not because they have truly developed medication tolerance, but because their original pain that was once controlled has now worsened—thus causing the increased pain. The process of true opioid tolerance typically takes place over a slow period of many months to years.

Topiceutical (Topical) Pain Agent   This is a term for analgesic medication that is applied right to a patient's painful skin area *topically*, usually in the form of a gel, like Voltaren gel, as a compounded pain cream—typically using several active agents with different mechanisms of action—or patch form, like 5% Lidoderm. There is a lot of research and science that supports this pain relief method and there are FDA-approved and non-FDA approved topiceutical choices that can alleviate pain. Topiceuticals have been shown to be effective, safe, tolerable, and shown to have little to no systemic or full body side effects. In comparison, the other pain medication relief delivery methods are *pharmaceutical*—oral, nasal, rectal, transcutaneous, and intravenous medication pathways—and *interventional* with injectable medication techniques using steroid and local anesthetic.

Transcutaneous Electrical Nerve Stimulation (TENS)   This is a pain relief modality that produces electro-analgesia pain relief through electrodes applied to the skin. TENS involves a small electrical stimulus coming from a battery powered device resulting in the blockage of pain messages from the skin to the brain. It works off what is commonly referred to as the *gate theory or counter-irritant mechanism* of pain relief, like acupuncture, where stimulating non-painful nerves in the skin can block the actual painful nerve fiber transmission that proceeds into the spinal and brain nervous system. TENS is safe, noninvasive, and affordable. TENS is often used in a physical therapy program and for patients to use at home.

Transdermal   This is a term for analgesic medication that is put on the skin and is absorbed through the skin into the blood stream for its systemic full body effect. The Duragesic fentanyl patch is an example of a transdermal opioid narcotic medication that is applied to the skin every two-to-three days.

Transforaminal   This is the anatomical term typically used for the roundish opening where the spinal nerves exit the sides of the spine. This can be an area of nerve root compression and inflammation causing sciatica-like symptoms. A *transforaminal* epidural steroid injection (TF ESI) can be fluoroscopically X-ray guided into this area with a small-gauge procedure needle through the skin to decrease sciatica pain, with relief that can last for weeks to months. The other epidural injection approaches include *interlaminar*—a midline technique across the lamina part of the posterior bony spine—and the *lumbosacral or caudal technique*—an approach to the epidural space just above the tailbone.

Trigeminal Nerve   This is the name of the largest cranial nerve in the head out of the twelve total cranial nerves that exist and is responsible for the painful condition of trigeminal neuralgia when this nerve is irritated or compressed.

Trigeminal Neuralgia   This is a type of neurologic pain condition involving tenderness and swelling of the trigeminal nerve resulting in intense sharp, shooting, lightning-like pain in the scalp, cheek, or chin. Medications, interventional procedures, and surgical options for care are all available to control this difficult neuropathic pain state if patients suffer with frequent pain episodes.

Trigger Point   This is the name given to an area in a tight muscle or disrupted connective tissue that is hypersensitive to pressure. Trigger points can either be active or inactive. An inactive or *latent* trigger point is typically sore when you press it, but is does not actively radiate pain away from that point. An active trigger point radiates pain in a characteristic fashion and it is these muscle spots that best respond to trigger point injections (TPIs) with local anesthetic, to break the active spasm pain cycle and allow patients to better rehabilitate. TPIs are often followed up with applications of heat and ice, whatever feels better to the patient, and active stretching of the affected muscle groups.

Trigger Point Injections (TPIs)   This is a safe outpatient office-based minimally invasive procedure to relax active painful muscle trigger points. Local anesthetic with or without other additives is injected into the trigger point areas to break the spasm cycle and allow further healing and rehabilitation. TPIs can give patients relief for hours, days, or for weeks. TPIs can be repeated periodically, typically weekly, or monthly in the short run and then as needed for flare ups of spasm for longer-term care, as part of a multidisciplinary pain management program—medications, physical therapy with modalities of heat and ice, TENS unit and ultrasound, along with massage and acupuncture, and other techniques like yoga.

Triptans   This is a class of drugs for the *abortive* treatment of migraines with a quick onset for acute pain attacks that act on a certain class of serotonin receptors (5-HT receptors) in the brain. Triptans help relieve other symptoms of migraine besides the pain itself, such as nausea, vomiting, and sensitivity to light and sound. Triptans can be effective in relieving migraines for many patients, but they do not prevent further attacks or lessen their frequency. Many *chronic migraine* sufferers also take *prophylactic* migraine medications on a regular basis, including topiramate (Topamax), amitriptyline (Elavil), propranolol (Inderal), valproic acid (Valproate), gabapentin (Neurontin), and others.

Trochanteric Bursitis   This a painful condition caused by inflammation of the *"bursa"* on the outside the hip caused by injury or repetitive overuse activity that can eventually lead to chronic and debilitating hip pain. Minimally invasive ultrasound-guided bursa injections of steroid and local anesthetic can be offered to treat persistent symptoms, especially if medical treatment with rest, nonsteroidal anti-inflammatory medication, ice and heat, and physical therapy fails.

U

Ulcer   This is the term for an area of tissue erosion most commonly in the skin, as a decubitus ulcer or vascular ulcer in the legs, or on the lining of the gastrointestinal (GI) tract presenting as a stomach or duodenal ulcer. Classically, taking nonsteroidal anti-inflammatory drug medications (NSAIDs), like Motrin and Aleve, for a prolonged period can put patients at risk of developing gastritis and ulcer formation.

Ultrasound   This is a therapeutic modality used in physical therapy to relieve muscle strain and osteoarthritis pain. Ultrasound works by using high frequency sound waves to warm injured tissues and promote healing. Ultrasound is also used to obtain images inside the body. Ultrasound is often used for interventional pain management guidance in performing various joint injection therapy, certain peripheral nerve blocks, and tendon and bursa injections, where the imaging can help provide more accurate procedure needle placement.

V

Vascular Pain   This is a type of visceral and somatic pain where vascular disease or injury to blood vessels can cause vasculitis and ischemic pain, especially in the hands and legs, but also within a bodily organ, like painful ischemic bowel disease. *Peripheral vascular disease (PVD)* in the legs can cause vascular claudication calf pain when patients walk even short distances. Skin breakdown and ulcer disease can occur with severe cases and lead to gangrene pain. Patients with certain ulcers that are nonoperative may be candidates for the spinal cord stimulation (SCS) device to help restore blood flow and oxygen in healing tissues, with the hope of controlling pain and healing the ulcers.

Vegetative Depression   This is the psychiatric term for physical symptoms commonly associated with depression, such as fatigue, weight change, loss of libido, and insomnia. Patients need control of the psychological depression symptoms as importantly as control of the actual physical pain problem they are experiencing.

Vertebra   This is the anatomical term for the bony segments that make up the spinal column. There are 33 total vertebrae, including 7 in the cervical (neck) area, 12 in the thoracic (mid-back), 5 in the lumbar (low back), 5 in the sacral (buttock area), and 4 in the coccyx (tail bone area). Any one of these areas can give rise to pain in the spine and surrounding nerves due to injury or a disease process.

Vertebral Discs   This is the anatomical term for the rounded collagen-containing spinal structures between each vertebral body that serve mainly as shock absorbers. Discogenic pain is common in patients with *degenerative disc disease (DDD)* with internal disc disruption (IDD) due to irritation and disruption of the basivertebral nerves that exist in the back of spinal discs, and from leaking disc substances that typically cause a lot of inflammatory-related spinal nerve pain.

Vertebroplasty   This is the name of a minimally invasive surgical procedure, much like kyphoplasty, for the repair of vertebral fractures and compression due to osteoporosis or trauma. Through a small tube, medical cement is directly injected into a bone fracture area to keep it from worsening. Orthopedists, neurosurgeons, and certain interventional pain specialists perform this procedure.

Visceral Pain   This is one of the subtypes of pain of the major nociceptive pain category that arises from internal organs, and can feel crampy, pressure-like, or colicky. Patients with gallstones, kidney stones, or pancreatitis can feel this type of pain. This is opposed to somatic pain, which is a subtype of nociceptive pain that arises from bones and muscles. Together, somatic, and visceral pains make the major pain type, known as nociceptive pain, which is pain that arises from receptors called *nociceptors* that exist in skin, bone, muscle, organs, and other tissues.

Viscosupplementation   This is a procedure in which viscous fluid substance—derived from either the rooster comb or chicken cartilage and commonly referred to as *gel shots*—is injected directly into a joint space commonly for FDA-approved treatment of osteoarthritis knee, but also for shoulder and hip pain and immobility in selected patients. A series of 3–5 weekly office-based injections every six months is typical care for these pain patients, based on clinical response. There are different types of viscosupplements, like Synvisc, Supartz, Euflexxa, and others, and it is up to the treatment team which ones they prefer for an individual patient.

Vulvodynia   This is a type of dysfunctional pain, like TMJ, migraines, IBS, fibromyalgia, which involves pain around the vulva or the front of the vaginal canal that arises from different possible etiologies, including muscle spasm, nerve injury, recurrent yeast infections, sexual trauma, and other reasons. It can be difficult to treat, but the mainstay of treatment is medications, pelvic floor exercises, and other symptomatic care approaches.

W

Waddell's Signs   These are physical examination signs in a low back pain patient evaluation described by an orthopedic doctor named Gordon Waddell many decades ago, that are thought to be an indication of a *psychological component* to a patient's pain. They are considered nonorganic or non-physical signs. They are behavioral responses, like overreaction to the physical examination where a patient excessively grimaces, trembles, or excessively verbalizes his or her pain reactions. These signs have been used to accuse back pain patients of malingering—sometimes unfairly—but this is not common.

Whiplash   This is the common term for a neck pain injury that occurs with motor vehicle accidents, where the neck experiences a sudden acceleration and deceleration force, where classically the neck hyperextends backward and hits the head rest. The muscles, ligaments, cervical facet joints and cervical spinal discs of the neck are the common pain sources following this type of injury. Whiplash is usually an acute, short-term pain condition, but can linger into a chronic pain problem, if not treated sufficiently at the initial time of a patient's accident or injury.

Wind-Up Pain   This is a term that describes pain that arises from nerve cells in the spinal cord that release certain chemicals that *intensify* a pain signal which affects the strength of the pain signal that reaches the brain. All these constant intense nerve sensations can result in a pain phenomenon known as *sensitization*. Once wind-up pain is established it can be more difficult to treat the patient's pain condition, and usually requires a multimodal and multidisciplinary pain management approach to get persistent discomfort under better control. Therefore, it is important to treat acute pain problems aggressively, like severe postoperative pain, to keep this wind-up phenomenon and sensitization process from creating a chronic pain state out of the initial severe acute pain state.

Withdrawal Symptoms   This is a term that describes abrupt physical or psychological symptoms that occur after sudden drug withdrawal, including sweating, tremor, nausea, anxiety, insomnia, and pain. This withdrawal is typical of opioid narcotics, but can occur with other nonnarcotic medications, like antidepressants, antineuropathics, and antihypertensives.

X

X-Ray   This is the common term for a type of black-and-white radiology picture, also known as a *plain film*, that many patients need as part of their medical evaluation looking for bodily damage or pathology including bone(s), the chest, the abdomen, soft tissue, and muscle, or checking an implantable device or post-surgical site. X-rays are often a *first line of radiologic imaging* in a patient workup to aid in the diagnosis of a painful condition due to an accident or injury, like acute back and neck pain conditions, or from persistent joint pain in the shoulder, hip, or knees, for example. Another use of X-ray is for fluoroscopic guidance when performing interventional pain management procedures, like epidural steroid injections (ESIs) or spinal facet and sacroiliac joint injections, to help ensure safety, accuracy, and patient comfort during the injection procedure.

Y

Yoga   This is a mind-body complementary medicine technique utilizing meditation, body postures and breathing techniques to help manage chronic pain. Yoga, as well as Pilates, can provide an excellent self-directed therapy for patients who are well motivated to keep themselves in the best shape as possible.

Z

Ziconotide   This is the name of a calcium-channel blocker medication with analgesic and neuroprotective effects that can help relieve chronic intractable pain, when given intrathecally in the spinal fluid using a continuous infusion implantable spinal pump device. The FDA-approved brand name of ziconotide is Prialt. This is an advanced type of pain control for severe intractable neuropathic pain.

Zovirax   This is the pharmaceutical brand name for the drug acyclovir, which is used to treat cases of acute shingles, or herpes zoster.

Zygapophysial Joint   This is the medical term for the *facet joints of the spine*, which are the paired synovial connecting joints for each vertebral level, offering spine stabilization with certain twisting and turning motions. These facet joints—existing in the cervical, thoracic and lumbar spine—are a common source of spinal inflammatory and mechanical pain when they become inflamed and degenerated, or traumatically injured.

INDEX

ABOUT THE AUTHOR

Peter A. Kechejian, MD, CPE (Dr. K) is a board-certified **Pain Management Specialist and Certified Pain Educator** who for the last twenty-five years has been taking care of pain patients on Long Island, New York.

He is the creator of the U.S. registered and trademarked **Pain is the PITS Program** for the medical treatment of chronic pain. Dr. K is also the **President and CEO of PITS Program, LLC**, a Texas-based pain management educational company. For over two decades Dr. K has been a passionate educational pain management speaker on Long Island and has produced video and podcast multi-media pain management program presentations for both the public and for healthcare professionals.

His hope is that the **Pain is the PITS Program** will be the first universally recognized chronic pain management educational methodology in America, easy for all to understand and follow. The program will bring the patient and their pain management team together for the best assessment and management of pain and will help answer the *Opioid Crisis* question in this country by providing an integrative, more balanced approach to treatment options for chronic pain. The **PITS Program** care approach will maximize a patient's comfort, function, and overall quality of life, without the need to keep escalating opioid narcotic levels for pain treatment therapy. In the end, following the **PITS Program** *philosophy of care* should also help to reduce the occurrences of addiction in America.

A graduate of **Georgetown University School of Medicine** in Washington, D.C., he completed his residency in **Anesthesiology and a Fellowship in Pain Management** at the **University of Massachusetts Medical Center** (now UMass Memorial Health Care), in Worcester, Massachusetts. He was the former **Director of Pain Management** for the **Anesthesia Residency Teaching Program at the Nassau University Medical Center-NUMC** (formerly, **Nassau County Medical Center**), in East Meadow, New York. While at NUMC, he was a **Clinical Assistant Professor of Anesthesiology** through **SUNY at Stony Brook, University Hospital and Medical Center**, in Stony Brook, New York.

After his formal academic teaching years, he spent the next ten years in the **North Shore-Long Island Jewish Health (NSLIJ) Health Care System** (now the **Northwell Health System**), working with **North American Partners in Pain Management (NAPPM)** as an **Interventional Pain Specialist and Director of Oncology Pain Services** for the group practice in Syosset, New York. Prior to this, he was **Adjunct Clinical Assistant Professor-Department of Surgery**, to the faculty of the **New York College of Osteopathic Medicine of New York Institute of Technology**, teaching pain management for the **Family Practice Residency Program**, at the Plainview Hospital campus, in Plainview, New York. He was also involved with the didactic teaching of interventional pain management for the **Palliative Care Fellowship Program at North Shore University Hospital**, in Manhasset, New York.

He is a member of the **International Association for the Study of Pain**, the **American Society of Interventional Pain Physicians**, and other professional organizations. He is board-certified in **Pain Management** and **Anesthesiology** through the **American Board of Anesthesiology** and is a **Certified Pain Educator** through the **American Society of Pain Educators**.

Currently, his pain management practice is focusing on the safe minimally invasive outpatient medical and interventional techniques for the treatment of acute and chronic neck and back spine pain conditions with **Total Orthopedics and Sports Medicine**, a New York-based medical group, utilizing the **Pain is the PITS Program** *philosophy* as an educational patient *adherence* guide for the best multidisciplinary integrative clinical care that America has to offer.

Dr. Kechejian and his wife of 31 years Dr. Joanne Massina Kechejian, an Internal Medicine physician, have four children and live on Long Island. In his spare time, he enjoys chess and traveling with his family. He used to enjoy golf at the club, but his family made him give it up while trying to get this book published!

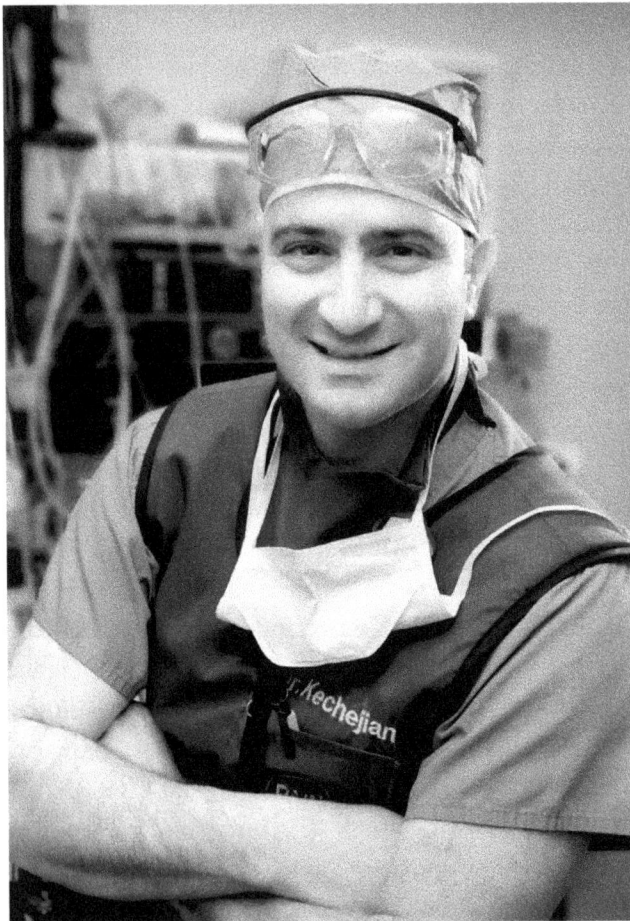

"Feel Better and Live your Life, Because Pain is the PITS!"

—Dr. K

ACKNOWLEDGMENTS

This book would not be possible if it were not for my many mentors and colleagues who through the last 30 years have given me the best possible residency and pain fellowship training, great academic teaching experiences, and all the clinical patient care opportunities that led to the development of the **PITS Program**. Special thanks to **Dr. Donald Stevens** for my initial pain training fellowship, during which he emphasized the importance of developing a good history and physical exam on my patients.

I am grateful to **Dr. Kenneth Freeze** for my Clinical Assistant Professor appointment as Director of Anesthesia Pain Management for a county hospital teaching program. I also wish to thank **Dr. John Stamatos** for advancing my clinical interventional pain treatment skills, in a robust healthcare system that first inspired me to create the early **Pain is the PITS Program** idea. In addition, I appreciated **Dr. Timothy Groth** giving me the opportunity to expand the **PITS Program** through the media. I am most grateful at this point to **Dr. Charles Ruotolo** for helping to finally get this important educational book information out to the public, and to the many health professionals that take care of pain sufferers.

I am very grateful to all of you, and the many along the way who I have not mentioned, like all the nurses (RNs and NPs), Physician Assistants (PAs) and medical assistants (MAs), and X-ray techs, and the front office staff. Special thanks to all my patients that agreed to be treated under the **Pain is the PITS Program** *philosophy of care* in its earliest days. The waters were dark, and uncharted back then, but many of them have gone on to enjoy more productive and less painful lives, with less opioid dependence.

I would like to thank my editor **Gerard Fitzpatrick** for recognizing the importance of this book as an educational program tool for the millions of pain sufferers in this country. Through his vision and helping me toward self-publishing, these millions will now have access to an easy to understand and follow pain management system of care that will dramatically improve their lives.

Lastly, but the most important of all, I would like to thank my family. My thoughtful and supportive wife Joanne has inspired me, and challenged me, through the many years it took to develop the **P-I-T-S** *acronym concept* and this book formation. She is the glue that kept me focused, and keeps our family together and thriving. To our children: Pete, Kate, Caroline, and Emma…thank you for your endless encouragement in helping make **P-I-T-S** a reality. Without all of you, I would never have had the mindset or the motivation to establish the **PITS Program** as a true legacy wellness program for this great country of ours, and get it to the finish line. I love you!

www.ingramcontent.com/pod-product-compliance
Lightning Source LLC
Chambersburg PA
CBHW052111020426

42335CB00021B/2716